Palliative Care in Amyotrophic Lateral Sclerosis

Second Edition

Palliative Care in Amyotrophic Lateral Sclerosis

From Diagnosis to Bereavement

Second Edition

Edited by

David Oliver
Consultant Physician in Palliative Medicine,
Wisdom Hospice, and Honorary Senior Lecturer
at the Kent Institute of Medicine and Health Sciences,
University of Kent, UK

Gian Domenico Borasio
Professor and Acting Chairman,
Interdisciplinary Center for Palliative Medicine,
and Head of the Motor Neurone Disease Research Group,
Department of Neurology, University of Munich, Germany

Declan Walsh
Professor and Director,
The Harry R Horvitz Center for Palliative Medicine,
Cleveland Clinic, USA

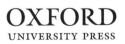
OXFORD
UNIVERSITY PRESS

OXFORD
UNIVERSITY PRESS

Great Clarendon Street, Oxford OX2 6DP

Oxford University Press is a department of the University of Oxford.
It furthers the University's objective of excellence in research, scholarship,
and education by publishing worldwide in

Oxford New York

Auckland Cape Town Dar es Salaam Hong Kong Karachi
Kuala Lumpur Madrid Melbourne Mexico City Nairobi
New Delhi Shanghai Taipei Toronto

With offices in

Argentina Austria Brazil Chile Czech Republic France Greece
Guatemala Hungary Italy Japan Poland Portugal Singapore
South Korea Switzerland Thailand Turkey Ukraine Vietnam

Oxford is a registered trade mark of Oxford University Press
in the UK and in certain other countries

Published in the United States
by Oxford University Press Inc., New York

© Oxford University Press 2006

The moral rights of the author have been asserted
Database right Oxford University Press (maker)

First published 2006

British Library Cataloguing in Publication Data

Data available

Library of Congress Cataloging in Publication Data
Palliative Care in Amyotrophic Lateral Sclerosis : from diagnosis to bereavement / edited by David Oliver, Gian
Domenico Borasio, Declan Walsh. – 2nd ed.
p. ; cm.
Includes bibliographical references and index.

ISBN-13: 978-0-19-921293-4 (hbk : alk. paper)
ISBN-10: 0-19-921293-7 (hbk : alk. paper)
ISBN-13: 978-0-19-857048-6 (pbk. : alk. paper)
ISBN-10: 0-19-857048-1 (pbk. : alk. paper)

1. Amyotrophic lateral sclerosis. 2. Palliative treatment. I. Oliver,
David, FRCGP. II. Borasio, Gian Domenico. III. Walsh, Declan.
[DNLM: 1. Amyotrophic Lateral Sclerosis–therapy. 2. Palliative Care. WE 550 P167 2006]
RC406.A24P352 2006
616.8'3–dc22
2006023591

Typeset by SPI Publisher Services, Pondicherry, India
Printed in Great Britain
on acid-free paper by
Biddles Ltd., King's Lynn, Norfolk

1 3 5 7 9 10 8 6 4 2

Contents

Preface

Although new treatments for amyotrophic lateral sclerosis (ALS)/motor neurone disease are being developed, these at present offer only the potential to
slow the disease process. Therefore a palliative care approach to the care of the
patient and their family is at the centre of good clinical practice in ALS. This
book aims to consider the various aspects of palliative care for patients with
ALS, based on the most recent research in the field. This edition has been
updated to include research and publications from the past five years and we
have added new chapters on ethical issues, spiritual care, decision-making and
nursing care.

The palliative care approach to the care of ALS is outlined and the role of the
multidisciplinary team emphasized. The international authorship allows a
comparison of the differences across cultures, social circumstances, health
care systems and nations. All contributors are clinicians involved in the care
of people with ALS and they are able to provide clear guidelines of the care
throughout the disease process, from the telling of the diagnosis to death. An
evidence-based approach, grounded in day to day care of patients, is used.
A short case history starts the majority of chapters, focusing the reader on the
clinical application of the research.

The book aims to provide a reference for all involved in the care of patients
with ALS, including neurologists, general physicians, rehabilitationists,
paramedical staff, general/family practitioners and specialist palliative care
teams. The care of a patient with ALS, and their family, is often a challenge,
but one all should take up so that patients can live life as fully as possible.

Throughout the book amyotrophic lateral sclerosis (ALS) has been used
rather than motor neurone disease, as the name ALS is recognized inter-
nationally and motor neurone disease is restricted to certain countries.

We would like to thank all involved in the production of this volume,
especially Catherine Barnes, Georgia Pinteau, Bethan Lee, and Clare Caruna
from Oxford University Press and the colleagues who have made comments
throughout the publication process.

DJO, Rochester, UK
GDB, Munich, Germany
DW, Cleveland, Ohio, USA
April 2006

List of Contributors

Gian Domenico Borasio, Interdisciplinary Centre for Palliative Medicine, and Head of the Motor Neurone Disease Research Group, Department of Neurology, University of Munich, Germany

Linda Centers, OTR/L, Eastern State Hospital, Kentucky, USA

Lauren Elman, Penn Neurological Institute, Philadelphia, USA

Dallas Forshew, ALS Center at UCSF, San Francisco, USA

Donal Gallagher, Wisdom Hospice, Kent, UK

Alison Garrett, Physiotherapy Department, King's College Hospital, London, UK

Deborah Gelinas, Forbes Norris MDA/ALS Center, California Pacific Medical Center, San Francisco, USA; Nashoba Valley Medical Center, Ayer, USA

Laura Goldstein, Department of Psychology, Institute of Psychiatry, London, UK

Ulrike Hammerbeck, Motor Nerve Clinic, Institute of Psychiatry, London, UK

Phil Hankins, ALS Patient (deceased)

Amanda Harris, Wisdom Hospice, Kent, UK

Wendy Johnston, University of Alberta, Canada

Jos Kerkvliet, Disablement Services Centre, Medway Maritime Hospital, Kent, UK

Chris Kingsnorth, Country Services, Independent Living Centre of WA, Nedlands, Western Australia, Australia

Robert Lambert, the Pastoral Service, McGill University Health Centre, Montreal, Canada

Rebecca Lyall, King's College Hospital, London, UK

Leo McCluskey, Penn Neurological Institute, Philadelphia, USA

Ann McMurray, Wisdom Hospice, Kent, UK

Maryanne McPhee, Speech Pathology Department, Bethlehem Healthcare, South Caulfield, Victoria, Australia

Barbara Monroe, St Christopher's Hospice, London, UK

David Oliver, Wisdom Hospice and Kent Institute of Medicine and Health Sciences, University of Kent, UK

Dieter E. Pongratz, Friedrich-Baur Institute, Ludwig Maximilians University, Munich, Germany

Mario Prosiegel, Neurologisches Krankenhaus München (NKM), Munich, Germany

Amanda Scott, Speech Pathology Department, The Alfred, Prahran, Victoria, Australia

Christopher Shaw, Department of Neurology, Institute of Psychiatry, London, UK

Richard Sloan, Joseph Weld Hospice, Dorchester, UK

Nigel Sykes, St Christopher's Hospice, London, UK

Raymond Voltz, Department of Neuroimmunology, Ludwig-Maximilians University, Munich, Germany

Edith Wagner-Sonntag, Neurologisches Krankenhaus München, Munich, Germany

Chapter 1

Amyotrophic lateral sclerosis/ motor neuron disease

Christopher Shaw

The aim of this chapter is to answer the question 'What is amyotrophic lateral sclerosis (motor neuron disease)?' The first section will include an account of the typical clinical presentation and diagnostic work-up of a patient with ALS and a brief description of the conditions that cause or mimic motor neuron degeneration. The second section will cover the pathological features of ALS and what is understood of its pathogenesis from molecular genetic and cell biology research. Lastly, therapies designed to alter the course of the disease will be discussed.

What do we mean by motor neuron disease?

The term 'motor neuron disorders' covers a range of conditions in which the motor neuron cell bears the brunt of the disease process. Clinical, pathological and, more recently, molecular genetic studies have helped distinguish many of these from typical motor neuron disease. Amyotrophic lateral sclerosis (ALS) is the name used in most parts of the world – in the United Kingdom and other Commonwealth countries it is known as motor neuron disease and in the United States it is often known as Lou Gherig's disease, after the famous baseball player who died of ALS.

It was originally thought to be a muscular condition until Charcot in 1869 published clinico-pathological studies which correctly identified motor neuron degeneration as the cause of muscle wasting.[1] The features that distinguish this disorder from others affecting the motor system are the combination of upper and lower motor neuron degeneration (the neurological pathways are shown in Figure 1.1).

Lower motor neurons (LMN) reside in the spinal cord and brainstem and project out in peripheral nerves to make direct contact with and activate muscle fibres. When LMN's degenerate the muscles they activate become weak, wasted and fasciculate (twitch). Upper motor neurons (UMN) reside in the motor cortex in the frontal lobes of the brain and they projec*

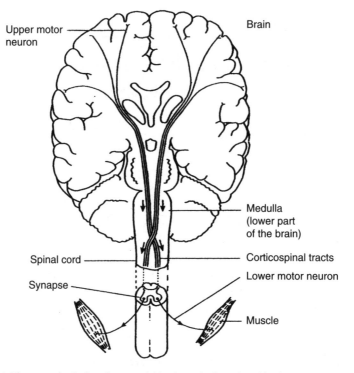

Fig. 1.1 The neurological pathways within the spinal cord and brain.

down to and activate the lower motor neurons. When UMN's degenerate muscles become spastic and the deep tendon reflexes are exaggerated. The plantar responses may be extensor rather than flexor, also called Babinski's sign – the big toe goes up rather than curling down when the sole of the foot is scratched. Most patients with ALS have a mixture of UMN and LMN signs, however, when only lower motor neuron features are present the condition may be called progressive muscular atrophy (PMA) while a pure upper motor neuron syndrome is known as primary lateral sclerosis (PLS). Pathological studies suggest that these syndromes are all forms of ALS but lie at the ends of a clinical spectrum. Interestingly both of these variants are associated with a slower disease progression and longer survival.

The diagnosis of ALS is essentially a clinical one and supportive evidence is obtained by a range of investigations. Typically it presents with progressive weakness and wasting of the muscles controlling limb movement, speech, swallowing or breathing. Motor neurons controlling eye movement and sphincters of the bladder and bowel are usually spared as are neurons in the sensory and autonomic nervous systems. Diagnostic criteria for ALS were established at a conference in the Spanish castle El Escorial and have been

Table 1.1 Revised El Escorial Criteria for the Diagnosis of Motor Neuron Disease/
Amyotrophic Lateral Sclerosis

- **Must be** progressive, have fasciculation and near normal motor nerve conduction
- **Must not** have cognitive, parkinsonism, sensory, visual, autonomic, sphincter involvement.

Suspected MND/ALS	Possible MND/ALS	Lab probable MND/ALS	Clin probable MND/ALS	Clin definite MND/ALS
LMN and UMN signs >= I region only	LMN and UMN signs in I region only	LMN and UMN signs in I and EMG >= 2 regions	LMN and UMN signs in 2 regions	LMN and UMN signs in 3 regions

recently updated[2] (Table 1.1). They are principally used as inclusion criteria in therapeutic trials but emphaisze the importance of detecting UMN and LMN signs in multiple regions to establish a more definite diagnosis of ALS.

Motor neuron disorders that mimic ALS

There are many different disorders of the motor neuron that may be mistaken for ALS. Given the very poor prognosis for most patients it is vital that the diagnosis be correct and all possible alternatives excluded. The most common mimic is spinal cord and/or nerve root compression due to degeneration of the vertebrae and discs in the spine. This can present with painless muscle wasting, weakness and fasciculation in one or more limbs. Detailed views of the spinal cord and nerve roots by magnetic resonance imaging (MRI) scanning are essential in every patient suspected of having ALS. MRI may also reveal rarer intrinsic cord lesions such as a spinal cord tumour or syrinx (benign cyst). Another condition that requires careful consideration is multifocal motor neuropathy (MMN). It is an autoimmune disorder where antibodies selectively attack the motor nerves and usually presents as an asymmetrical weakness of the upper limbs. MMN is often associated with patches of reduced electrical conduction in motor nerves, demonstrated by careful nerve conduction studies, and anti-GM1 ganglioside antibodies in the serum.[3] This mimic of ALS is not lethal and can improve following immunosuppressive treatment, such as intravenous human immunoglobulin.

Kennedy's disease, or spinobulbar muscular atrophy (SBMA), is a rare but significant cause of misdiagnosis in ALS. It is a pure lower motor neuron syndrome that solely affects adult males. It causes slowly progressive muscle wasting with prominent involvement of the tongue and tremor of the outstretched hands. Other features include testicular atrophy and gynaecomastia (breast enlargement), due to low androgen levels.[4] Nerve conduction studies commonly show a sensory neuropathy even though there may be no evidence of sensory loss on examination. The mutation is an expanded CAG nucleotide repeat sequence in the androgen receptor gene on the X chromosome.[5] The CAG triplet encodes for the amino acid glutamine and the expansion mutation makes the androgen receptor protein unfold and accumulate, which is toxic to motor neurons.

Even rarer is the autosomal recessive condition spinal muscular atrophy (SMA). Although SMA usually presents in infancy or childhood, a minority of adults develop a slowly progressive, pure lower motor neuron syndrome with wasting, weakness and absent reflexes, labelled SMA type IV because of the late onset.[6] The survival motor neuron gene (*SMN*) gene is found to be deleted or disrupted in more than 95 per cent of all SMA cases.[7]

Many other conditions need to be considered in the differential diagnosis, such as multiple sclerosis and hereditary spastic paraplegias which can cause UMN signs. Muscle twitching without focal wasting is a feature of the benign fasciculation syndrome as well as disturbed thyroid and parathormone disorders so a metabolic screen should be undertaken (Table 1.2).

Table 1.2 Conditions mimicking amyotrophic lateral sclerosis

Condition	Diagnostic screening tests
Spinal disease causing cord and/or nerve root compression (myelo-radiculopathy)	Magnetic resonance imaging (MRI) scans
Autoimmune neuropathies including multifocal motor neuropathy (MMN)	Nerve conduction studies, anti-ganglioside antibodies, protein electrophoresis
Spino-bulbar muscular atrophy (SBMA, also known as Kennedy's disease)	Genetic test for androgen gene CAG expansion mutation
Multiple Sclerosis	MRI of the brain and cerebrospinal fluid immunoglobulin electrophoresis
Hereditary spastic paraplegia	Electromyography (EMG, no evidence of LMN disease), gene testing
Benign fasciculation syndrome	EMG (no evidence of LMN disease)
Myopathies (eg: inclusion body myositis)	Muscle biopsy
Spinal muscular atrophy	Gene testing
Diabetic amyotrophy	Glycosylated haemoglobin
Thyrotoxicosis	Thyroid hormone assay
Hyperparathyroidism	Calcium, phosphate
Gangliosidoses	White cell enzyme hexosaminidase levels

The clinical course of typical ALS

In the majority of people with ALS muscle weakness begins insidiously in one limb (85 per cent), causing weakness of grip or the foot to catch on the pavement. Affected muscles become progressively more wasted and fasciculate as lower motor neurons in the spinal cord degenerate and die. Sometimes muscle cramps or spasms precede wasting and weakness, which may reflect early UMN involvement. Spasticity may accompany weakness and eventually all of the limbs become affected. In a minority of people symptoms begin in the throat (15 per cent) with slurred speech or difficulty swallowing.[8] Bulbar symptoms arise when LMN's in the brainstem (previously known as the bulb), degenerate and cause wasting and weakness of the tongue and pharyngeal muscles, often referred to as 'progressive bulbar palsy' (Figure 1.2). Sometime UMN signs affect the throat resulting in nasal and slurred speech due to poor elevation of the soft palate and spasticity of the tongue accompanied by a brisk jaw jerk and often referred to as 'pseudobulbar palsy'. These two syndromes are also variants of ALS and are usually accompanied by motor neuron symptoms and signs. Approximately 90 per cent of patients with limb-onset disease will eventually develop bulbar symptoms, and only a small minority, more commonly men, have solely spinal disease.

ALS causes significant disability early and relentlessly progresses so that most patients ultimately lose the ability to walk, feed and toilet themselves, speak and swallow. A particular cruelty is that intellectual function is usually spared so that patients are fully aware of their circumstances but are trapped in bodies that no longer work and are isolated by an inability to interact or communicate. Frank dementia can occur in 5–10 per cent of patients leading to abnormal behavioural and language problems – see Chapter 4c. Respiratory weakness due to thoracic and high cervical spinal cord involvement is almost universal prior to death. Often respiratory weakness is underestimated because the patient's mobility is compromised and a drop in the ventilatory capacity to 60 per cent of predicted may be asymptomatic. Death is usually due to respiratory failure and mean survival from symptomatic onset is on average three years. Only 25 per cent of patients survive five years and 10 per cent are alive at ten years.[9] Elderly female patients who have a bulbar onset of symptoms have a significantly poorer prognosis.

How can the diagnosis of ALS be made?

ALS is uncommon and the diagnosis can be difficult. Most general practitioners will encounter only one case in a working lifetime. For this reason they

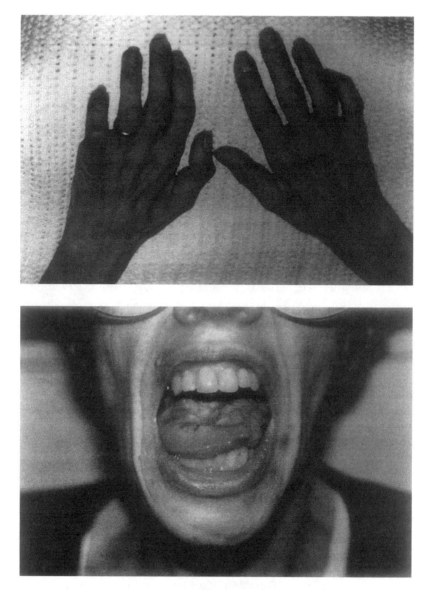

Fig. 1.2 Clinical appearance of amyotrophic lateral sclerosis. Note the pronounced muscle wasting of the patient's hands and tongue.

may not recognize the earliest symptoms or signs so that patients may be referred to specialists in rheumatology, orthopaedics or otolaryngology before they see a neurologist. While the symptoms and signs on examination may be suggestive of ALS there is no simple 'test for ALS'. Furthermore, as the implications are so profound, neurologists may delay discussing the possibility of ALS until they are absolutely certain of the diagnosis. These factors contribute to a considerable delay from the time of first symptom to diagnosis.

The investigations that are most useful are those that exclude other conditions that mimic ALS (Table 1.2). The most important is magnetic resonance imaging (MRI) of the spine or head to exclude an extrinsic or intrinsic lesion. Nerve conduction studies are essential to exclude a generalized or multifocal neuropathy and search for nerve entrapment and conduction block. Electromyography (EMG) is necessary to confirm evidence of acute lower motor neuron loss, particularly in regions not symptomatically affected and to exclude myopathy. Typical EMG features of ALS are spontaneous fibrillations and slow frequency fasciculations (0.3Hz) with unstable and complex motor unit potentials on voluntary activation. Muscle biopsy and spinal fluid studies are usually unnecessary unless the presentation is very atypical and an alternative diagnosis, such as a degenerative muscle or inflammatory neurological disease such as multiple sclerosis is suspected.

Who gets ALS?

For reasons that are not known males develop ALS more frequently than females with a ratio of approximately 1.7:1.[10] Males are more likely to have a younger age at onset. The mean annual incidence of ALS is approximately 1–2 per 100,000 per year, which is roughly half that of multiple sclerosis in the UK. Because of the relatively short survival of patients with ALS the prevalence rate is only about 3–7 per 100,000. The prevalence appears to be fairly consistent despite geographical, socio-economic and racial differences. High risk foci exist in the Kii Peninsular in Japan and the Pacific island of Guam where it is often associated with Parkinsonism and dementia. The incidence in Guam has been has been falling over the last three decades, which suggests that exposure to an environmental agent may be responsible: however, many case-control studies have failed to identify a particular toxin or infection that might be a risk factor for ALS. Epidemiological studies outside of Guam suggest that a history of previous musculoskeletal injury[11] and occupations with a high degree of electrical exposure or electric shock[12] appear to significantly increase the risk of ALS. The effect is relatively small with an odds ratio between 2 and 3.[9] The association with increased age is clear however, as there is a steep rise in incidence after the age of 50 which continues to increase in age-adjusted analyses.

What happens to motor neurons in ALS?

Although muscular and anterior spinal root atrophy is striking at post-mortem, the brain and spinal cord usually look reasonably normal. The

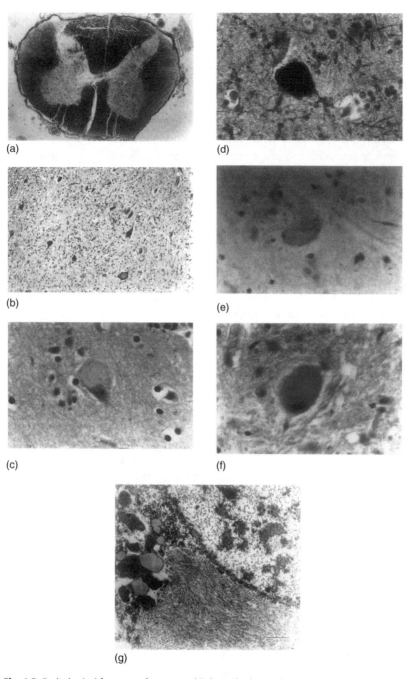

Fig. 1.3 Pathological features of amyotrophic lateral sclerosis by light and electron microscopy. Spinal cord in cross section showing a low number of motor neurons in the anterior horn (a). At low powered magnification motor neurons in the cord appear swollen or shrunken (b). At higher power a variety of aggregates can be seen including hyaline inclusions (c), and those that immunolabel with antibodies to neurofilaments (d) and ubiquitin showing the characteristic thread-like skeins (e) and Lewy body-like and proximal axonal inclusions (f). Transmission electron microscopy reveals that the cell body is packed with neurofilaments, lipofuscin and other protein aggregates (g, scale bar = 1 μm).

minor changes externally are in contrast to the dramatic changes that occur at a microscopic level. Charcot[1] was one of the first to describe the abnormal appearance of neurons within the spinal cord. The characteristic features are of often severe motor neuron loss with proliferation and hypertrophy of neighbouring astrocytes (supporting brain cells). The few surviving motor neurons are either shrunken or swollen and have a variety of protein aggregates (cytoplasmic inclusions) and axonal degeneration (Figure 1.3). Similar changes are seen in the large upper motor neurons in the cerebral cortex (Betz cells) although there is increasing evidence that neuronal loss is common in other, non-motor, regions of the cortex.[13]

One of the earliest changes and most specific for ALS are thread-like protein aggregates within motor neurons that appear to block the proximal axon.[14] These can be identified by staining tissues for a protein called ubiquitin. When proteins are damaged or mutated they are often targeted for degradation by the cell through the attachment of ubiquitin. Ubiquitinated inclusions occur in several late-onset neurodegenerative diseases such as Parkinson's and Alzheimer's disease, where they act as a molecular rubbish bag that helps recycle unwanted cellular proteins. For reasons that still unknown this recycling process breaks down and may contribute to neurodegeneration.

Molecular genetics and ALS: clues from SOD1

For many years our understanding of the underlying cause(s) of ALS was confined to a description of the cellular pathology and using neurotoxins to model these effects in animals. There were many hypotheses but the most important clues to the pathogenesis of ALS have come from molecular genetics. Although the majority of motor neuron disease occurs sporadically, in approximately 5–10 per cent of cases other members of the family are affected. Most commonly familial ALS is a dominant disorder, being passed down through the generations. Linkage to a region on chromosome 21 was reported in 1991[15] and two years later mutations in the copper/zinc superoxide dismutase (*SOD1*) gene were discovered.[16] SOD1 is a powerful antioxidant catalytic enzyme responsible for neutralizing potentially harmful free-radicals produced as a result of normal cellular activity. To date more than 110 different mutations have been described, mostly due to a single base change causing a single amino-acid substitution,[17] (Figure 1.4). Mutations in *SOD1* are found in approximately 20 per cent of familial and 3 per cent of apparently sporadic cases.[18] The clinical symptoms, signs and pathology of patients with *SOD1* mutations are indistinguishable from non-*SOD1* ALS cases.[19]

Mice bred to over-express the mutant human *SOD1* gene develop adult-onset motor neuron degeneration and progressive paralysis.[20] Mice

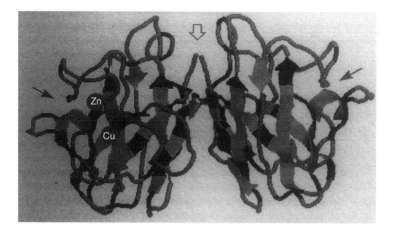

Fig. 1.4 The SOD1 molecule and ALS causing mutation sites. This cartoon demonstrates how tightly SOD1 is coiled on itself. Two ions, zinc and copper, bind to SOD1, which in turn binds to itself to form a homodimer (white arrow). The reduced copper ion lies at the base of an active channel (dark arrows) where it reduces superoxide radicals to hydrogen peroxide by the Fenton reaction. Mutations associated to ALS (black bands) can occur throughout the molecule and the precise mechanism of their toxicity to motor neurons has not been determined.

lacking SOD1 or over-expressing normal human SOD1 are healthy, proving that motor neuron death is due to a toxic property of the mutant protein and not a loss of normal SOD1 function. The catalytic activity of SOD1 is entirely dependant on the copper ion bound at the base of the active channel. Early studies on the biochemical effects of SOD1 mutation suggested that mutations would alter the shape of the active channel and could increase the production of hydroxyl radicals (OH^-) and peroxynitrite ($ONOO^-$), which may damage cellular lipids, proteins and DNA.[21] If toxicity was due to abnormal catalytic activity one would predict that the toxic effects of the mutations would be abolished if copper binding could be prevented making the enzyme inactive. Experiments which prevented the delivery of copper (by knocking out the copper delivery molecule,[22] or preventing its binding to SOD1[23] showed that SOD1 which was Cu free and enzymatically inactive was just as toxic to motor neurons as before. An alternative mechanism was proposed when aggregates of SOD1 were detected in the spinal cord, which is the site of degeneration.[24]

Hypotheses about the pathogenesis of ALS

There are a great number of disease mechanisms postulated to play a role in ALS. Although viral infection, toxin exposure and autoimmunity have been

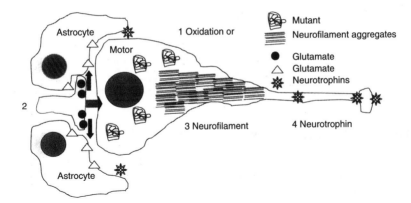

Fig. 1.5 ALS pathogenesis: summary of hypotheses. The only proven cause of ALS is mutant SOD1 but the precise mechanism of toxicity is unknown and *SOD1* mutations are found in only a minority of patients. Neurofilament and ubiquitinated inclusions are the hallmark of ALS but it is still uncertain whether their aggregation is in itself toxic or a failed attempt at protection. The hypotheses are not mutually exclusive and include; (1) oxidative injury due to free radicals such as O^-, NO^-, NOO^- and OH^-, (2) excitotoxicity due to a failure of glutamate transport leading to excess glutamate, (3) disruption of neurofilament transport and (4) neurotrophin deficiency.

implicated, an extensive body of research has failed to support these hypotheses. This section concentrates on those mechanisms for which there is greatest experimental evidence: excitotoxicity, oxidative injury, cytoskeletal disruption and loss of neurotrophic support (summarized in Figure 1.5). Each has its protagonists citing observational and experimental research but none are mutually exclusive. Given the heterogeneity of genetic susceptibility it may be that a primary dysfunction of any one of several biochemical systems converge to a common pathway and that each of these mechanisms may contribute to motor neuron cell death.

Glutamate and neuronal excitotoxicity

The finding that neurotransmitters and their chemical analogues which activate neurons can also harm them, prompted a great deal of research into their role in the pathogenesis of many neurodegenerative diseases. The excitotoxic hypothesis in ALS has centred around the handling of the amino acid glutamate. When an electrical impulse arrives at a presynaptic terminal it depolarizes the cell membrane, causing the release of glutamate at the synapse. Glutamate is the principal neurotransmitter used by neurons projecting to the motor neurons in the cortex and spinal cord. Glutamate is potentially toxic and the brain contains more than 1,000 times the amount of glutamate necessary to kill every neuron. Therefore the strict regulation of glutamate levels is of vital importance and is principally the task of neighbouring astrocytes. Only a small proportion of the glutamate released at the synapse binds to receptors; the remainder is taken up and removed from the synaptic cleft by excitatory amino acid transporters (EAAT) (see Figure 1.5).

Does glutamate excitotoxicity play a role in ALS?

Given that glutamate is so potently toxic to neurons what evidence is there that its regulation is disturbed in ALS? In one study, levels of glutamate were found to be increased up to threefold in the cerebrospinal fluid (CSF) in 80 per cent of ALS patients compared to controls.[25] One of the glutamate trans-porters, EAAT2, is expressed solely on astrocytes, and is reported to be selectively reduced in the motor cortex and spinal cord of up to 70 per cent of sporadic ALS patients.[26] However other laboratories report that glutamate is increased in the cerebrospinal fluid in only a minority of patients (30 per cent)[27] and that decreased EAAT2 protein is only found in the spinal cord.[28] Thus, glutamate induced toxicity may contribute to, but is unlikely to be solely responsible for, motor neuron degeneration.

Free radicals, oxidative stress and ALS

During normal oxidative metabolism several species of free radicals containing reduced oxygen ions are produced (O^-, NO^- and OH^-). Free radicals are capable of damaging proteins, lipids and nucleic acids and are thought to contribute to the normal ageing of cells. All cells have a range of self-protective antioxidant molecules to mop up free radicals and mechanisms to identify and remove oxidized cellular components. Protein oxidation has been detected in the motor cortex and spinal cord in patients with ALS[29] and mutant SOD1 transgenic mice.[30]

Another potential oxidative toxin to cells is peroxynitirite, (NOO^-). This free radical can bind to the amino acid tyrosine, a major component of many proteins to form 3-nitrotyrosine. Evidence of NOO^- injury and 3-nitrotyrosine has been described in tissue in sporadic and familial ALS,[31] and mutant SOD1 transgenic mice.[32] Moreover, dramatically increased levels of 3-nitrotyrosine have been detected in the CSF of patients with sporadic ALS.[33] While these increases are non-specific and occur in other neurodegen-erative diseases, they do suggest that the nitrosylation of proteins is occurring at a greatly increased rate in ALS supporting the case that oxidative stress contributes to motor neuron degeneration.

Cytoskeletal disruption and motor neuron degeneration

Motor neurons are the biggest cells in the body and in the majority of people they function perfectly throughout a normal lifespan. Following the identification of neurofilament (NF) aggregates within motor neurons, a role for this structural protein in the pathogenesis of ALS has been postulated. Neurofilaments are linked together to form the internal scaffolding for neurons, and in particular maintaining their axonal diameter. They are aligned with microtubules which are the highways along which organelles such as mitochondria, vesicles and proteins are transported. Mice transgenic for a point mutation (single spelling mistake) in the mouse NF light chain[34] or over-expressing of normal human NF heavy chain[35] develop motor neuron degeneration with some pathological similarities to ALS. When mice deficient of neurofilaments crossed with mutant *SOD1* mice the onset of motor neuron degeneration and death is significantly delayed.[36] While mutations in the NF genes have not been found in familial MND/ALS cases, deletions in the tail domain of the NF-H gene were detected in 10 sporadic cases.[37,38] Collectively this work suggests that neurofilament aggregation may play a contributory role to motor neuron injury, but it is not a primary or essential mechanism in the pathogenesis of ALS.

Neurotrophic factors and neurodegeneration

The discovery that selected populations of neurons are dependent on specific neurotrophic factors, both during early development and for long-term survival, has prompted research into their role in the pathogenesis and treatment of neurodegenerative diseases. While embryonic dorsal root ganglion neurons have an absolute requirement for a range of neurotrophins, this is not the case for motor neurons. Ciliary neurotrophic factor (CNTF) and insulin-like growth factor (IGF) do enhance the survival of embryonic motor neurons grown in culture and both CNTF and brain-derived neurotrophic factor (BDNF) will rescue facial motor neurons following axotomy.[39] Furthermore, CNTF can retard motor neuron degeneration in the progressive motor neuronopathy (pmn) mouse.[40] A relative decrease in CNTF expression in the anterior spinal cord and nerve growth factor (NGF) in the motor cortex in ALS have been described in ALS tissue at post-mortem but it is difficult to distinguish cause and effect. While it is an attractive hypothesis that defective neurotrophin generation by target cells or their retrograde transport in axons will result in neurodegeneration, clear evidence in human disease states is lacking. However, neurotrophins may still have a role in increasing the survival of ailing neurons and a great deal of experimental work in this field is currently underway and several phase III clinical trials.

Drugs that alter survival in ALS

In a recent survey of published therapeutic trials in ALS recorded in the Cochrane Controlled Trials Register (CCTR) 57 studies were identified using 31 different treatments.[41] Of these only the glutamate release inhibitor riluzole has shown a statistically significant effect on survival in a multicentred, double-blind, controlled trial of 957 patients.[42] There was a three-month delay in the time to death or tracheostomy in the active treatment group compared to controls during the 18-month trial period. Clinical trials of other agents that influence the glutaminergic pathways are nearing completion. Of the neurotrophic agents IGF, CNTF and BDNF have all been trialled using a subcutaneous route of administration without a statistically significant effect on survival.[43,44] Another important tool in screening drug efficacy is the mutant SOD1 transgenic mouse. Interestingly, the glutamate release inhibitors riluzole and gabapentin were shown to delay disease progression and Vitamin C delayed disease onset but not survival[45] while the copper chelator d-penniciliamine and mitochondrial substrate creatine improve both onset and survival.[46,47] Questions still remain about how valid mutant SOD1 transgenic mice are as a model of ALS, but the obvious advantage is that hundreds of drugs can be screened with no risk to patients providing considerable savings in expenditure and time.

Conclusion

Charcot was the first to attempt to answer the question 'What is motor neuron disease?' His observations helped to define the essential clinical and morphological pathological features of motor neuron degeneration. The molecular basis of these abnormalities has been characterized and neurofilamentous, ubiquitinated and other neuronal inclusions provide a pathological hallmark for the diagnosis of ALS. Recent advances in molecular genetics and cell biology have transformed hypotheses of causation based on speculation to those based on fact. Now, 135 years after Charcot, we have our first proven cause of ALS (mutant SOD1) and a modestly effective treatment (riluzole). We still have only a few pieces of the jigsaw puzzle and further clues are urgently needed if we are to translate insights into the pathogenesis of ALS into effective treatments. The very fact that the therapeutic door has been prised open gives researchers, clinicians and those living with ALS hope that drugs capable of slowing down or halting disease progression will soon be developed.

References

1. Charcot J. M., Joffroy A. (1869) Deux cas d'atrophie musculaire progressive avec lesions de la substance grise et des faisceaux antero-lateraux de la moelle epiniere. *Archives of Physiology, Neurology and Pathology* 2: 744.

2. Brooks B. R., Miller R. G., Swash M., Munsat T. L. (2000) El Escorial revisited: revised criteria for the diagnosis of amyotrophic lateral sclerosis. *Amyotroph Lateral Scler Other Motor Neuron Disord* 1: 293–9.

3. Pestronk A., Cornblath D. R., Ilyas A. A., Baba H., Quarles R. H., Griffin J. W. *et al.* (1988) A treatable multifocal motor neuropathy with antibodies to GM1 ganglioside. *Ann Neurol* 24: 73–8.

4. Harding A. E., Thomas P. K., Baraitser M., Bradbury P. G., Morgan-Hughes J. A., Ponsford J. R. (1982) X-linked recessive bulbospinal neuronopathy: a report of ten cases. *J Neurol Neurosurg Psychiatry* 45: 1012–19.

5. La Spada A. R., Wilson E. M., Lubahn D. B., Harding A. E., Fischbeck K. H. (1991) Androgen receptor gene mutations in X-linked spinal and bulbar muscular atrophy. *Nature* 352: 77–9.

6. Dubowitz V. (1995) Chaos in the classification of SMA: a possible resolution. *Neuromuscul Disord* 5: 3–5.

7. Lefebvre S., Burglen L., Reboullet S., Clermont O., Burlet P., Viollet L. *et al.* (1995) Identification and characterization of a spinal muscular atrophy-determining gene [see comments]. *Cell* 1995; **80**: 155–65.

8. Haverkamp L. J., Appel V., Appel S. H. Natural history of amyotrophic lateral sclerosis in a database population. Validation of a scoring system and a model for survival prediction. *Brain* 118: 707–19.

9. Kondo K. (1995) Epidemiology of motor neuron disease. In Leigh P. N. and Swash M. (eds) *Motor Neuron Disease. Biology and Management*, pp. 19–33. London: Springer-Verlag.

10. Chancellor A. M., Warlow C. P. (1992) Adult onset motor neuron disease: worldwide mortality, incidence and distribution since 1950. *J Neurol Neurosurg Psychiatry* 55: 1106–15.

11. Kondo K., Tsubaki T. (1981) Case-control studies of motor neuron disease: association with mechanical injuries. *Archives of Neurology* 38: 220–6.

12. Deapen D. M., Henderson B. E. (1986) A case-control study of amyotrophic lateral sclerosis. *Am J Epidemiol* 123: 790–9.

13. Maekawa S., Al-Sarraj S., Kibble M., Landau S., Parnavelas J., Cotter D. *et al.* (2004) Cortical selective vulnerability in motor neuron disease: a morphometric study. *Brain* 127: 1237–51.

14. Leigh P. N., Dodson A., Swash M., Brion J. P., Anderton B. H. (1989) Cytoskeletal abnormalities in motor neuron disease. An immunocytochemical study. *Brain* 112: 521–35.

15. Siddique T., Figlewicz D. A., Pericak Vance M. A., Haines J. L., Rouleau G., Jeffers A. J. *et al.* (1991) Linkage of a gene causing familial amyotrophic lateral sclerosis to chromosome 21 and evidence of genetic-locus heterogeneity [published errata appear in *N Engl J Med* 1991 4 325(1): 71 and 1991 15 325(7): 524] [see comments]. *N Engl J Med* 324: 1381–4.

16. Rosen D. R. (1993) Mutations in Cu/Zn superoxide dismutase gene are associated with familial amyotrophic lateral sclerosis. *Nature* 362: 20–21.

17. Andersen P. M., Sims K. B., Xin W. W., Kiely R., O'Neill G., Ravits J. *et al.* (2003) Sixteen novel mutations in the Cu/Zn superoxide dismutase gene in amyotrophic lateral sclerosis: a decade of discoveries, defects and disputes. *Amyotroph Lateral Scler Other Motor Neuron Disord* 4: 62–73.

18. Shaw C. E., Enayat Z. E., Chioza B. A., Al-Chalabi A., Radunovic A., Powell J. F., *et al.* (1998) Mutations in all five exons of SOD-1 may cause ALS. *Annals of Neurology* 43: 390–4.

19. Shaw C. E., Enayat Z. E., Powell J. F., Anderson V. E., Radunovic A., al-Sarraj S. *et al.* (1997) Familial amyotrophic lateral sclerosis. Molecular pathology of a patient with a SOD1 mutation. *Neurology* 49: 1612–16.

20. Gurney M. E., Pu H., Chiu A. Y., Dal Canto M. C., Polchow C. Y., Alexander D. D. *et al.* (1994) Motor neuron degeneration in mice that express a human Cu,Zn superoxide dismutase mutation [see comments] [published erratum appears in *Science* 1995 14 269(5221): 149]. *Science* 264: 1772–5.

21. Beckman J. S., Carson M., Smith C. D., Koppenol W. H. (1993) ALS, SOD and peroxynitrite [letter]. *Nature* 364: 584.

22. Subramaniam J. R., Lyons W. E., Liu J., Bartnikas T. B., Rothstein J., Price D. L. *et al.* (2002) Mutant SOD1 causes motor neuron disease independent of copper chaperone-mediated copper loading. *Nat Neurosci* 5: 301–7.

23. Wang J., Slunt H., Gonzales V., Fromholt D., Coonfield M., Copeland N. G. *et al.* (2003) Copper-binding-site-null SOD1 causes ALS in transgenic mice: aggregates of non-native SOD1 delineate a common feature. *Hum Mol Genet* 12: 2753–64.

24. Wang J., Xu G., Borchelt D. R. (2002) High molecular weight complexes of mutant superoxide dismutase 1: age-dependent and tissue-specific accumulation. *Neurobiol Dis* 9: 139–48.

25. Rothstein J. D., Martin L. J., Kuncl R. W. (1992) Decreased glutamate transport by the brain and spinal cord in amyotrophic lateral sclerosis [see comments]. *N Engl J Med* 326: 1464–8.

26. Rothstein J. D., Van Kammen M., Levey A. I., Martin L. J., Kuncl R. W. (1995) Selective loss of glial glutamate transporter GLT-1 in amyotrophic lateral sclerosis. *Annals of Neurology* 38: 73–84.

27. Shaw P. J., Forrest V., Ince P. G., Richardson J. P., Wastell H. J.(1995) CSF and plasma amino acid levels in motor neuron disease: elevation of CSF glutamate in a subset of patients. *Neurodegeneration* 4: 209–16.

28. Fray A. E., Dempster S., Williams R. E., Cookson M. R., Shaw P. J. (2001) Glutamine synthetase activity and expression are not affected by the development of motor neuronopathy in the G93A SOD-1/ALS mouse. *Brain Res Mol Brain Res* 94: 131–6.

29. Shaw P. J., Ince P. G., Falkous G., Mantle D. (1995) Oxidative damage to protein in sporadic motor neuron disease spinal cord. *Annals of Neurology* 38: 691–5.

30. Andrus P. K., Fleck T. J., Gurney M. E., Hall E. D. (1998) Protein oxidative damage in a transgenic mouse model of familial amyotrophic lateral sclerosis. *Journal of Neurochemistry* 71: 2041–8.

31. Beal M. F., Ferrante R. J., Browne S. E., Matthews R. T., Kowall N. W., Brown R. H., Jr. (1997) Increased 3-nitrotyrosine in both sporadic and familial amyotrophic lateral sclerosis [see comments]. *Annals of Neurology* 42: 644–54.

32. Ferrante R. J., Shinobu L. A., Schulz J. B., Matthews R. T., Thomas C. E., Kowall N. W., *et al.* (1997) Increased 3-nitrotyrosine and oxidative damage in mice with a human copper/zinc superoxide dismutase mutation. *Annals of Neurology* 42: 326–34.

33. Tohgi H., Abe T., Yamazaki K., Murata T., Ishizaki E., Isobe C. (1999) Remarkable increase in cerebrospinal fluid 3-nitrotyrosine in patients with sporadic amyotrophic lateral sclerosis. *Annals of Neurology* 46: 129–31.

34. Lee M. K., Marszalek J. R., Cleveland D. W. (1994) A mutant neurofilament subunit causes massive, selective motor neuron death: implications for the pathogenesis of human motor neuron disease. *Neuron* 13: 975–88.

35. Cote F., Collard J. F., Julien J. P. (1993) Progressive neuronopathy in transgenic mice expressing the human neurofilament heavy gene: a mouse model of amyotrophic lateral sclerosis. *Cell* 73: 35–46.

36. Couillard-Despres S., Zhu Q., Wong P. C., Price D. L., Cleveland D. W., Julien J. P. (1998) Protective effect of neurofilament heavy gene overexpression in motor neuron disease induced by mutant superoxide dismutase. *Proceedings of the National Academy of Sciences of the United States of America* 95: 9626–30.

37. Al-Chalabi A., Powell J. F., Russ C. R., Leigh P. N. (1997) Novel deletions in the heavy eurofilament subunit tail in patients with amyotrophic lateral sclerosis. *Neurology* 48: SS349.

38. Figlewicz D. A., Krizus A., Martinoli M. G., Meininger V., Dib M., Rouleau G. A. *et al.* (1994) Variants of the heavy neurofilament subunit are associated with the development of amyotrophic lateral sclerosis. *Human Molecular Genetics* 3: 1757–61.

39. Giehl K. M., Tetzlaff W. (1996) BDNF and NT-3, but not NGF, prevent axotomy-induced death of rat corticospinal neurons *in vivo*. *European Journal of Neuroscience* 8: 1167–75.

40. Sendtner M., Schmalbruch H., Stockli K. A., Carroll P., Kreutzberg G. W., Thoenen H. (1992) Ciliary neurotrophic factor prevents degeneration of motor neurons in mouse mutant progressive motor neuronopathy [see comments]. *Nature* 358: 502–4.

41. Parton M. J., Lyall R., Leigh P. N. (1999) Motor neuron disease and its management. *J R Coll Physicians Lond* 33: 212–18.

42. Lacomblez L., Bensimon G., Leigh P. N., Guillet P., Meininger V. (1996) Dose-ranging study of riluzole in amyotrophic lateral sclerosis. *Lancet* 347: 1425–31.

43. Anonymous (1999) A controlled trial of recombinant methionyl human BDNF in ALS: The BDNF Study Group (Phase III). *Neurology* 52: 1427–33.

44. Borasio G. D., Robberecht W., Leigh P. N., Emile J., Guiloff R. J., Jerusalem F. *et al.* (1998) A placebo-controlled trial of insulin-like growth factor-I in amyotrophic lateral sclerosis. European ALS/IGF-I Study Group. *Neurology* 51: 583–6.

45. Gurney M. E., Cutting F. B., Zhai P., Doble A., Taylor C. P., Andrus P. K. *et al.* (1996) Benefit of vitamin E, riluzole, and gabapentin in a transgenic model of familial amyotrophic lateral sclerosis. *Annals of Neurology* 39: 147–57.

46. Hottinger A. F., Fine E. G., Gurney M. E., Zurn A. D., Aebischer P. (1997) The copper chelator d-penicillamine delays onset of disease and extends survival in a transgenic mouse model of familial amyotrophic lateral sclerosis. *European Journal of Neuroscience* 9: 1548–51.

47. Klivenyi P., Ferrante R. J., Matthews R. T., Bogdanov M. B., Klein A. M., Andreassen O. A. *et al.* Neuroprotective effects of creatine in a transgenic animal model of amyotrophic lateral sclerosis. *Nat Med* 5: 347–50.

Chapter 2

Palliative care

David Oliver

Summary

Palliative care aims to improve the quality of life of both the person with ALS and their family, by the careful, multidisciplinary assessment of the problems that are experienced – physical, psychosocial and spiritual. This care should be provided by all health and social care professionals but there may be a need for more specialist services, to help in the care of more difficult issues.

Case history

Mr S was a 45-year-old man, cared for by his wife, who had two children from her earlier marriage and a four-year-old daughter from this relationship. He had been a very active man, working as a hairdresser until he had developed weakness of his hands and then legs as a result of ALS. As he deteriorated he became restricted to a wheelchair and communication was very difficult. His wife found it increasingly hard to care for him, as well as the family, and he was admitted to the hospice for a period of assessment. During this time his wife expressed her concerns that she could not cope if he came home again. After much discussion and support for the family and staff it was agreed that he would return home, with increased support and regular readmission for respite care. Communication was helped by new communication aids, following assessment by the speech and language therapist, and his drooling was eased by regular anticholinergic medication. His wife and children received regular support from the social work and nursing teams. The children were involved and supported as he deteriorated and after his death at home there was ongoing support for the funeral and in bereavement.

Palliative care is defined as:

An approach that improves the quality of life of patients and their families facing problems associated with life-threatening illness, through the prevention and relief of suffering, early identification and impeccable assessment and treatment of pain and other problems, physical, psychosocial and spiritual.[1]

The only treatment that can currently be offered for people with ALS will at best delay the progression of the disease process, and is not curative, so it can be argued that the mainstay of the care of these patients is palliative from the time of diagnosis.[2]

The aim of palliative care is to look at the 'whole patient' in the context of their social support system, which is usually their family. This holistic approach is crucial in the care of someone with ALS and is relevant from the time of investigation, before the diagnosis has been confirmed and throughout the progression of the disease.

It is important to stress that palliative care:

- Affirms life and regards dying as a normal process
- Neither hastens or postpones death
- Provides relief from pain and other distressing symptoms
- Integrates the psychological and spiritual aspects of patient care
- Offers a support system to help the family cope during the patient's illness and in their own bereavement
- Uses a team approach to address the needs of patients and their families, including bereavement counselling, if indicated
- Will enhance quality of life, and may also positively influence the course of the illness.[1]

In the past there have been many debates, especially in the care of cancer patients, about the differing roles of curative and palliative treatment. It has been suggested that curative treatment should be continued until no further benefit can be obtained and at this point palliative care should be instituted. The timing of this sudden switch in the care of the patient can be very variable and may occur very late in the disease process, when death is imminent, and this may deny the patient supportive care, such as the control of symptoms or psychosocial care. There is now a greater awareness of the need for an integrated approach to the care of a patient with a potentially incurable disease, particularly when the trajectory of the disease progression may be very variable and unsure.

Within neurology there is an increasing appreciation that palliative care is appropriate for patients with certain neurological disorders. The Ethics and Humanities Subcommittee of the American Academy of Neurology, has stated that 'neurologists understand and apply the principles of palliative care'. ALS is seen as one of the progressive and incurable neuromuscular diseases where this approach may be appropriate and 'optimal medical care depends on determining the most appropriate means of achieving those goals for each patient'.[3] Studies have shown that there has been an improvement in the care of people with ALS and over 90 per cent are able to die peacefully.[4,5]

However, there is often a reluctance to accept the progressive nature of the disease and patients and their families receive over-optimistic ideas concerning its nature and progression. Doctors have little training in either the breaking of bad news or palliative care and may find it difficult to provide patients with this information.[6,7] As a result the care of the patient and family may be less than optimal, with symptoms remaining unrelieved and psychosocial concerns never addressed or only partly recognized until near to death, when the possibilities of resolution are limited. As ALS is a disease of progressive loss and increasing disability it is essential that all aspects of care are addressed as early as possible:

- physical aspects, such as the control of symptoms
- psychological aspects, such as the fears and concerns about the disease
- social aspects, involving families and those close to the patient
- spiritual aspects, the areas concerning the meaning of life and the fears for the future.

It is very difficult to address the more profound concerns of the patient if communication is limited due to loss of speech. Earlier intervention, when the patient is more easily understood and communication aids are not necessary, allows better interaction and communication.

There may be barriers in the provision of palliative care – and these may be from the health care professionals and/or the patient and family.[2] Many professionals still see their role as the cure and alleviation of disease, whereas in reality the majority of patient care involves the palliation of symptoms and disability. All health care professionals need to accept the limitations of the care that can be given and approach patients and their families in a positive, but realistic, way. This particularly applies to the care of people with ALS, who face continual losses as the disease progresses and may require a great deal of help in coping with these losses and the ensuing changes in their lifestyle.

The negative attitudes of the health care professionals may profoundly influence the patient and family, and these attitudes may be difficult to change – as they are often related to the discomfort in dealing with dying patients, lack of acceptance of the inevitability of symptoms, disengagement when 'active' treatment is not possible and ignorance about palliative care.[2] There is a need for greater education in the principles of palliative care for all health professionals and awareness of the symptomatic treatments that can be offered to people with ALS.[8] All too often palliative care is seen as applying only to the final stages of the disease, whereas end-of-life discussions and care will start at an earlier stage and early intervention may alleviate physical and psychological distress throughout the disease progression.[2]

Many people with ALS will require more specialized help. This may be provided by a specialized neurological team, a disability or rehabilitation team or specialist palliative care services. Whichever model is used a specialized multidisciplinary team approach is essential, with the many different disciplines working collaboratively together in maximizing the care offered to the patient and family. There may be limitations as to team involvement in the care, for instance in the USA specialist palliative care services only receive Medicare funding for the last six months of life. However the need for specialized multidisciplinary care extends throughout the disease process, and may be for many years. It is essential that the same palliative care principles are provided by all the services throughout the patient's care pathway.

Specialist palliative care

In the UK many specialist palliative care providers are involved in the care of people with ALS. A survey in 2003 showed that at least 90 per cent of the inpatient units were involved in the care of this patient group.[9] The involvement varied, with units providing care

- ◆ throughout the disease, from the time of diagnosis
- ◆ respite care as the disability progressed
- ◆ terminal care, in the final weeks or days of life.

However, the units responding appeared to be involved later in the disease progression and involvement from the time of diagnosis was unusual – only 8 per cent of the responding units. The majority of units were involved later in the disease progression – for the palliation of symptoms (88 per cent) or in the terminal phase (32 per cent).[9] This can hinder the provision of palliative care as the team will meet initially with a person with more severe symptoms and often restricted communication.

The specialist palliative care services may provide care and support in different ways:

- ◆ at home, with the support of the multidisciplinary team, in collaboration with the General Practitioner (Family Physician) and community nurses
- ◆ in an inpatient palliative care unit or hospice, for symptom control, respite care or terminal care
- ◆ in a day hospice, providing care for the day, allowing respite for carers and the opportunity for multidisciplinary assessment, involvement in

rehabilitation and other activities, complementary therapies and socialization

◆ in hospital, with a palliative care team providing advice and support to patient and family and the health care professionals

◆ specialist psychosocial care from social workers, counsellors and psychologists

◆ care after the patient's death, with bereavement support and counselling for families.

This specialist palliative care follows the patient and the aim should be to provide a seamless service, wherever the patient is at that particular time. The specialist nature of the care is ensured by the close involvement of the multidisciplinary team, including:

◆ Medical practitioner, in particular a consultant in palliative medicine

◆ Nursing specialist

◆ Social worker

◆ Speech and language therapist

◆ Occupational therapist

◆ Physiotherapist

◆ Chaplain and others trained in providing spiritual care and support

◆ Clinical psychologist

◆ Dietitian

◆ Pharmacist

◆ Complementary therapists, e.g. providing aromatherapy or massage.

All the members of the team should be working primarily within specialist palliative care, have been trained and be receiving ongoing support and training in this area of expertise.

Specialist palliative care aims to look at the positive aspects of a person's life and abilities and to enable patients and their families to remain as active as possible. For many people, including health care professionals, a hospice may be seen merely in terms of terminal care and is sometimes seen very negatively.

Several studies have shown the needs of patients with ALS and the role of hospices and specialist palliative care providers in the care of this patient group.[5,10–12] O'Brien et al.[13] found that only 15 per cent of patients had been referred for symptom control although many had uncontrolled symptoms, which could benefit from the multidisciplinary assessment of the palliative care team. Although many symptoms may be experienced by the person with

ALS during the disease progression they can be managed effectively, and choking to death and severe distress at the end of life are very rare.[5,13]

Ethical dilemmas

In the care of a person with ALS there may be many ethical dilemmas to be faced. There are decisions to be made about treatment that can alter the life of the patient. As treatments, such as riluzole, are developed to slow the progression of the disease process, there will be increasing ethical debates on the effectiveness and appropriate use of these new, and usually expensive treatments. There are other decisions about treatment interventions, such as gastrostomy feeding or ventilatory support, that affect the prognosis and the survival of the patient. The appropriateness of these treatment options will need careful discussion, and it may be very difficult to discuss such issues with patients and families. Both the benefits and risks do need to be discussed. This may include discussion about the possibility of becoming 'locked in' and unable to move or communicate for someone contemplating ventilatory support (see Chapter 9a). At the same time there needs to be a full assessment of the palliative care needs of the patient and family so that palliative care can continue alongside the more active care. This often occurs in the care of patients with cancer, as there are needs for symptom control and psychosocial support while oncological treatments, such as chemotherapy, are continued. There is a need for close collaboration between neurological services and palliative care providers to ensure the patient is offered the maximum number of treatment possibilities.

Palliative care services can be involved in these processes and the need for accurate and responsible communication is very much part of the role offered by palliative care. Close collaboration is helpful and some neurological centres are suggesting the involvement of palliative care services earlier in the disease progression so that this collaboration can be fostered. It is suggested in some centres that all patients being considered for non-invasive ventilation should have specialist palliative care team contact so that the discussions about the future, and how to cope when ventilatory function deteriorates further, can be instituted by a local service who can support the patient at this time. This aims to overcome the risk of invasive ventilation being instituted in an emergency situation, by a hospital team with little knowledge of the patient, when the patient and family have already discussed this issue earlier and decided not to be considered for ventilation.[14]

ALS patients face many of these issues and fears, particularly of pain and choking. Many influential textbooks and books on diseases still talk of death from ALS being distressing and due to choking, even though there is much evidence that with good symptom control this is unlikely.[5,13] In the UK there have been two court cases brought by people with ALS, Annie Lindsell and Diane Pretty, who asked the courts to allow administration of medication when their distress was such that they no longer wished to live. After several court hearings it was felt that there was no case and the action was dropped. The arguments were based on fears of choking and respiratory distress, and as the cases were of high profile within the media many other patients with ALS have come to fear their own deaths.

Palliative care aims to help and support the patient and family and does not intend to shorten life. With the control of distress many patients feel more positive and life may even be extended. There may be rare occasions when the shortening of life may be a foreseeable consequence of treatment but the intention is never to shorten life. On occasions patients may decide against procedures or treatments that could prolong their lives, for instance a feeding gastrostomy or ventilatory support. As long as the patient is able to make this decision clearly the health care team should provide support to the patient, and family, with this decision and help in minimizing distress by the provision of good palliative care.[3]

There may be increasing challenges with the discussion of these issues, as the prevalence of cognitive change appears to be greater than once was thought – with evidence of frontal lobe changes in up to 65 per cent of people with ALS and dementia in up to 10 per cent. The decisions regarding treatment options will need to be made earlier in the disease progression, while the person is competent, although at this time the shock of the diagnosis of ALS and facing all the losses of the disease may make it difficult for a person with ALS to contemplate and discuss these issues. It may, however, be possible to discuss the person's preferences soon after diagnosis in a more general way and in this way raise the issues. The use of the 'Ethics Questionnaire' or 'Patient Preference Tool' has been suggested,[15,16] although some patients may decline these discussions – up to 30 per cent in one study.[17] Speaking earlier of these issues may allow further discussion later and the development of an advance directive (in the USA and Europe) or an advanced decision to refuse treatment (in the UK) which will clarify their wishes.

The patient with ALS faces many challenges and many losses as the disease progresses. These affect the family and close carers as well, and the health care professionals involved with the care may also be affected by these losses. Palliative care from a multidisciplinary team, working collaboratively with all the other services involved in the care, help the patient, and family, to continue to function as effectively as possible, with the aim of ensuring that the quality of life can be as good as possible.

References

1. World Health Organization (2002) *Palliative care* www.who.int/cancer/palliative/definition/en/accessed 5 January 2006.

2. Kristjanson L. J., Toye C., Dawson S. (2003) New dimensions in palliative care: a palliative approach to neurodegenerative diseases and final illness in older people. *Med J Australia* 179, S41–S43.

3. The American Academy of Neurology, Ethics and Humanities Subcommittee. (1996) Palliative care in neurology. *Neurology* 46, 870–2.

4. Mandler R. N., Anderson F. A., Miller R. G. *et al.* (2001) The ALS Patient Care Database: insights ino end-of-life care in ALS. *Amyotroph Lateral Scler Other Motor Neuron Disord* 2, 203–8.

5. Neudert C., Oliver D., Wasner M., Borasio G. D. (2001) The course of the terminal phase in patients with amyotrophic lateral sclerosis. *J Neurol* 248, 612–16.

6. Fallowfield L. J., Lipkin M., Hall A. (1998) Teaching senior oncologists communication skills: results from phase 1 of a comprehensive longitudinal program in the UK. *J Clin Oncol* 16, 1961–8.

7. Fallowfield L. J., Jenkins V. A., Beveridge H. A. (2002) Truth may hurt but deceit hurts more: communication in palliative care. *Palliat Med* 16, 297–303.

8. Mitsumoto H., Bromberg M., Johnston W. *et al.* (2005) Promoting excellence in end-of-life care in ALS. *Amyotroph Lateral Scler Other Motor Neuron Disord* 6, 145–54.

9. Oliver D., Webb S., Sloan R., Sykes N., Smith J. (2003) Specialist palliative care involvement in the care of people with motor neurone disease. Poster presentation at the 14th International Symposium on ALS/MND, Milan 2003.

10. O'Brien T.,Welsh J., Dunn F. G. (1999) ABC of palliative care: Non-malignant conditions. *BMJ* 316, 286–9.

11. Oliver D. (1996) The quality of care and symptom control – the effects on the terminal phase of MND/ALS. *J Neuro Sci* 139 (Suppl.), 134–6.

12. Borasio G. D., Voltz R. (1997) Palliative care in amyotrophic lateral sclerosis. *J Neurol,* 339, 967–73.

13. O'Brien T., Kelly M., Saunders C. (1992) Motor neurone disease: a hospice perspective. *BMJ* 304, 471–3.

14. Parton M. J., Lyall R., Leigh P. N. (1999) Motor neuron disease and its management. *J R Coll of Physicians of Lond* 33, 212–18.

15. Das A. K., Mulley G. P. (2005) The value of an ethics history? *J R Soc Med* 98, 262–6.

16. Murtagh F. E. M., Thorns A. (2006)Evaluation and ethical review of a tool to explore patient preferences for information and involvement in decision making. *J Med Ethics* 32, 311–5.

17. Murtagh F. E. M., Thorns A. (2005) Taking an 'ethics history' – letter. *J R Soc Med* 98, 442–3.

Chapter 3a

Communication:

breaking the news

Richard Sloan, Dieter E. Pongratz, and
Gian Domenico Borasio

Case history

During a hospital admission, Michael had just been diagnosed with amyotrophic lateral
sclerosis. He noticed that his neurologist seemed in a rush to get away after telling him on
the open ward and the nurses seemed embarrassed. However, Michael didn't care much as
he was relieved to be told that he could now go home.

Not having heard of ALS before, he and his wife looked it up together on the Internet.
The first phrase they saw was '. . . an inevitably fatal disease with an average life expectancy
of 2–3 years from diagnosis'. It was a Friday evening and Michael's general practitioner
wasn't around to talk about it until the Monday. Michael and his wife recall that weekend
as the worst of their lives.

On the Monday morning, they booked an appointment to see the general practitioner. He
hadn't yet received any information from the hospital and, having not seen a case of ALS since
medical school, wasn't able to answer the many questions that Michael and his wife had. After
several weeks at a follow-up appointment, the neurologist painted a gloomy picture of
increasing disability, breathing and swallowing problems, leading to death. One phrase
particularly stuck in Michael's mind – that, apart from a drug to slow the process down, the
doctor said 'I am afraid there is nothing else we can do.' This completely devastated him. He
felt as if he had been cast adrift to face an awful death full of suffering for him and his family.

Introduction

Telling the diagnosis to patients with amyotrophic lateral sclerosis (ALS) is a
daunting task for any neurologist. Obviously, breaking the news in ALS is not
a procedure that can be standardized. However, proven techniques exist to
reduce the trauma to the patient and ease the burden on the doctor, thus
reducing the risk of burnout and the tendency to 'pull away' from the patient.
Such communication skills are of fundamental importance to clinical practice

and should be more prominent in medical teaching. The way the patient is told the diagnosis is now recognized to be the first and one of the most delicate steps in palliative care.

The task of telling a patient that they have ALS generally falls to the neurologist diagnosing it. Whilst the messenger can get blamed for bad news, there is anecdotal and research-based evidence that it is not always performed optimally.[1,2] Because of the poor prognosis there has been reluctance in the past to tell the patient the whole truth. Often, the patient was given 'reassuring' statements, while the relatives were informed more fully, with the addendum 'there is nothing more that can be done for him or her'. This practice still exists, although most clinicians now respect the ethical principle of patient autonomy.

The majority of patients do want to have information on their condition, even if it is life-threatening.[3,4] Without this, the stress they suffer through uncertainty is often worse than knowing they will die. One in five patients with cancer develop full-blown psychiatric disorders.[5] The main predictive factor for this is the way in which bad news is broken.[6] The feeling of hopelessness present on both sides when the diagnosis of ALS is disclosed should not lead to withholding information that might be essential for the patient's life-planning.[7] Breaking the news is an ongoing process throughout the course of the disease: it is not just limited to the communication of the diagnosis (which in itself is a multi-step procedure), but encompasses all the aspects of the information flow from the physician to the patient regarding the disease process, thus including good as well as bad news. This chapter offers some suggestions on how to achieve this.

Background

Johnston and co-workers[2] interviewed 50 patients about their experiences of being told they had ALS. Most patients saw the providing of a label for their condition as a positive thing – 'at least I now know what I have to contend with'. Negative aspects included being told too late – 'I could have used the past year better if I had known it might have been my last'; being told the diagnosis without the option of having a relative present; lack of privacy (e.g. in the open wards); being told in vague or confusing terms; and too much detail all at once. Although there was no evidence that poor communication at the time of diagnosis was responsible for prolonged mood disturbance, patients may well have undergone unnecessary psychological trauma at the time they were told. A summary of the findings is shown in Table 3a.1.

Table 3a.1 Communicating the diagnosis of ALS

Most people see positive aspects on being told the diagnosis, especially as it provides a label for the condition

People prefer the diagnosis to be communicated in a direct, empathetic style

Being able to ask questions is important

Doctors should guard against giving too pessimistic a message all at once

Information on where to get further help (e.g. from a patients' association) is important at the time of diagnosis

People generally prefer to be told with someone else present

After Johnston et al.[2]

Table 3a.2 Why breaking bad news is difficult for doctors

Fear of the messenger getting blamed for bad news

Perceived lack of time

Lack of training

Fear of causing distress

Fear of being asked difficult questions

Fear of not having all the answers

Invoking fears of one's own mortality

After Buckman.[11]

Lack of adequate communication skills also leads to stress in doctors.[8] Burn-out is more likely amongst consultants who feel insufficiently trained in communication skills.[9] As the Health Service Commissioner for the UK[10] (1991) points out, improvement in communications between health care workers, patients and relatives would result in a marked reduction in the number of complaints reported to him. Table 3a.2 outlines the reasons why breaking bad news is difficult.

What to tell

Minimum information

After the diagnosis is firmly established, the patient should be informed that they have a progressive disease of the motor nerves, for which no curative therapy is available. The name of the disease must be told and explained to avoid confusion, for example, with multiple sclerosis. If the family history is negative, it is reassuring for patient and family to know that their children are unlikely to be at risk. Positive aspects (e.g. no pain, no disturbances in sensation, continence etc.) should be stressed, as well as the availability of effective palliative measures for practically all symptoms of ALS.[12] Current research efforts, and where available, the possibility of taking part in clinical studies of new drugs should be pointed out as a means to foster hope.

Beginning of the disease

Patients often suspect a connection between the outbreak of the disease and a specific event (e.g. accident, operation, private or professional crises etc.). This question should be addressed, and patients should be told that the disease starts many years if not decades before the first symptoms appear. Since at least 50 per cent of the spinal motor neurons have to degenerate prior to clinical manifestation, it is impossible to establish when the disease began in any single patient, even with a large degree of approximation.

Prognosis

Many ALS patients ask directly about their remaining lifespan since, at the time of diagnosis, they have usually witnessed the progression of the disease for several months if not years. The answer to this question should include the information that there are no sudden relapses, that periods of relative stabilization may occur and that rare remissions have been observed. The patients should be told that the course of ALS may vary between months and decades (e.g. Stephen Hawking), making a firm statement on prognosis all but impossible for any single patient. In our experience, many patients appreciate a rough approximation, for example, 'I think you have probably got several months rather than several years left.' This allows them to plan the rest of their lives and is more helpful than an outright refusal to speculate. However, if a patient explicitly asks for available statistics, they have the right to know. Sensitive questioning about suicidal thoughts may be advisable if the patient appears depressed. Such acknowledgement reduces rather than increases suicidal attempts.

Available therapies

Since 1996, the first substance with a modest life-prolonging effect in ALS has been on the market (riluzole).[13] Subject to availability of reimbursement for this drug, an open discussion on its pros and cons should take place. Patients must know that they will not notice any improvements in function due to riluzole. The possible side effects (nausea, asthenia, dizziness) should be mentioned. This discussion avoids raising false hopes, which might otherwise eventually lead to disillusion and frustration.

Unconventional treatments

It is all too understandable that patients with ALS start looking for help outside the boundaries of 'classical' medicine. This topic should therefore be addressed the first time the diagnosis is told. Patients should be reassured that their physician does not object to their trying homeopathic medication, acupuncture etc., if they so wish. However, patients and families must be warned that some alternative methods (e.g. 'fresh cell therapy' or snake toxins) may be dangerous to their health, while others may entail serious financial consequences for the benefit of charlatans and common criminals (including, sadly, some physicians).

Patients' associations

Patients can obtain invaluable help (indeed, more than their doctors can usually offer) from the ALS patients' associations, which are present in almost every major country in the world and are grouped together in the Alliance of ALS/MND associations (a list with addresses and contact details can be found on the Internet at http://www.alsmndalliance.org). It is therefore essential to inform patients and families from the beginning about the existence of these associations, provide them with the relevant addresses and telephone numbers, and explicitly encourage them to get in touch with the association.

Second opinion

Many patients, when confronted with a diagnosis like ALS, will want a second opinion. Again, this is more than understandable and should be accommodated by the physician who is breaking the news. Possible tertiary referral centres should be discussed with the patient. This can strengthen the doctor–patient relationship and help to avoid the patient self-referring from one doctor to another.

If the diagnosis is only suspected

What has been said so far presupposes an unequivocal clinical diagnosis of ALS, i.e. 'probable' or 'definite' ALS according to the El Escorial criteria of the World Federation of Neurology.[14] If these criteria are not met, the physician will obviously take a more careful approach, depending on the degree of clinical certainty. The offer of information on possible differential diagnoses and the diagnostic plan can reduce the stress of not being told anything. However, if the El Escorial criteria for 'possible' ALS are fulfilled, information on appropriate palliative measures, available drug options and therapeutic studies should be considered as these patients rarely turn out to have something else.

Discussing mechanical ventilation and the terminal phase

For many ALS patients, the onset of dyspnoeic symptoms marks a turning point during the course of their disease. Often, the first dyspnoeic bouts happen after choking on food, on exertion or during sleep. At the beginning of clinically manifest involvement of the respiratory muscles, anxiety is usually the most prominent symptom during dyspnoeic attacks (which therefore respond very well to short-acting benzodiazepines, e.g. lorazepam 0.5–1 mg sublingually). If the subject has not been discussed previously, the following factors should be the trigger for the offer to talk to the patient about the terminal phase of the disease: when the first dyspnoeic symptoms appear: symptoms of chronic nocturnal hypoventilation develop; a rapid drop in FVC below 50 per cent occurs.[15] The reason for this recommendation is that almost all patients, when questioned at this stage, report fears of 'choking to death'. In our experience, describing the physiological mechanism leading to terminal hypercapnic coma and the resulting peaceful death in sleep will relieve these fears in most cases. Patients and relatives must also be informed that the array of medications available in the terminal phase, if correctly applied, do prevent suffering.[16] This information needs to be reiterated in subsequent visits.

At this stage, patients should be asked whether they would wish to be intubated and ventilated in the event of terminal respiratory insufficiency. Patients who have been informed about the possible subsequent clinical course, which may end up in a 'locked-in' syndrome on an intensive care unit,[17] will usually decline such a procedure. This refusal must be documented by the physician and is often best incorporated into a living will (see Chapter XX on advance directives). The consequences of such a decision must be discussed with patient, family and the family physician (e.g. concerning the use of medications in the terminal phase for relieving distressing physical or psychological symptoms).[18]

How to tell

Maguire and co-workers (1986) have outlined the factors to be considered when breaking bad news (Table 3a.3), which will be discussed in detail below.

Table 3a.3 The stages in breaking bad news

Setting
Finding out what the patient already knows or suspects
Finding out how much more they want to know
Firing the warning shot
Providing information in stages (the hierarchy of euphemisms)
Acknowledging and responding to the patient's reaction to the news
Contract for the future
Reinforcement of information

Modified from Maguire et al.[19]

They define three underlying objectives in the process:

1. Do not withhold information if the patients wants it.

2. Do not impose information if the patient does not want it.

3. Gauge and respond to the patient's reaction to the news.

The setting

In some countries, for example the United States, diagnostic procedures for ALS are usually performed in an outpatient setting, while in others (e.g. Germany and the UK), patients are usually referred to a neurology department for inpatient work-up once ALS is suspected. The latter procedure gives the physician the possibility of a step-wise offering of information over several days, thereby allowing the patient to reflect overnight and ask additional questions. If the diagnosis is told in an outpatient setting, a short-term follow-up visit should be scheduled.

Privacy is essential, so that both doctor and patient can feel free to discuss difficult issues without feeling self-conscious that others are listening in. Although traditional, disclosure of personal medical details on the open ward is a breach of confidentiality which would be universally condemned in any other clinical setting. Even if the patient is immobile, with planning, it should be possible to transfer them to a quiet room. There should be no interruptions. The phone should be off the hook and bleeps handed to someone else for taking messages. The manner in which the news is broken is just as important as the words used.[20] Warmth, eye contact, empathy and lack of medical jargon are considered important by patients.

Patients often say that they would have liked to have had the option of having someone else with them when the news was broken, such as a relative or nurse. This may be helpful for picking up pieces afterwards. The patient can also check out with the other person details they may not have taken in fully the first time. When it is known that results of investigations are likely to be through by a certain day, the patient should be asked in advance if they would like someone else there with them.

Roger Carus, a patient who wrote about his experience of being diagnosed with ALS in the mid-1970s, found out inadvertently whilst in hospital for investigations. He was not sure whether or not his wife had been told the diagnosis by his neurologist and recalls 'I spent two of the most agonising weeks of my life trying to find out whether she knew or not.'[1]

Cross-cultural differences should be recognized and taken into account when delivering the diagnosis.[21] In some countries, such as Japan, it is customary for the patient to delegate any decision concerning e.g. end-of-life issues to the family and the physician, although a trend towards more open discussion has taken place in recent years.[22]

Finding out what the patient knows or suspects

To launch straight into an explanation of the diagnosis can be disastrous. Finding out what the patient understands so far helps gauge the pace of the consultation and where the patient is starting from. Some patients may genuinely have no idea that there is anything seriously wrong. Others may be terrified that they are going to die next week. 'What have you made of things so far?' is a good opening question.

Finding out how much more they want to know

Although the majority will want more information, a small minority would be devastated if told bad news at any stage. 'Some people wish to know everything about their health and others just what the doctor's treatment plan is. Which camp do you fall into?' Those who habitually cope by using denial will relate to the latter and be spared unnecessary distress.

Firing a warning shot

Where the patient is asking for more information, it is still important to signal that difficult news is coming before disclosing it. This lessens the blow for those still relatively unsuspecting. 'I'm afraid that the results of your investigations are not what I was hoping for.' There should then be a pause during which the doctor gauges the patient's reaction. If they look shocked, ask what is going through their mind. If in doubt as to whether to continue, ask whether they want more information or time to think about it. Where the patient says 'What do you mean, not what you were hoping for?', this is a clear request for more information and it is right to proceed.

Providing information in stages

It is better to give the patient small pieces of information at a time and check whether they have understood before going on to the next bit of detail – 'Does this make sense to you?' or 'Do you want me to go over that again?' To conduct a monologue only find out that the patient froze after the first sentence is a waste of everyone's time. Again, if the patient looks shocked, ask what is on their mind and check out whether they are ready to go on or not.

A good technique for delivering information stepwise is known as the 'hierarchy of euphemisms': small pieces of information of increasing seriousness are told to the patient, with pauses in between for the patient to digest them. This avoids extreme distress and the patient 'switching off' to any further explanation through shock. For example: 'The tests we have performed show you have a problem with the nerves which transmit instructions to the muscles'; 'The nerves are gradually being destroyed so that your muscles can't work properly'; 'The condition you have got is called amyotrophic lateral sclerosis, or motor neurone disease'; 'Unfortunately, there is no known cure at the moment, although there is a drug (riluzole) which modestly slows the deterioration down'; 'Yes, the disease is eventually fatal.'

Where the diagnosis is inevitably fatal, this may be too much to handle straight away. Unless they ask directly, it may be better to offer to see the patient again and find out how much more information they are ready for.

Acknowledging and responding to the patient's reaction to the news

In order not to impose information that the patient is not yet ready for, the doctor pauses at each step to gauge whether they are ready for further information. If the patient looks shocked or cries, the messenger's response is crucial. Carrying on through embarrassment will appear uncaring to the patient who will be unable to take anything more in anyway. 'This must be shocking news' acknowledges that this is an understandable reaction in the circumstances. Try to find out exactly what the source of their distress is – 'Can you bear to tell me what's going through your mind right now?' This allows them to decline if it is too difficult to talk about. The answer may seem obvious, but will be different for different people, based on previous concepts and experiences. It is an opportunity to address misunderstandings. If the patient is expressing undue pessimism, such as thinking they are going to die next week, appropriate reassurance can be given that this is not the case.

Contract for the future

It is important at the end of the consultation to make specific arrangements for the patient to be seen again and have the opportunity to clarify or ask more. Where there is no definitive medical treatment, it is tempting to tell the patient they don't need to come back again but this can be very frightening. Offering to see the patient again yourself conveys to patients the feeling that they are being supported, not abandoned.

Phrases like 'I'm afraid there's nothing more we can do' leave patients devastated, presuming falsely that they are condemned to intractable suffering. We have found it helpful to demonstrate concern for the patient by informing them of sources of help and support, as outlined above, and arranging a short-term follow-up meeting. Further exploration of the emotional impact of the diagnosis can be provided by a specialist member of staff, such as a social worker, either straight away or a few days later in the patient's own home.[23] Often, patients tend to forget information, even if they have fully understood it when it was first told. It is therefore important, on each clinic visit, to re-check where the patient stands and to move on jointly from there.

Reinforcement of information

Evidence from the cancer literature suggests that patients might profit from being handed out an audiotape of the consultation or receiving a letter outlining the consultation in lay terms, with a preference for the former.[24] This approach has not yet been tested in ALS patients. Data from a small sample[25] show that a large proportion of patients and relatives felt that they received no or insufficient information from their physician at the time of diagnosis. A brochure containing general information on ALS in lay terms was regarded to be informative by almost all patients and relatives. Therefore, handing out written information after the consultation will be helpful in most cases. However, it might be advisable to ask patient and relatives whether they feel that they are ready for it or whether they would prefer to receive the material at a later stage.

Collusion

Collusion is defined as a secret agreement to conspire to deceive. In health care, it usually takes the form of a relative asking the doctor or nurse not to tell the patient they have a serious illness or a poor prognosis. Ethically, this is unjustifiable as the patient has the right to know information about themselves. Alternatively, patients may ask professionals not to tell relatives or children of their illness. Although this too eventually causes problems, by contrast, it is ethically justifiable as the patient has the right to decide who, other than those professionally involved in their care, has access to confidential medical information about themselves.[26]

The colluder's motive is usually the protection of loved ones from distressing news. This instinctive action, well-meaning though it is, usually results in more distress in the long run – both for the patient who may become isolated and anxious on becoming less well, and for the colluder, as secrets become harder to maintain in the face of that deterioration.[26] If not recognized or addressed, the situation also becomes more stressful for the professionals involved. They become torn between the duty to be truthful to the patient and incurring the wrath of the colluder. It is easy for an unsuspecting doctor or nurse, unaware of the collusion, to innocently disclose information and feel castigated by everyone.

Often, because of lack of training, professionals don't confront the collusion and everyone ultimately suffers the consequences.

There are, however, guidelines to prevent the situation escalating.[19] They are based on two fundamental ethical premises which were already mentioned above:

1. patients have the right to medical information about themselves if they want it:
2. patients have the right to decline medical information about themselves if they do not want it.

The guidelines aid negotiation with the colluder to find out which category the patient is in. Because the protective instincts of the colluder are very strong, it is crucial to first understand and openly acknowledge why they are doing it. This prevents a confrontation developing and wins them over so that you can then negotiate checking out with the patient if there is anything else they wish to know. The colluder can then be helped to see the potential downsides of their well-meaning actions.

Guidelines for dealing with collusion

1. Ascertain from the colluder why they have chosen to do it and acknowledge their reasons – if they fear the patient going to pieces, do they have any evidence from the past that this might indeed happen?

Where there is justified concern, the doctor would rightly be more cautious in his subsequent dialogue with the patient.

2. Find out the cost to the colluder of the collusion – colluders may not acknowledge the stress on themselves or the strain on their relationship with the patient. 'How have things changed between you since he got his illness?' 'How are you sleeping?'

3. Discuss the down side to collusion for patient and colluder – although relatively easy to maintain at first, collusion usually becomes more and more stressful with time.

4. Negotiate with the colluder to see the patient on your own to find out how they are feeling about their situation and whether there is anything else they wish to know – promise that you won't force information on them that they don't ask for. However, most patients do want to know in time and, if asked, you would give honest answers. If the colluder denies access to the patient, it would be potentially confrontational to insist. It may be better to remain vigilant and use future opportunities as they present themselves to remind the colluder of the escalating stress as it develops.

5. Interview the patient alone. If they are in denial and do not want any more information, allow them to maintain this coping mechanism, saying that they can always ask anything in the future if they wish to. More often, they will appreciate the opportunity to find out more, but may have been keeping quiet because of the imposed block to communication – colluding with the collusion. Many patients will have worked out for themselves that their illness is a serious one by the awkwardness of family and professionals. Patients often express relief when things are finally out in the open. Offer to talk with them and their family to share what has just been discussed.

6. Talk with patient and family together. This models open communication within the family and gets over the fear of how to break the ice.

The concept of hope

When faced with adversity, humans often avoid going to pieces by holding out hope for better days. In the case of serious illness, hope for a cure may persist, even when this is highly unlikely. Professionals should be wary of killing all hope – this may remove the patient's main coping mechanism and risks rejection of the messenger. Nor should professionals be over-optimistic either as this jeopardizes trust when reassurances turn out to be false.

The skill for the health care professional is in helping the patient adjust their goals realistically to their situation at a pace which is acceptable to them. This may mean consoling the person who is finally realizing that they are never going to regain full functional capacity whilst giving them realistic hope that mobility can still be maintained to a lesser degree in a wheelchair.

For those coming to realize their mortality from a neurological disease, the pledging of continuing support whatever happens is important in maintaining hope for a comfortable, peaceful death.

Conclusion

Whilst breaking the news in ALS will never be easy, proven techniques exist to reduce the trauma to the patient and ease the burden on the doctor. Such communication skills are of fundamental importance to clinical practice, and should be given as much prominence as clinical skills in both undergraduate and postgraduate teaching.[27] The way the patient is told the diagnosis is now recognized to be the first and one of the most important steps in palliative care.[28] There is increasing research evidence of optimal communication skills, how to acquire and retain them, and the beneficial effects they have on patient psychological well-being.[29,30] To quote from Caplan:[31]

The increased number of diagnostic and treatment options makes even more crucial the physician's skill in managing illness and the art of communicating with patients and their loved ones. There but for the grace of God go we all, for all of us and our families are, or will eventually become, patients.

Acknowledgement

This chapter incorporates material from a paper published in the 1998 Supplement of the *Journal of Neurological Sciences* devoted to the 8th International Symposium on ALS/MND.[25] We thank the publishers of the *Journal of Neurological Sciences* for their permission to use the material.

References

1. **Carus R.** (1980) Motor neurone disease: a demeaning illness. *BMJ* 80, 455–6.

2. **Johnston M., Earll L., Mitchell E., Morrison V., Wright S.** (1996) Communicating the diagnosis of motor neurone disease. *Palliative Medicine* 10, 23–34.

3. **Ley P.** (1998) *Communication with Patients: Improving Communication, Satisfaction and Compliance.* Croom Helm, London.

4. **Silverstein M. D., Stocking C. B., Antel J. P., Beckwith J., Roos R. P., Siegler M.** (1991) Amyotrophic lateral sclerosis and life-sustaining therapy: patients' desire for information, participation in decision making, and life-sustaining therapy. *Mayo Clinical Proceedings*, 66, 906–13.

5. **Parle M., Jones B., Maguire G. P.** (1996) Maladaptive coping and affective disorders in cancer patients. *Psychological Medicine* 26, 735–44.

6. Fallowfield, L. J., Hall, A., Maguire, G. P., Baum, M. (1990) Psychological outcomes of different treatment policies in women with early breast cancer outside a clinical trial. *BMJ* **301**, 575–80.

7. Meininger V. (1993) Breaking bad news in amyotrophic lateral sclerosis. *Palliative Medicine* **7** (Suppl. 2): 37–40.

8. Davis H., Fallowfield L. (1991) *Counselling and Communication in Health Care*, Wiley, Chichester.

9. Ramirez A. J., Graham J., Richards M. A., Cull A., Gregory W. M. (1996) Mental health of hospital consultants: the effects of stress and satisfaction at work. *Lancet*, **347**, 724–8.

10. Health Service Commisssioner (1991) *Third Report for Session 1990–91*. HMSO, London.

11. Buckman R. (1996) *How to Break Bad News*. Papermac, London.

12. Borasio G. D., Voltz R. (1997) Palliative care in amyotrophic lateral sclerosis. *Journal of Neurology* **244** (Suppl. 4): S11–S17.

13. Lacomblez L., Bensimon G., Leigh P. N., Guillet P., Meininger V. (1996) Dose-ranging study of riluzole in amyotrophic lateral sclerosis. *Lancet* **347**, 1425–31.

14. Brooks B. R. (1994) El Escorial World Federation of Neurology criteria for the diagnosis of amyotrophic lateral sclerosis. *Journal of Neurological Sciences* **124** (Suppl.): 96–107.

15. Mitsumoto H., Bromberg M., Johnston W., Tandan R., Byock I., Lyon M., Miller R. G., Appel S. H., Benditt J., Bernat J. L., Borasio G. D., Carter A. C., Clawson L., Del Bene M. L., Kasarskis E. J., LeGrand S. B., Mandler R., McCarthy J., Munsat T., Newman D., Sufit R. L., Versenyi A. (2005) Promoting excellence in end-of-life care in ALS. *Amyotrophic Lateral Sclerosis and Other Motor Neuron Disorders* **6**, 145–54.

16. O'Brien T., Kelly M., Saunders C. (1992) Motorneurone disease: a hospice perspective. *BMJ* **304**: 459–60.

17. Hayashi H., Shuuichi K., Kawada A. (1991) Amyotrophic lateral sclerosis patients living beyond respiratory failure. *Journal of the Neurological Sciences*, **105**, 73–78.

18. Voltz R., Borasio G. D. (1997) Palliative therapy in the terminal stage of neurologic disease. *J Neurology*, **244** (Suppl. 4): S2–S10.

19. Maguire P., Falkner A. (1988) Communicating with cancer patients: 2 – handling uncertainty, collusion and denial. *BMJ* **297**: 907–9.

20. Brewin T. B. (1992) Three ways of giving bad news. *Lancet* **337**: 1207–9.

21. Silani V., Borasio G. D. (1999) Honesty and hope: announcement of diagnosis in ALS. *Neurology*, **53** (Suppl. 4): S37–S39.

22. Borasio G. D., Gelinas D. F., Yanagisawa N. (1998a) Mechanical ventilation in ALS: a cross-cultural perspective. *Journal of Neurology* **245** (Suppl. 2): S7–S12.

23. Ackerman G. and Oliver D. J. (1997) Psychosocial support in an outpatient clinic. *Palliative Medicine* **11**, 167–8.

24. Tattersall M. H., Butow P. N., Griffin A. M., Dunn S. M. (1994) The take-home message: patients prefer consultation audiotapes to summary letters. *Journal of Clinical Oncology* **12**, 1305–11.

25. Borasio G. D., Sloan R., Pongratz, D. E. (1998b) Breaking the news in amyotrophic lateral sclerosis. *Journal of the Neurological Sciences* **160** (Suppl. 1): S127–S133.

26. **Benson J, Britten N.** (1996) Respecting the autonomy of cancer patients when talking with their families: qualitative analysis of semistructured interviews with patients. *BMJ* **313**: 729–731.

27. **Kidd J, Patel V, Peile E, Carter Y.** (2005) Clinical and communication skills: Need to be learnt side by side. *BMJ* **330**(7488): 374–5.

28. **Doyle D., O'Connell, S.** (1996) Breaking bad news: starting palliative care. *Journal of the Royal Society of Medicine* **89**, 590–1.

29. **Stewart M. A.** (1995) Effective physician-patient communication and health outcomes: a review. *Can Med Assoc J* **152**: 1423–33.

30. **Maguire P, Pitceathly C.** (2002) Key communication skills and how to acquire them. *BMJ* **325**: 697–700.

31. **Caplan L. R.** (1990) *The Effective Clinical Neurologist.* Blackwell Scientific, Oxford.

Decision making

Wendy Johnston

Introduction

Prognosis and quality of life have steadily improved for patients with ALS, due in part to improved nutrition and respiratory support, as well as the modest benefit of riluzole. However, treatment is limited and inevitably decisions about accepting or forgoing life-sustaining therapies will be made. Requests for assisted suicide and/or euthanasia may form part of the discussion of decisions for the end of life. Management of ALS therefore requires developing individualized advance care planning, particularly addressing specific decisions regarding respiratory and nutritional support. The medical, psycho-social and spiritual context for each individual and family as well as medical, community and financial resources will influence both the decisions and their implementation. Emerging data regarding cognitive deficits and depression in ALS patients, both of which can influence decision-making, must also be addressed in anticipation of end-of-life care.

What are 'decisions for the end of life'?

Any decision to limit or forgo a life-sustaining intervention, to accept symptom relief over life-prolonging therapy, or to hasten death is a decision for the end of life (EOL). Specific goals may include completion of tasks, reconciliation of conflicts, or determining a legacy. The preferred location of death and presence of loved ones are important considerations. Planning for EOL necessitates an understanding at some level that death, while perhaps not imminent, is the likely outcome of disease progression. Decisions may be disease-specific, for example, whether to forgo mechanical ventilation via tracheostomy in ALS, or value driven, such as the desire to die at home. Each decision will be subject to variables particular to the individual and their milieu.

It is incumbent on clinicians treating ALS to make decisions too. They must acknowledge that their own values and traditions may influence the presentation of information for decision-making. Interventions recommended in published guidelines are subject to limitations and pressures of the medical system in which they practice. Conflict may arise when values clash. Clinicians wish to do no harm, and also fear censure and legal difficulties related to the provision of end-of-life care. While death and dying are not ethical issues per se, the ethics of withdrawing and withholding care, and the use of medications that putatively hasten death are unclear to many practitioners.

What are advance directives, and when should advance directives be prepared?

Advance directives (AD) are the documented preferences of the patient for the type and timing of medical interventions. Generic advance directives would appear to be of limited utility, and major studies have documented that AD are frequently overridden or ignored. However, disease-specific, detailed ADs help guide physicians, especially in conjunction with ongoing discussions with the patient and designated proxy decision-maker.[1]

The timing of the discussion of EOL issues and advance care planning with patients and their families has to strike a balance between the desire for knowledge, and the need to make timely decisions about life-sustaining therapies. The timing and manner of disclosure of the diagnosis can have a lasting impact on the patient and family.[2,3] While there are expert opinions as to when to address EOL issues in ALS, no studies have assessed the impact of timing on outcomes (such as unwanted invasive ventilation) or quality of life of patient or caregivers. A recent survey of German neurologists and ALS patients (15 in each group) found both groups adopted a 'wait and see' approach to living wills, waiting for symptoms of respiratory failure to emerge before completing a generic, not an ALS-specific form.[4] Both neurologists and patients in this study perceived AD as a harbinger of imminent death. The authors conclude that the goals of preparing AD were not met in this cohort. However both the American[5] and European[6] practice guidelines advocate the preparation of AD as well as designating a proxy decision-maker, and to review the content with both at least every six months. The ALS CARE database, largely reflecting major multidisciplinary clinics in the US and Canada, shows the majority utilize ADs and that the AD is respected.[7]

The ALS Peer Workgroup identified six triggers for discussion of EOL issues:[8]

1. The patient or family asks
2. Severe psychological, social or spiritual distress or suffering

3. Pain requiring high doses of analgesic medication

4. Dysphagia requiring feeding tube

5. Dyspnea or symptoms of hypoventilation, or FVC of 50 per cent or less

6. Loss of function in two body regions.

End of life care should be addressed routinely as part of discussions about prognosis, or when considering interventions that could have a low probability of success. More urgent discussions should be prompted by concerns that death is imminent (as perceived by the physician, patient or family) or that disease progression has been severe. An expressed desire to die, queries about assisted suicide and interest in hospice or palliative care must be dealt with immediately. Severe suffering is an emergency that demands medical intervention.[9]

The failure to address advance care planning leads to unplanned interventions, particularly mechanical ventilation.[10,11,12] Overall, the use of tracheostomy and mechanical ventilation is low in the US,[13,14] at 4 per cent or less. In spite of the advent of the AAN Practice Parameters advocating the use of non-invasive ventilation (NIV) for symptomatic management of respiratory failure, use of even NIV remains low.[13] This could reflect a lag in knowledge, but could also reflect the values and attitudes of the medical practitioners providing the care. Variability in rates of mechanical ventilation in ALS patients in Illinois was related to physician attitudes in the medical centres where the patient were managed.[11] Physicians 'frame' the discussion of mechanical ventilation in chronic lung diseases in either a positive or negative way[15] depending on their perception of the patient's quality of life, and the potential reversibility of respiratory failure. This has not been evaluated for ALS patients, but it is possible that the physician's own attitudes to NIV and long-term ventilation may be the main determinants of the likelihood for their use. The variability in use of riluzole in different centers as reported in the ALS CARE database likely reflects framing of the information presented for ostensibly patient-centred decision-making.[13]

Patient autonomy in decision-making can only be assured when the available information is presented neutrally, but fully. The resources available to support the decisions must be understood, as well as the family and community support. Advance care planning should be firmly grounded in the values of the individual, who in turn should understand the consequences of the decisions, both for themselves and their family. Values of the individual may not reflect the mainstream; exploring the spiritual and cultural values of the person with ALS and their family should be integral to the decision-making process, and should be established before crises occur. When cultural differences appear to preclude patient-centred decision-making, or appear at odds with the values of the clinicians, consultation with an institutional ethics committee, community leaders or spiritual counsellors of the individual may resolve potential conflict.

How do cognitive dysfunction and depression affect decision-making capacity of ALS patients?

Competence, also called decision-making capacity, reflects the ability to make autonomous choices. The central abilities required are that the patient must be able to:

1. Communicate a choice.
2. Understand the relevant information.
3. Appreciate the situation and its consequences.
4. Manipulate the information rationally.

Communication itself is a challenge in ALS. Alternative and augmented communication techniques may be needed, and can be time-consuming. In addition, communication about preferences for treatment is not an event but a process that occurs over time, and preferences may change as the patient experiences progression of disease.[16] Patients must understand the relevant information, which encompasses the risks, benefits and burdens of alternative courses of treatments available, including the risk of death. Patients 'appreciate' their situation when they can apply information to themselves. For example, depressed patients may not be able to appreciate benefits of treatment if they are too hopeless to imagine that an intervention such as a gastrostomy tube might improve the quality of their life.[17] Reasoning behind the decision must be logical and understandable, even when the clinician does not agree with the decision. Impairments in appreciation and rationality are most often found in patients with major psychiatric disorders such as psychosis, mania or depression.[18]

Unlike patients with other terminal illnesses, ALS patients often retain decision-making capacity up until the final hours of life. However, intact decision-making abilities cannot be taken for granted. Delirium, depression and cognitive impairments are the most common reason for a lack in decision-making capacity. Delirium is found in up to 90 per cent of cancer patients in hospices during the final weeks of life and universally interferes with decision-making capacity. Family caregivers of 50 ALS patients who died reported that 26 per cent were confused in the final month of life (Ganzini, personal communication). Among ALS patients, dehydration, hypercarbia, infections and other organ system dysfunction may all contribute to delirium. Medications commonly used at the end of life that may cause delirium include anticholinergics, benzodiazepines and opioids. Ironically, at times, patients whose wishes are not known will require ventilation or hydration in order to recover capacity to make these decisions.

Frank dementia in ALS patients is not common, but recent research reveals that many ALS patients suffer from cognitive impairment. In some studies, impairment in executive function, and other frontal lobe-mediated domains, was found in half of the study participants.[19] The relationship between these impairments and decision-making capacity in ALS patients has not been studied. In studies of patients with schizophrenia and Alzheimer's disease, it is frontal impairment, even more than memory impairment or psychiatric symptoms, which is most associated with reduced capacity to make medical decisions. The frontal lobe is especially important in the ability to flexibly consider and weigh alternatives, to apply one's values and goals, and to appreciate the relevant information. In ALS frontal dysfunction appears progressive, underscoring the importance of beginning discussions about values and goals early in the course of the illness.

Estimates of the prevalence of depression in ALS vary between 10–48 per cent,[20–23] and did not increase in a prospectively followed group in hospice in the last months of life.[22] However, when present, symptoms of depression that have an impact on decision-making ability include hopelessness, pessimism, low self-esteem and suicidality. Mild to moderate depression did not influence decisions. However, with effective treatment of severe depression, elderly patients were more likely, when presented hypothetical scenarios of illness, to prefer life-sustaining treatments. Patients with severe depression who would decline treatment were hopeless, overestimated the risks and burdens of treatment and underestimated the benefits.[17]

Patients accept or decline treatment through the process of informed consent. Choices must be voluntary and without undue influence from others. Clinicians must assure that patients have adequate and balanced information. There are two situations in which informed consent is not required. First, patients may waive their right to make an informed decision, and ask that their decision be made by their family, or even their physician. Second, informed consent is not required for emergencies.[24] However, failure to determine and clearly document goals of care in advance can result in inappropriate use of emergency interventions. Even when patients have advance directives, these are often overridden, ignored or never communicated in emergency settings.

What is the best response to requests for physician assisted suicide or euthanasia?

The re-emergence of the 'right to die' social movement in the mid-twentieth century, and its rise to prominence, parallels the development of successful medical interventions to extend life, as well as the legal milestones sanctioning the right of individuals (or their proxy decision-makers) to refuse or withdraw life-sustaining measures.[25] Patients with ALS have featured prominently in legal challenges, as well as individuals represented in the press and on television.

Patients with ALS seem to be more likely to request and complete physician-assisted suicide (PAS) or euthanasia than those with other terminal diseases such as cancer.[26] Interest in assisted suicide is high[20] and sustained[27] in Oregon where PAS has been legal since 1998, Recent studies in New York[28] and Germany[29] indicate a high level of interest in hastening death even in those patients enrolled in a hospice, or under the care of physicians with palliative care training.

The debate about the ethics of PAS and euthanasia centres on interpretation of basic principles of medical practice that superficially do not conflict: the imperatives to relieve suffering, respect patient autonomy and to do no harm. Medical ethicists have written in support of PAS and euthanasia for patients with ALS[30] and in opposition.[31] It is therefore not surprising that a survey of neurologists reveals a range of attitudes, as well as persistent concerns about the morality and legality of withdrawal of life support and the use of medications that sedate or potentially depress respiratory function.[32]

The American Academy of Neurology and other professional organizations specifically condemn PAS and euthanasia.[33] Yet 44 per cent of neurologists surveyed indicated willingness to perform PAS if legalized, and 13 per cent would do so under current conditions.[34] The European Federation of Neurological Sciences guidelines do not address the issue of dealing with requests for assisted death, despite the legality of the practice in at least three countries in Europe.[6]

In the wake of legalizing PAS in Oregon, studies of the apparent motivation of those requesting or completing PAS suggest that loss of autonomy, control and independence, and the inability to pursue pleasurable activities play a role, more than physical symptoms.[34,35] In addition, fear of future suffering and higher levels of hopelessness (but not depression) as well as fixed characteristics of the individual, including male gender, higher educational and socio-economic status and potentially modifiable factors including religiosity were also significantly associated with interest in PAS.[20] In contrast, a request for PAS in the last month of life did correlate with higher pain scores and insomnia.[36] Interest in, or requests for PAS may reflect a number of concerns. These queries should be approached as the opening to discuss end-of-life issues in general.

An ongoing study of ALS patients in the hospice setting[28] revealed a significant interest in hastening death in nearly 20 per cent. The decision to hasten dying was expressed consistently before death. Those who hastened dying reported poorer mood and less religiosity; they are more likely to have depressive symptoms of clinical significance, feel less in control and more hopeless. Although the numbers are small (10 of 53 expressed a desire to hasten death, 3 hastened dying) this careful prospective study is the first to identify factors that might predict interest in hastened death, and factors that may be modified by improved care.

Medical records of patients dying of ALS in the Netherlands between 1994 and 1999 were examined, with 72 per cent of the attending physicians responding to the survey,[37] 20 per cent of patients with ALS, died as a result of PAS (3 per cent) or euthanasia (17 per cent). The choice of physician-assisted death was positively associated with dying at home, and negatively associated with anxiety and importance placed on religion. Other variables (age, income, educational level, disease or care-related) were not associated with choosing physician-assisted death. 'The frequency of feelings of pain, despair, fear, choking and anger were felt to be similar in the two groups of patients.'[37] Two deaths by euthanasia were of unconscious patients who had not explicitly requested it, although one had an advance directive requesting physician-assisted death. The study did not directly survey patients, using the physician's recollection and records.

This study yields other interesting information about death and ALS. No end of life decision was made in 54 (27 per cent) of those who died, and in 37 (18 per cent) 'such decisions could not be made because the patients died suddenly', although 9/37 had advance directives requesting physician-assisted death. Therefore 40 per cent of patients studied died without having made any decisions. Although tracheostomy was present in 3 per cent and NIV used in 16 per cent no comment is made about withdrawal of respiratory support nor how such cases were classified. Guidelines for withdrawal of respiratory support from ventilator-dependent patients provide specific recommendations that include both sedation and analgesia,[38,5] however, it is possible that euthanasia may have been used instead.

In general, requests for assisted suicide and euthanasia do not persist, but persistent requests are challenging for physicians, even where there is a legal framework for the query. Interviews with physicians in Oregon who received these requests demonstrated that they are emotionally difficult both for physicians who might participate in PAS as well as those who feel they cannot.[9,40] The physician should be ready to listen thoroughly and assure the patient that no matter what the final decision, the physician is available to the patient through the illness, even if he or she cannot – or will not – prescribe a lethal medication.[41,42] Some physicians reported a sense of hopelessness and failure after receiving a request. At other times, too much empathy and identification with the patient will lead to failure to look thoroughly for alternatives. In our experience, patients who persist in wanting assisted suicide have strong needs for control, negative views of the future, and strong dislike of being dependent on others – all areas in which ALS particularly affects people. There is the risk that too much medical intervention may result in the patient feeling more dependent. Every effort to improve the patient's independence and avoid institutionalization should be made, even if safety in the home is not optimal.[39]

Summary and conclusions

The discussion of end-of-life issues would appear to be fraught with ethical challenges and difficult choices. The potential for conflict exists, and may lead clinicians to avoid open discussion and advance care-planning. Yet people with ALS and their loved ones can achieve good quality of life. Informing and guiding patients and their families through the decision-making process to a peaceful death should be integral to medical practice.

References

1. Mower W. R., Baraff L. J. (1993) Advance directives – effect of type of directive on physicians' therapeutic decisions. *Archives of Internal Medicine* 153: 375–81.
2. Borasio G. D., Sloan R., Pongratz D. E. (1998) Breaking the news in amyotrophic lateral sclerosis. *J Neurol Sci* 160 (Suppl. 1): 127–33.
3. McCluskey L., Casarett D., Siderowf A. (2004) Breaking the news: A survey of ALS patients and their caregivers. *ALS and other Motor Neuron Dis* 5: 131–5.
4. Burchardi N., Rauprich O., Hecht M., Beck M., Vollmann J. (2005) Discussing living wills. A qualitative study of a German sample of neurologists and ALS patients. *J Neurol Sci* 237 (1–2): 67–74.
5. Miller R. G., Rosenberg J. A., Gelinas D. F. *et al.* (1999) ALS Practice Parameters Task Force. Practice parameter: the care of the patient with amyotrophic lateral sclerosis (an evidence-based review). Report of the quality standards subcommittee of the American Academy of Neurology. *Neurology* 52: 1311–23.
6. Andersen P. M., Borasio G. D., Dengler R. *et al.* (2005) EFNS task force on management of amyotrophic lateral sclerosis: guidelines for diagnosing and clinical care of patients and relatives. *Eur J Neurol* 12 (12): 921–38.

7. Mandler R. N., Anderson F. A. Jr, Miller R. G., Clawson L., Cudkowicz M., Del Bene. M. (2001) The ALS Patient Care Database: insights into end-of-life care in ALS. *Amyotroph Lateral Scler Other Motor Neuron Disord* 2 (4): 203–8.

8. Mitsumoto H., Bromberg M., Johnston W. *et al.* (2005) Promoting excellence in end-of-life care in ALS *Amyotroph Lateral Scler Other Motor Neuron Disord* 6 (3): 145–54.

9. Borasio G. D. and Miller R. G. (2001) Clinical characteristics and management of ALS. *Sem Neurol* 21: 155–66.

10. Kaub-Wittemer D., von Steinbuchel N., Wasner M., Laier-Groeneveld G., Borasio G. D. (2003) Quality of life and psychosocial issues in ventilated patients with amyotrophic lateral sclerosis and their caregivers. *J Pain Symptom Manage* 26: 890–6.

11. Moss A. H., Casey P., Stocking C. B., Roos R. P., Brooks B. R., Siegler M. (1993) Home ventilation for amyotrophic lateral sclerosis: outcomes, costs and patient, family and physician attitudes. *Neurology* 43: 438–43.

12. Oppenheimer E. A. (1994) Respiratory management and home mechanical ventilation in amyotrophic lateral sclerosis. In Mitsumoto H., Norris F. (eds) *Amyotrophic Lateral Sclerosis*, 139–62. New York, Demos.

13. Bradley W. G., Anderson F., Bromberg M., Guttman L., Harati Y., Ross M., Miller R. G. (2001) Current management of ALS: comparison of the ALS CARE Database and the AAN Practice Parameter. *Neurology* 57: 500–4.

14. Albert S. M., Murphy P. L., Del Bene M. L., Rowland L. P. (1999) Prospective study of palliative care in ALS: choice, timing, outcomes. *J Neurol Sci* 169: 108–13.

15. Sullivan K. E., Hebert P. C., Logan J., O'Connor A. M., McNeely P. D. (1996) What do physicians tell patients with end-stage COPD about intubation and mechanical ventilation? *Chest* 109: 258–64.

16. Silverstein M. D., Stocking C. B., Antel J. P. (1991) Amyotrophic lateral sclerosis and life-sustaining therapy: patients' desires for information, participation in decision-making and life-sustaining therapy. *Mayo Clin Proc* 66: 906–13.

17. Ganzini L., Lee M. A., Heintz R. T., Bloom J. D., Fenn D. S. (1994)The effect of depression treatment on elderly patients' preferences for life-sustaining medical therapy. *American Journal of Psychiatry* 151: 1631–6.

18. Appelbaum P. S., Grisso T. (1995) The MacArthur Treatment Competence Study I, II, III. *Law and Human Behavior* 19: 105–74.

19. Ringholz G. M., Appel S. H., Bradshaw M., Cooke N. A., Mosnik D. M., Schulz, P. E. (2005) Prevalence and patterns of cognitive impairment in sporadic ALS. *Neurology* 65: 586–90.

20. Ganzini L., Johnston W. S., McFarland B. H., Tolle S. W., Lee M. A. (1998)Attitudes of patients with amyotrophic lateral sclerosis and their caregivers toward physician-assisted suicide. *N Engl J Med* 339: 967–73.

21. Rabkin J. G., Wagner G. J., Del Bene M. (2000) Resilience and distress among amyotrophic lateral sclerosis patients and caregivers. *Psychosomatic Medicine* 62: 271–9.

22. Rabkin J. G., Albert S. M., Del Bene M. L., O'Sullivan I., Tider T., Rowland L. P., Mitsumoto H. (2005) Prevalence of depressive disorders and change over time in late-stage ALS. *Neurology* 65: 62–7.

23. Kubler A., Winter S., Ludolph A. C., Hautzinger M., Birbaumer N. (2005) Severity of depressive symptoms and quality of life in patients with amyotrophic lateral sclerosis. *Neurorehabil Neural Repair.* **19** (3): 182–93.

24. Ganzini L., Volicer L., Nelson W. A., Fox E., Derse A. R. (2004) Ten myths about decision-making capacity. *Journal of the American Medical Directors Association* **5**: 1–5.

25. McInerney F. (2000) 'Requested death': a new social movement. *Social Science and Medicine* **50**: 137–54.

26. Ganzini L., Block S. (2002) Physician-assisted death – a last resort? *N Engl J Med* **34** (6): 1663–5.

27. Ganzini L., Silveira M. J., Johnston W. S. (2002) Predictors and correlates of interest in assisted suicide in the final month of life among ALS patients in Oregon and Washington. *J Pain Symptom Manage* **24**: 312–17.

28. Albert S. M., Rabkin J. G., Del Bene M. L., Tider T., O'Sullivan I., Rowland L. P., Mitsumoto H. (2005) Wish to die in end-stage ALS. *Neurology* **65**: 68–74.

29. Neudert C., Wasner M., Borasio G. D. (2003) Attitudes towards life-prolonging treatments and active euthanasia in German patients with amyotrophic lateral sclerosis. *ALS and other Motor Neuron Dis* **4** (Suppl.): 41.

30. Loyal L. (2000)The case for physician-assisted suicide and active euthanasia in amyotrophic lateral sclerosis. In Brown R. H., Meininger V., Swash M. (eds) *Amyotrophic Lateral Sclerosis*, pp. 423–39. London, Martin Dunitz.

31. Bernat J. (2001) Ethical and legal issues in palliative care. *Neurol Clin.* **19**: 969–87.

32. Carver A. C., Vickrey B. G., Bernat J. L. *et al.* (1999) End-of-life care: a survey of US neurologists' attitudes, behaviour, and knowledge. *Neurology* **53**: 284–93.

33. American Academy American Academy of Neurology Ethics and Humanities Subcommittee (1998) Assisted suicide, euthanasia, and the neurologist. *Neurology* **50**: 596–8.

34. Ganzini L., Nelson H. D., Schmidt T. A., Kraemer D. F., Delorit Mam Lee M. A. (2000) Physicians' experience with the Oregon Death with Dignity Act. *N Engl J Med* **342**: 557–63.

35. Sullivan A. D., Hedberg K., Hopkins D. (2001) Legalized physician-assisted suicide in Oregon 1998–2000. *N Eng J Med* **344**: 605–7.

36. Ganzini L., Johnston W. S., Silveira M. J. (2002) The final month of life in patients with ALS. *Neurology* **59**: 428–31.

37. Veldink J. H., Wokke J. H. J., van der Wal G., de Jong J. M. B. V., van den Berg L. H. (2002) Euthanasia and physician-assisted suicide among patients with amyotrophic lateral sclerosis in the Netherlands. *N Eng J Med* **346**: 1638–44.

38. Borasio G. D., Voltz R. (1998) Discontinuation of mechanical ventilation in patients with amyotrophic lateral sclerosis. *J Neurol* **245**: 717–22.

39. Ganzini L., Dobscha S. K., Heintz R. T., Press N. (2003) Oregon physicians' perceptions of patients who request assisted suicide and their families. *Journal of Palliative Medicine* **6**: 381–90.

40. Dobscha S. K., Heintz R. T., Press N., Ganzini L. (2004) Oregon physicians' responses to requests for assisted suicide: A qualitative study. *Journal of Palliative Medicine* **7**: 450–60.

41. Bascom P. B., Tolle S. W. (2002) Responding to requests for physician-assisted suicide: 'these are uncharted waters for both of us . . .'. *JAMA* **288**: 91–8.

42. Werth J. L. Jr, Benjamin G. A. H., Fenn D. S., Gordon E. D., Stutsman J. R., Bates A., Bascom P. B., Tolle S. W. (2002) A patient requesting physician-assisted suicide. *JAMA* **288**: 1984.

Chapter 3c

Advance directives

Gian Domenico Borasio and Raymond Voltz

Summary

The consideration of advance directives (AD) is increasing in many parts of the world, allowing the wishes of patients to be clear, even if they are not able to express them due to the progression of the disease. Discussing and formulating an advance directive in ALS can be a difficult and time-consuming effort and physicians and health care professionals may feel inadequately prepared for this task. However, we need to understand the role of the advance directive and a checklist is given at the end of this chapter to enable professionals to be at greater ease with some of these discussions.

Advance directives are increasingly recognized as an important tool for safeguarding patient autonomy at a stage when the patient cannot be asked directly about their preferences, as is often the case in the terminal phase of many diseases including ALS. However, there is no clear evidence that advance directives improve quality of life in any disease.[1] Specifically, advance directives did not improve patient-physician communication or decision-making in two studies involving cancer patients.[2,3] On the other hand, educating physicians about ADs significantly increased the frequency of their use and improved the physician's attitude towards ADs.[4] Importantly, physicians are more likely to follow detailed therapy- and disease-specific advance directives that are supported by a discussion with the patient and a proxy designation rather than general-type advance directives.[5]

It is clear from several studies that both physicians and patients do want to utilize ADs.[6] Interestingly, although patients want to start the discussion about ADs earlier than their physicians, both patients and physicians believe that it should be the doctor who initiates discussion.[7] Unfortunately, this often does not take place.[8] In addition, a cross-cultural study found large variations in the use of an AD between the USA, Europe and Japan,[9] despite a uniformly positive attitude towards ADs in health care professionals.[10] A recent qualitative study underscored the importance of early patient-physician communication on ADs.[11]

In a sample of ALS patients receiving mechanical ventilation, 96 per cent of patients had completed or wished to complete an AD.[12] The same study showed that ALS patients who had completed an AD were significantly more likely to have communicated their preference to stop ventilation to their family and physician than patients without an AD. A separate study in a general ALS population showed that the great majority (81 per cent) of ALS patients want "as much information as possible". Importantly, a significant proportion of surveyed patients (8 of 26) changed their preferences for life-sustaining measures (e.g., ventilators) over a six-month period.[13] In a study on the last month of life in ALS patients,[14] caregivers reported that 86 per cent of patients had a living will, 76 per cent had a health care power of attorney, and 88 per cent had at least one of these advance directives. Half of the caregivers reported that the advance directive was helpful, and half reported that it had "no effect on care". Four patients received cardiopulmonary resuscitation including two for whom the primary goal of care was to relieve pain and discomfort even if it meant shortening life.

Thus, available evidence and clinical experience results in the following guidelines for AD in ALS:

1. The physician, not the patient, should initiate discussion of AD in ALS. Such a discussion should be attempted with all patients.

2. The discussion must be result of an intensive and long-standing communication between the involved health care professionals, patients, and relatives.

3. The discussion needs to be initiated well in advance of the terminal phase (at the latest when first dyspneic symptoms appear – see Chapter 3a, Communication: breaking the news).

4. The AD should be as detailed and therapy-specific as possible. It should include clear statements about life-sustaining and invasive treatments (e.g. percutaneous endoscopic gastrostomy, tracheostomy).

5. The family, particularly the primary caregiver, should be closely involved in the process.

6. Cultural differences need to be recognized and taken into account when discussing and formulating the AD.

7. A health-care proxy should be appointed according to local laws and regulations. He or she should also sign the AD.

8. A copy of the AD should be forwarded to the home physician and the local hospital's intensive care unit.

9. All professionals involved in the care of the patient, including nurses, counsellors, hospice staff etc., should be informed about the AD.

10. Once established, the AD should be periodically re-evaluated and re-signed by patient and proxy at six-month intervals.

With the advent of new therapies and new methods for life prolongation, the importance of ADs will undoubtedly increase in the future. Care must be taken to comply with local laws and regulations, which may vary greatly between countries and states. In some ethnical groups, it may be appropriate to initiate the discussion with the family first.[15] However, the final decision should reside with the patient unless they prefer otherwise.

Discussing and formulating an AD in ALS can be a difficult and time-consuming effort. Often, physicians feel inadequately prepared for this task, and fear legal consequences especially with regard to decisions involving refusal or withdrawal of life-sustaining treatments. Collaboration with hospice institutions can be of invaluable help.[16] A checklist which may be helpful for the planning of end-of-life decisions is shown below. Suggestions for ALS-specific advance directives have been published,[17] but are still a matter of controversy.[18] More education and research is needed in this area to develop accepted guidelines and increase patients' and physicians' awareness of the importance of AD for preservation of patient autonomy at the end of life.

Checklist for planning of end-of-life decisions and advance directives in ALS

Contents

1. Medical therapy decisions

- Disease-modifying treatments (riluzole, creatine etc.): when to stop them?
- Non-invasive ventilation
- Percutaneous entero-gastrostomy
- Cardio-pulmonary resuscitation
- Invasive ventilation
- Antibiotics
- Nutrition
- Hydration
- Heparin
- Specific emergency treaments: dyspnea, pain.

(*Continued*)

Checklist for planning of end-of-life decisions and advance directives in ALS *(continued)*

2. Locus of care

- ◆ Stay at home?
- ◆ Admission to hospital?, which hospital?
- ◆ Hospice care?

3. Net of care and support

- ◆ For example family, friends, emergency phone numbers, physicians, nurses, social worker, other professionals, technical help, hospice group, proxy.

4. Psychological coping

- ◆ Devices for communication (e.g. alphabet chart, communcator)
- ◆ Professional help in telling a loved one?
- ◆ Spiritual help?

5. Personal organizatory

- ◆ Financial?
- ◆ Will?
- ◆ Funeral details?

6. Advance directives

- ◆ Proactive for specfic AD
- ◆ Does patient give oral AD?
- ◆ Does patient want information on written AD?

7. Appointing a proxy

- ◆ Informal or implicit appointment?
- ◆ Want information on formal appointment?

B. How to proceed

1. Advance directives

- ◆ Informed consent by patient
- ◆ Must be result of an intensive and longstanding communication between health care professionals, patients, and relatives
- ◆ Note oral ADs in medical record
- ◆ Help in written AD:

(Continued)

Checklist for planning of end-of-life decisions and advance directives in ALS *(continued)*

- must know patient well
- patient must be fully informed about diagnosis, prognosis, options
- patient must be mentally clear (statement of treating physician included)
- as specific and individualized as possible
- regular revision
- avoid influencing wording, but give all information necessary
♦ Witness present and signing
♦ Excluding prosecution of physician following AD may enhance acceptance.

2. Appointing a proxy

♦ Must be result of an intensive and long-standing communication between health care professionals, patients, and relatives
♦ Has patient informally or implicitly named a proxy already?
♦ Help in formally appointing a proxy according to national laws:
  - proxy must be trustworthy, fully informed, present
  - check conflict of interests
  - regular revision and discussions
♦ Witness present and signing.

3. Accompanying measures

♦ Compliance with national laws
♦ Signature of witness, caregivers, relatives, physicians
♦ Statement of treating physician (+ hospice worker):
  - patient has signed AD in my presence
  - patient is fully informed about disease and meaning of AD
  - patient has discussed AD with other professionals and relatives
  - patient does not show signs of depressive syndrome or other mental impairment
  - patient is informed about possibility of withdrawal of AD at any time
♦ Statement of all other treating physicians including the home physician:
  - acknowledging receipt of copy of the AD and willingness to comply with it

(Continued)

> **Checklist for planning of end-of-life decisions and advance directives in ALS** *(continued)*
>
> ◆ Statement of patient:
> – fully informed about disease and meaning of AD
> – has discussed AD with other professionals and relatives
> – is informed about possibility of withdrawal of AD at any time
> – I want my physician to have no/slight/moderate/much leeway in the actual decision
> – statement of relative/proxy:
> – fully informed about contents of AD and willing to comply with it.
>
> Modified from Voltz *et al.*[9]

References

1. Miller R. G., Rosenberg J. A., Gelinas D. F., Mitsumoto H., Newman D., Sufit R. *et al.* (1999). Practice parameter: the care of the patient with amyotrophic lateral sclerosis (an evidence-based review): report of the Quality Standards Subcommittee of the American Academy of Neurology: ALS Practice Parameters Task Force. *Neurology*, 52: 1311–23.

2. Teno J. M., Lynn J., Connors A. F., Jr, Wenger N., Phillips R. S., Alzola C. *et al.* (1997) The illusion of end-of-life resource savings with advance directives. SUPPORT Investigators. Study to Understand Prognoses and Preferences for Outcomes and Risks of Treatment. *Journal of the American Geriatrics Society* 45: 513–18.

3. Schneiderman L. J., Pearlman R. A., Kaplan R. M., Anderson J. P., Rosenberg E. M. (1992). Relationship of general advance directives instructions to specific life-sustaining treatment preferences in patients with serious illness. *Archives of Internal Medicine* 152: 2114–22.

4. Reilly B. M., Wagner M., Magnussen C. R., Ross J. H., Papa L., Ash J. (1995) Promoting inpatient directives about life-sustaining treatments in a community hospital. Results of a 3-year time-series intervention trial. *Archives of Internal Medicine* 155: 2317–23.

5. Mower W. R., Baraff L. J. (1993) Advance directives – effect of type of directive on physicians' therapeutic decisions. *Archives of Internal Medicine* 153: 375–81.

6. Davidson K. W., Hackler C., Caradine D. R., McCord R. S. (1989) Physicians' attitudes on advance directives. *Journal of the American Medical Association* 262: 2415–19.

7. Johnston S. C., Pfeifer M. P., McNutt R. (1995) The discussion about advance directives. Patient and physician opinions regarding when and how it should be conducted. End of Life Study Group. Archives of Internal Medicine 155: 1025–30.

8. McDonald E. R., Hillel A., Wiedenfeld S. A. (1996) Evaluation of the psychological status of ventilatory-supported patients with ALS/MND. *Palliative Medicine* 10: 35–41.

9. Voltz R., Akabayashi A., Reese C., Ohi G., Sass H. M. (1998a). End-of-life decisions and advance directives in palliative care: a crosscultural survey of patients and health care professionals. *Journal of Pain and Symptom Management* 16: 153–62.

10. **Voltz R., Akabayashi A., Reese C., Ohi G., Sass H.-M.** (1999) Attitudes of health care professionals towards clinical decisions in palliative care: A cross-cultural comparison. *Journal of Clinical Ethics* **10**: 309–15.

11. **Burchardi N., Rauprich O., Hecht M., Beck M., Vollmann J.** (2005) Discussing living wills. A qualitative study of a German sample of neurologists and ALS patients. *J Neurol Sci* **237**: 67–74.

12. **Moss A. H., Oppenheimer E. A., Casey P., Cazzolli P. A., Roos R. P., Stocking C. B.** *et al.* (1996) Patients with amyotrophic lateral sclerosis receiving long-term mechanical ventilation: Advance care planning and outcomes. *Chest* **110**: 249–55.

13. **Silverstein M. D., Stocking C. B., Antel J. P.** (1991) Amyotrophic lateral sclerosis and life-sustaining therapy: patients' desires for information, participation in decision making and life-sustaining therapy. *Mayo Clinical Proceedings* **66**: 906–13.

14. **Ganzini L., Johnston W. S., Silveira M. J.** (2002) The final month of life in patients with ALS. *Neurology* **59** (3): 428–31.

15. **Blackhall L. J., Murphy S. T., Frank G., Michel V., Azen S.** (1995) Ethnicity and attitudes toward patient autonomy. *Journal of the American Medical Association* **274**: 820–5.

16. **Voltz R., Raischl J., Borasio G. D.** (1998b). A disease-specific advance directive for ALS patients. Presentation at the 9th International Symposium on ALS/MND, Munich, Germany.

17. **Benditt J. O., Smith T. S., Tonelli M. R.** (2001) Empowering the individual with ALS at the end-of-life: disease-specific advance care planning. *Muscle Nerve* **24** (12): 1706–9.

18. **Bradley W. G.** (2002) Advanced care planning in ALS. *Muscle Nerve* **25** (6): 923.

Chapter 4a

Control of symptoms:

dyspnoea and respiratory symptoms

Rebecca Lyall and Deborah Gelinas

Case Report

Mr. DS was a 64-year-old supplier of car parts. In March 1998 he developed left foot drop, and in August, 1998 noted wasting of the muscles of his right hand. At that stage a diagnosis of ALS was made. In February 1999 he complained of excessive daytime sleepiness, and was often found sleeping at his desk at work. He complained of a 'muzzy' head in the morning. His appetite was reduced, and his wife was finding this stressful, as she observed that he was loosing weight. He was not particularly breathless, as by this time his left leg weakness had progressed, such that he was unable to walk and used a wheelchair to get around. His sniff nasal inspiratory pressure (SNIP) was reduced (-31cm H_2O, predicted -100cm H_2O). Ear lobe blood gases showed a pCO_2 of 6 kPa, pO_2 of 9.4 kPa and a bicarbonate of 30 mmol/l. A polysomnogram showed repeated arousals due to hypoventilation. He started to use non-invasive ventilation overnight. He had increased energy levels in the day and returned to a full day's work. His appetite improved and he began to put on weight. In January 2000 he began to notice dyspnoea after exertion, and also felt breathless after meals – he tended to put the ventilator on for a couple of hours after eating, and after exertion such as a shower. He was using the ventilator almost continuously for the three months prior to his death in August 2000. He still liked to shower, and would use sublingual lorazepam for relief of dyspnoea during his shower. He died peacefully at home, whilst still wearing the ventilator. Although he had difficulty clearing his secretions in the weeks prior to his death, he did not wish to use any other form of ventilatory support, and his secretions were managed with hyoscine patches and suction, that his wife applied. During the last few months of his illness, he was unable to attend the hospital. He had made contact with his local palliative care team in the months prior to his death, and was visited at home by community palliative care team. His wife was his sole carer.

Summary

Progressive loss of respiratory muscle function ultimately results in respiratory failure, the cause of death in the majority of amyotrophic lateral sclerosis

(ALS) patients. However, before respiratory muscle strength declines to a critical level, a number of symptoms can arise, generally insidiously. This chapter will describe the symptoms that arise from progressive respiratory muscle weakness and outline available management strategies.

Assessment of respiratory function

The respiratory muscles are traditionally subdivided into groups, according to their predominant function.

Inspiratory muscle function

The most important *inspiratory muscle* is the diaphragm which, at rest contributes over 70 per cent of minute volume. However, increasing ventilatory requirement, for example during exercise, involves activation of accessory muscles – namely, the intercostal muscles, scalenes, trapezii and sternocleidomastoid. A symptom of diaphragm weakness is orthopnoea (breathlessness when lying flat) as assuming a recumbent position displaces the contents of the abdomen, normally held in place by the diaphragm, into the thorax, thereby reducing lung volume. By the same mechanism dyspnoea can occur when standing in deep water or bending over. However, orthopnoea is not a universal finding and may be absent in the presence of severe generalized respiratory muscle weakness, when abdominal wall weakness prevents supine upward displacement of the diaphragm. As respiratory muscle weakness becomes more generalized, patients may notice exertional dyspnoea, however this may be under-recognized if mobility is curtailed by limb weakness. Patients describe dyspnoea on talking and that speech volume declines, with the cough and sneeze becoming audibly weaker. Dyspnoea at rest occurs when global inspiratory muscle weakness is profound and by this stage patients are close to hypercapnic ventilatory failure.

It is often not appreciated that in many patients the first manifestation of significant respiratory muscle weakness may not be dyspnoea, but symptoms arising from the presence of sleep-disordered breathing. Hypoventilation may occur during sleep when overall respiratory muscle strength remains sufficient for daytime ventilation.[1,2] Initially, hypoventilation occurs in rapid eye movement (REM) or 'dreaming' sleep as the accessory muscles, particularly the intercostal muscles, are less active in this sleep stage.[3] Ventilation then becomes exclusively dependent on the diaphragm, which, if weak, is further disadvantaged by the supine position. As weakness progresses, episodes of hypoventilation occur throughout sleep, causing repeated arousals and sleep fragmentation. Patients with nocturnal hypoventilation may complain of daytime sleepiness, increased frequency of and particularly vivid nightmares (as arousal in REM causes waking mid-dream), reduced ability to concentrate, mood disturbance and loss of appetite. Some patients report that a dry mouth wakes them as the increased respiratory effort can result in 'panting' at night. Other patients ascribe their arousal to urinary problems, however, nocturia frequently resolves with treatment of hypoventilation and is a symptom rather than cause of the sleep disturbance. In other patients, it is their bed-partners who are first aware of restless and disturbed sleep, and may report periods of apnoea or notice change of personality or mood. Eventually hypoventilation leads to significant nocturnal hypercapnia which gives rise to morning headache. It must be emphasized that the symptoms of nocturnal hypoventilation arise insidiously, often in the absence of daytime dyspnoea, and it is important that patients are questioned directly about such symptoms as these may not readily be volunteered. Hypersomnolence, lack of appetite and personality change can be wrongly attributed to depression, particularly in patients increasingly debilitated by other aspects of the disease. It should also be remembered that sleep may be disturbed in ALS without the presence of sleep-disordered breathing – patients can become uncomfortable at night for a number of reasons, for example immobility.[4]

The signs of inspiratory muscle weakness are subtle. Diaphragm weakness can cause paradoxical movement of the abdominal wall on inspiration – inward, instead of the normal outward motion. With progressive inspiratory muscle weakness, examination reveals markedly reduced chest movement, tachypnoea and use of the accessory muscles – often all that can be seen moving are the muscles of the neck.

Expiratory muscle function

The abdominal muscles are predominantly *muscles of expiration*. Working in coordination with the muscles of the upper airway, their most important contribution is the generation of an efficient cough. ALS patients with significant abdominal muscle weakness may complain that they are unable to clear secretions, or may develop a recurrent cough. Pooling of secretions in the oropharynx and ineffective attempts to clear secretions will repeatedly trigger the cough reflex. In general, expiratory muscle weakness does not occur in isolation, but we have seen expiratory muscle weakness predominate in patients with severe lower limb weakness.

There may be few signs of expiratory muscle weakness – patients may report abdominal distension, but often the most useful bedside indicator is to simply ask patients to perform a voluntary cough, revealing audible abnormality. However, as the generation of an efficient cough requires coordination of inspiratory, expiratory and upper airway muscles, an ineffective cough may arise in a number of ways and will be discussed in further detail below.

Upper airway function

There are many muscles involved in the efficient function of the vocal cords and other structures of the upper airway. ALS may cause progressive weakness of this 'bulbar' musculature. Patients with significant bulbar weakness can experience sudden episodes of severe dyspnoea, and may notice this when attempting to swallow, particularly liquids. The sensation is often described as choking, and may be accompanied by a stridor-like sound. Abnormalities of the upper airway can be demonstrated by measuring the rate of air flow during inspiration and expiration – which can be represented graphically in a 'flow volume loop'.

The presence of upper airway dysfunction and abnormal vocal cord movement in ALS has been suggested by several studies in which flow volume loops have been utilized.[5–9] The abnormalities described have been either flow limitation or gross oscillations of flow (sawtooth pattern). The former may occur because of airway narrowing due to vocal cord weakness or paralysis. This can be accentuated by inability of the cords to withstand the distal negative inspiratory pressure generated in the thorax and be sucked inwards, rather than opening, during inspiration. The sawtooth abnormality may be due to 'fluttering' of the cords. Such flow volume abnormalities are frequently associated with bulbar dysfunction, and may even anticipate the appearance of bulbar signs.[8] In ALS the cricopharyngeal sphincter muscle becomes hyperreflexive and hypertonic, and the normal coordination of laryngeal closure with voluntary swallowing is lost.[10]

Patients with upper motor neurone bulbar signs particularly report the distressing symptom of choking,[11,12] and it has been suggested that in such hyperreflexic patients, the closure reflex may be triggered at a lower threshold, enhancing the risk of upper airway obstruction. The sensation of choking may be a manifestation of sudden upper airway obstruction as the larynx closes. These abnormalities may also underlie the flow volume loop findings described above, as spontaneous closure may occur. We have performed upper airway endoscopy on patients who described such symptoms, observing that the vocal cords involute rather than open during inspiration, and the airway aperture reduces with increasingly forceful inspiratory manoeuvres.[9]

In general, significant respiratory muscle weakness arises insidiously over many months. However, a more rapid onset of symptoms can be precipitated by, for example, pneumonia.

Investigations of respiratory function in ALS patients

Respiratory muscle weakness is inevitable in ALS. The presence or absence of symptoms is an insensitive way of determining respiratory muscle strength, and indeed symptoms often only occur when considerable weakness is present. As there are now a number of treatments available to ameliorate the consequences of weakness it is important for strength to be measured, so that such treatments may be offered in a timely fashion. A number of investigations can be used to evaluate respiratory muscle strength,[13] although an evidence-based review of the management of ALS patients published by the American Academy of Neurology[14] acknowledged that 'no evidence indicated the best test for detecting early signs of impending respiratory failure'. A useful screening test is the 'slow' vital capacity (VC) performed in the upright and supine positions. Diaphragm weakness is suggested by a greater than 25 per cent fall in VC on assuming a supine position.[15] A normal supine VC makes significant diaphragm weakness unlikely. ALS patients often have difficulty in achieving an adequate mouth seal around the mouthpiece causing leakage of air when breathing out, resulting in an underestimation of VC. The manoeuvres required to perform an erect and supine VC may be difficult to achieve by a wheelchair-bound patient but several recent studies[16–18] have shown that the test can be used to predict the presence of diaphragm weakness and correlates with respiratory symptoms in ALS.

Although measurement of maximal mouth pressures can give information about inspiratory and expiratory muscle strength, respectively, these tests also require efficient utilization of mouthpieces and if leaks are present strength can be similarly underestimated. A poor correlation has been found between the maximal inspiratory mouth pressure and diaphragm strength in ALS patients,[19] and this measurement is rarely used clinically. By contrast, the pressure produced at the nose during a maximal inspiratory manoeuvre, the sniff nasal inspiratory pressure or SNIP, is a useful screening investigation.[20,21] The predicted 'normal' value can be calculated.[22] Hand-held SNIP meters are available (Respiratory Pressure Meter, Micro Medical Ltd., Rochester, Kent, UK www.micromedical.co.uk). All these measures are volitional and require the patient to make maximal efforts if measurements are to reflect true muscle strength. If a patient achieves a result within the normal range then significant weakness is unlikely. Submaximal results can either indicate weakness or reflect the patient's difficulty in performing the test to maximum effect, for example, due to a mouth leak or reduced effort.

A cough is generated by inspiration of a volume of air, closure of the vocal cords, contraction of the expiratory muscles and generation of increased pressure in the thorax and finally, sudden opening of the cords, with subsequent explosive exhalation. Therefore, the production of an effective cough requires adequate inspiratory and expiratory muscle strength, the presence of a normally functioning upper airway and the ability to coordinate these muscle groups. Weakness in any muscle group can reduce cough effectiveness. No single test of cough effectiveness yet exists. Peak cough flow (PCF) can be measured. Patients cough into a peak flow meter – more commonly used to measure peak flow in asthma. Using measurements of PCF, Bach[23] has suggested a plan of 'cough management' for patients with ALS. An adequate cough produces a PCF greater than 160 l/min. If the patient cannot achieve this unaided, a mechanical cough device, delivering positive (insufflation), then negative (exsufflation) pressure is used to overcome such muscle weakness and the resulting PCF measured. If despite compensating for inspiratory and expiratory muscle weakness, a reduced PCF is still obtained, it is assumed that the ineffective cough is due to bulbar dysfunction, and patients are advised to undergo tracheostomy placement for adequate airway clearance.

More detailed tests of respiratory muscle strength, which do not involve patient effort (non volitional tests) are available in specialized respiratory laboratories.[13,19,24] However they may be difficult to obtain universally. A pragmatic approach is to screen for respiratory muscle weakness using SNIP. If a patient can achieve the predicted normal value then significant weakness is unlikely. However, in a symptomatic patient, a value less than predicted should be further investigated with blood gas analysis and nocturnal oximetry.

Blood gas analysis

Analysis of arterial blood gas tension is useful and can be easily, and relatively painlessly achieved from ear lobe capillary blood samples. As respiratory muscle weakness occurs, the first abnormality of the blood gas is mild hypoxia and hypocapnia, as patients hyperventilate to maintain oxygen saturation. Progressive respiratory muscle weakness results in hypercapnic ventilatory failure. Recent evidence suggests that the development of hypercapnia indicates a very poor prognosis. Measurement of venous chloride and bicarbonate can provide information on the presence or absence of hypercapnia without the need for arterial blood gas estimation. Prolonged carbon dioxide retention results in chronic respiratory acidosis. This is compensated for by renal excretion of hydrogen ions in exchange for bicarbonate ions, resulting in raised plasma bicarbonate, which in turn is compensated for by increased chloride excretion. Therefore, chronic hypercapnia will result in reduced venous chloride and raised venous bicarbonate. Two studies in ALS[25,26] have shown that venous bicarbonate rises and chloride falls to abnormal levels close to death. In the latter study, the mean (range) time from detection of abnormality to death was 2.2 (0.5–6) months, suggesting that the development of hypercapnia is a pre-terminal event.

Most ALS patients have normal lungs and by the time the blood gases show substantial hypoxia, in addition to hypercapnia, respiratory muscle weakness is profound, and the prognosis is likely to be limited to months or weeks. In ALS, it is unlikely that inspiratory muscle weakness is the cause of severe hypoxia in the absence of hypercapnia, and in this case a lung parenchymal cause, such as pneumonia or pulmonary embolus should be sought.

Overnight oximetry and polysomnography

Polysomnography gives detailed analysis of sleep. During polysomnography, measurements are made of oxygen and carbon dioxide levels, abdominal and thoracic movement, as well as the electroencephalogram from which sleep can be staged. Indications for a polysomnogram may include symptoms of sleep disturbance without evidence of daytime respiratory failure, in order to gather evidence of hypoventilation-related arousal and exclude non-respiratory muscle causes of sleep disturbance. If arousal due to hypoventilation is present, the sleep disturbance may be effectively treated with nocturnal ventilation, if not then other causes of sleep disturbance should be sought. However, to perform polysomnography, patients must be admitted to a sleep laboratory. A much simpler way to identify nocturnal hypoventilation is to measure nocturnal oxygen saturations using pulse oximetry. Many oximeters can store at least eight hours of data and patients can use the machines at home. A number of recent papers[27–29] have shown that they are useful for the management of ALS patients and can identify hypoventilation due to sleep-disordered breathing. It is our practice to assess patients with symptoms of sleep-disordered breathing by obtaining an ear lobe blood gas, SNIP and overnight oximetry. Evidence of respiratory muscle weakness and an abnormal oximetry is an indication for a trial of non-invasive positive pressure ventilation (NIPPV).

Treatments of the symptoms of respiratory muscle weakness

The treatments available for symptomatic respiratory muscle weakness have evolved hugely over the last decade. However, there still remains considerable disparity in the treatments that are offered to individual ALS patients. It is important to emphasize that no modality is universally superior and treatment should be tailored to the individual.

The symptoms of sleep-disordered breathing (SDB) can be very effectively treated with ventilatory support – both NIPPV and invasive ventilation. This modality will be described in greater detail below. An alternative way of managing SDB is to enable the patient to sleep in an upright position, thereby reducing the impact of the supine position on the weak diaphragm. Hypnotics may reduce restlessness during sleep but may exacerbate hypoventilation by reducing the drive to breathe and may result in worsening hypercapnia and morning headache.

The symptoms arising from vocal cord dysfunction can be difficult to treat. We have found that minimizing the impact of a poor swallow by emphasizing safer swallowing techniques such as the chin tuck, or use of alternative feeding strategies such as gastrostomy may reduce the frequency of episodes. Vigorous treatment of siallorhoea appears to be beneficial. We emphasize to patients that it is unlikely that the vocal cords will shut permanently and explain that the natural response of taking deeper breaths may actually prolong the episode. We have found that this explanation and reassurance helps patients and carers manage the symptom better. Sublingual lorazepam (0.5–1 mg) can reduce the panic that the symptom, not surprisingly, induces and thereby shorten the episode.

Dyspnoea may be alleviated by use of NIPPV. However, this may not be universally indicated or appropriate. Intermittent dyspnoea is effectively treated with short-acting benzodiazepines such as lorazepam or diazepam. Opiates may be useful. There is a risk that opiates reduce respiratory drive. However, we have found that if initiated at low dosage and titrated slowly, whilst vigilant for symptoms of increased drowsiness, headache or somnolence, opiates can be used for long periods effectively. Oxygen can relieve dyspnoea, although it can potentially suppress respiratory drive.

The symptom of ineffective cough can be a difficult one to palliate. The mechanism of an efficient cough has been described above. Cough can be 'assisted' in a number of ways. Physiotherapy techniques such as the assisted cough can be helpful when expiratory muscle weakness is the predominant problem. The patient breathes in as normal and abdominal thrusts are applied during the cough. The technique requires sufficient upper limb strength, and although patients can be taught to perform the manoeuvre independently, most benefit appears to occur when thrusts are applied by a carer. Mechanical cough devices are available. The mechanical insufflator–exsufflator (MI-E) delivers rapidly alternating positive and negative pressures via a facial mask. Recent studies[30,31] have quantified the magnitude of PCF enhancement afforded by these techniques. The latter study found MI-E produced greatest improvement, but the majority of patients studied had minimal bulbar dysfunction. Sancho[32] described collapse of the upper airway when the device was used in ALS patients with significant bulbar weakness. Bach[23] suggests a plan of 'cough management', described above, involving cough enhancement techniques including MI-E. When significant bulbar muscle dysfunction precludes production of PCF >160 l/min despite using MI-E, patients undergo tracheostomy placement for airway clearance. Although Bachs' group[23,28,32–35] report considerable anecdotal evidence for the efficacy of this approach, no study has yet compared these different methods of cough management in ALS. MI-E is not widely available. Recent surveys in the USA[36] and UK[37] found it used in only 5 per cent of American neuromuscular clinics, and no UK centres. Reduction of the tenacity of secretions using N-acetyl carbocisteine and increased fluid intake may help. Some patients find mouth and pharyngeal suction of secretions helpful, although others find that the technique precipitates choking. It is important to manage siallorheoa adequately (see Chapter 4d, p. 132, Chapter 7c, p. 218, Chapter 4b, p. 105), as pooling of saliva frequently triggers cough.

Treatment of respiratory muscle weakness with NIPPV

Ventilatory failure arising from progressive muscle weakness can be treated by either invasive (via tracheostomy, TV) or non-invasive ventilatory support. Non-invasive positive pressure ventilation (NIPPV) is a treatment modality whereby ventilation is delivered via a nasal or facial mask.[38,32] TV has been shown to prolong survival of ALS patients considerably.[32,39] NIPPV can improve the polysomnographic and blood gas abnormality associated with SDB,[40] relieve symptoms of sleep disturbance and breathlessness, improve appetite and make the voice louder,[41,42] improve cognitive function,[43] and reduce the morbidity of gastrostomy placement.[44–46]

NIPPV can be used when respiratory muscle weakness becomes profound and the patient incapable of ventilator free respiration, with Bach[23] reporting patients using 24-hour non-invasive ventilation for mean (+/− SD) of 17.2 +/− 35.4 months. Early reports showed improved survival with NIPPV.[32,35,47–49,23] The majority of these studies compared survival of patients using ventilation to those who either did not accept, or 'tolerate' NIPPV, and demonstrated prolonged survival in those using NIPPV. Kleopa and co-investigators (1999) offered NIPPV to all patients with a FVC less than 50 per cent predicted and compared survival in patients who either refused or were judged intolerant of NIPPV (less than four hours daily use) to those who used the treatment successfully (more than four hours per night). The mean (+/− SD) survival times from onset of NIPPV were significantly different and were respectively, 4.6 (+/− 12.7), 7.0 (+/− 6.7) and 14.2 (+/− 13) months, with the rate of decline of FVC slower in successful users. Subsequent studies reinforced the view that NIPPV improved survival and reported increasing acceptance of NIPPV by patients − with more than 70 per cent of patients to whom it was offered using NIPPV successfully,[50,51] compared to 49 per cent and 54 per cent respectively in earlier studies.[48,49] However, opponents of the use of NIPPV in ALS emphasized that these studies were not randomized, and using selected patients may have influenced the results. A recent study[52] randomized patients to receive NIPPV or 'standard care' and demonstrated both prolonged survival and quality of life in ventilator users.

The prevalence of both TV and NIPPV in ALS management has varied considerably both within and between countries.[41,53] A study of practice amongst ALS treating neurologists in the US[54] found 2.8 per cent and 15.7 per cent of patients on TV and non-invasive support respectively, whilst in the UK[37] the rates were lower, respectively 0.4 per cent and 5.5 per cent. Considerable heterogeneity exists regarding attitudes towards NIPPV, with three UK neurologists making 30 per cent of all referrals for treatment nation-wide, whilst 10 per cent of their colleagues judged there to be no role for NIPPV in the management of ALS.[37] Further evidence suggests that only a proportion of patients with respiratory dysfunction receive mechanical support − in a survey of over 2000 patients, Bradley et al.[55] found that only 28 per cent of patients with dyspnoea and 9 per cent with a FVC less than 40 per cent predicted were using NIPPV. This disparity of management may in part be due to financial considerations. However, the major cause of reluctance to offer NIPPV to patients is likely to be related to the progressive nature of ALS, and the fear that prolonged survival in the face of increasing disability may reduce, rather than enhance quality of life (QL).

Effect of mechanical ventilation on quality of life

Previously few data were available on the effects of mechanical ventilation on QL in ALS, and the majority was derived from uncontrolled, retrospective studies on patients treated with TV. In the main, these studies showed that patients valued the QL achieved. McDonald et al.[56] compared the psycho-logical status and QL of 18 ALS patients on TV (13 using TV for more than 20 hours a day) with non-ventilated ALS patients and found no significant difference in depression or hopelessness, and QL as measured by life satisfac-tion ratings was the same. Moss et al.[57] reported the views of 50 patients on long term TV. The majority were satisfied with their lives and would choose TV again (80 per cent), particularly those who were living at home rather than in an institution, and who had made the decision to go onto TV themselves rather than being placed on it during an emergency situation without prior discussion. Fifty-one per cent of patients living at home on TV wanted resuscitation in the event of a cardiac arrest compared with 23 per cent living in an institution. Initial data on QL in ALS patients receiving NIPPV showed an improvement in quality of life scores after commencement,[58,59] however these studies involved small numbers of patients and did not use controls, and may not have been representative of the general ALS population. A study of QL in a group of ALS patients started on NIPPV has been undertaken, and showed a statistically significant improvement in QL, despite increasing disability.[60] Most recently Bourke[52] demonstrated that patients randomised to receive NIPPV had significantly improved QL compared to those receiving 'standard care'.

Areas of controversy in NIPPV for ALS

The optimal time for initiation of ventilation is not precisely known. Discussion of disease progression and respiratory muscle weakness may provoke anxiety in patients and carers. However, failure to recognize impending ventilatory failure may result in patients being intubated and ventilated before their views on this treatment can be established. Acute ventilation has a poor outcome, with in one study, 29 per cent of patients dying in the intensive care unit, and 54 per cent requiring permanent tracheostomy.[61] The 'Practice Parameters' of the American Academy of Neurology[14] suggest initiation of NIPPV in the presence of respiratory symptoms or when the FVC is less than 50 per cent predicted. However, significant levels of SDB have been documented in patients with FVC of 61–73 per cent predicted,[40] suggesting that restricting the treatment to those with FVC less than 50 per cent predicted might potentially exclude some that could benefit. Published data from a study measuring survival and QL in patients prescribed NIPPV at FVC of less than 50 per cent predicted, compared to those receiving the intervention at the onset of nocturnal desaturation, irrespective of FVC, suggest that improved QL is seen in the latter group.[62]

The factors that influence the magnitude of the effect of ventilation on subsequent survival and QL are not clear. Of particular concern is the presence of significant bulbar weakness. There is a theoretical risk of increased aspiration with NIPPV, as the positive pressure can potentially blow upper airway secretions through an inadequately protected airway. Studies report differing effects of bulbar weakness on the response to NIPPV, with some suggesting poor tolerance of NIPPV[48,59,51] in the presence of severe bulbar weakness and others[49] finding bulbar symptoms did not influence acceptance. A recent paper[50] has emphasized the importance of secretion management in the successful use of NIPPV by patients with significant bulbar weakness. Most recently, Bourke et al.[52] found that patients with bulbar weakness using NIPPV noted improved sleep and reduced breathlessness but QL was not improved to the same extent as in patients with lesser bulbar weakness. Survival in bulbar patients using NIPPV was not significantly prolonged.

There are several possible reasons why patients with bulbar weakness may not achieve benefit from NIPPV. A number of bulbar patients do not tolerate NIPPV, and they also complain of frequent episodes intermittent of 'choking' breathlessness and stridor. In these patients abnormal flow volume loops were found and inward inspiratory vocal cord movement was seen at bronchoscopy. Polysomnography showed episodes of upper airway obstruction, presumably from the adducted vocal cords. Ventilators capable of delivering expiratory pressure can be used to try and overcome this obstruction, but NIPPV did not improve symptoms of breathlessness or sleep disturbance in these patients and in some cases precipitated episodes of stridor. Other bulbar patients with profound hypercapnia had minimal symptoms. Although the NIPPV improved nocturnal hypercapnia, patients did not feel better. It may be that such patients have a reduced drive to breathe due to brainstem involvement and although hypercapnic do not recognize this, hence the lack of symptoms. Some centres offer NIPPV to all bulbar patients with symptoms of sleep-disordered breathing or respiratory failure, vigorously treating secretions in order to improve acceptance. Such patients are advised that the risk of aspiration may be increased with NIPPV, and if the patient's swallowing is severely impaired we may suggest gastrostomy. If after full discussion, a patient does not want a gastrostomy but finds that NIPPV palliates their symptoms, then we do not withdraw it. Although many are enthusiastic about the benefits of NIPPV, it is important to emphasize to patients and carers that the treatment may not be helpful to everyone – if patients do not benefit from an initial trial, this can be discontinued, and perhaps try again at a later date. As patients and carers have become more aware of the potential improvement in survival with NIPPV, patients who do not feel that it improves either symptoms or QL significantly, have occasionally felt pressured to use it to prolong life.

Bach has emphasized the importance of adequate cough capacity both in the choice of mode of ventilation and the effect of NIPPV on survival.[23,28,33,35] He points out that NIPPV compensates for inspiratory muscle weakness but suggests that prolonged survival also requires attention to expiratory and bulbar muscle dysfunction. There are few data available as to the optimal management strategy of an ineffective cough. At the very least patients and carers should be taught the assisted cough technique and where benefit can be demonstrated, MI-E supplied. Further research needs to be done in this area, as the majority of patients may not find tracheostomy an acceptable way to manage secretions.

Practicalities of NIPPV in ALS

When discussing the use of NIPPV with patients and their carers, there are a number of points that need to be considered. First, it is important to be sure that the symptoms of sleep disturbance are due to respiratory muscle weakness, and therefore might be ameliorated by NIPPV. Second, it is important to make an assessment of the patient's home situation. Efficient ventilation requires careful mask application, and patients with significant upper limb and hand weakness are unlikely to be able to achieve this independently. ALS patients living alone may need to consider accepting a night-time carer. The amount of assistance available from external agencies will vary between health systems, and for example, in the UK, it is very difficult for social services to provide night-time care. It should be emphasized that NIPPV is very likely to prolong survival, and therefore patients are likely to experience increasing disability whilst using a ventilator. Additionally, ventilation does not prevent progressive respiratory muscle weakness, and therefore, it is our experience that patients who accept nocturnal ventilation, gradually begin to use the machine in the daytime to alleviate dyspnoea, as respiratory muscle strength declines. This leads to increasing ventilator use, and in our experience, most patients will eventually use 24-hour ventilation. Clearly this has implications for care provision. Although long-term 24-hour NIPPV has been described,[23] NIPPV is less efficient than TV, and at this stage TV may be considered. NIPPV is reported to be preferable to TV, both to patients and caregivers.[33] Tracheostomy care involves nursing input, and domiciliary use is thus expensive and may be burdensome to families,[41] and in some health systems rarely accomplished. Cazzolli and Oppenheimer[42] found that no ALS patients cared for at home with NIPPV required additional nursing input compared to 80 per cent of TV patients. However, the increased care burden of all forms of mechanical ventilation should not be underestimated.[64,65]

It is the practice in some centres to emphasize that patients may use the ventilator for daytime dyspnoea, but equally use of the ventilator does not preclude use of pharmacological means of symptom control. It is also stressed that patients may cease use of ventilation whenever they wish, and that drug treatments can be used to alleviate distressing symptoms during discontinuation. Although patients and their carers often find discussion of these issues surrounding ventilation distressing, the majority appreciate having a full understanding of the implications prior to commencement. It may be useful for patients to receive written information at the time of initial discussion – useful resources are available on the MNDA and ALSA web sites (see the web site list in the appendix).

Choice of ventilator

Many different ventilators suitable for home NIPPV use exist, but detailed review of the various models is beyond the scope of this chapter. Broadly speaking, non-invasive ventilators are programmed to deliver a set positive inspiratory pressure or volume, differing in magnitude during inspiration and expiration, via a nasal or full facial mask, or mouthpiece. It is essential that the ventilator can be programmed with a back-up rate capable of achieving adequate ventilation during apnoea or hypoventilation. Most can be triggered by the patient to deliver extra breaths, if required. Some ventilators have an integral battery, which can be used by ventilator-dependent patients who wish to go out for short periods of time.

Choice of interface

The interface, that is, the method of delivering ventilation can vary. Generally, the choices lie between nasal mask, a full-face mask, nasal cushions or mouthpiece. All of these come in a wide variety of sizes and designs. It is important to choose a system that is comfortable and can be easily applied for each individual, taking into consideration the degree of upper limb weakness. A number of patients will require a customized mask for an adequate fit. The nasal mask is usually the simplest to fit but skin abrasion on the bridge of the nose can occur. This occurs more frequently when patients use a ventilator for longer periods than overnight. Once a sore has developed this can be difficult to heal and prevention is the key. First, a well-fitting mask is essential as patients and carers frequently over tighten the straps in response to leaks, which can be uncomfortable, particularly if air goes into the eyes. Second, patients can use protective dressing on the bridges of the nose. If patients begin to use ventilation, both in the daytime and nocturnally it is helpful to use several different interfaces such as nasal mask, nasal cushions, or mouthpiece. To reduce the risk of mouth leak, which may decrease the efficiency of ventilation, patients can use a chin strap or full face mask.

Ventilator dependency and end-of-life issues

The fear of ventilator dependency and of patients reaching a locked-in state in which they are unable to communicate may have limited the widespread use of mechanical ventilation in the past. It has been suggested that the use of NIPPV (in contrast to TV) would avoid this situation as it was thought that the technique was not capable of sustaining ventilation when respiratory muscle weakness was such that ventilation was required for 24 hours. However there is now considerable evidence that patients can survive for many years with 24-hour NIPPV, particularly when techniques are used to achieve adequate clearance of secretions. Bach[23] reports a series of patients whose mean survival with 24-hour non-invasive ventilation was 3.9 years with a range of two months to 26 years. Some patients used NIV continuously. This requires the use of different interfaces and considerable skill from carers to prevent skin abrasions. Others may prefer to alternate NIPPV and pharmacological means to treat dyspnoea. Not all patients will use NIPPV continuously and some may die of pneumonia before using 24-hour ventilatory support.

Although patients and carers should be fully aware of all the options available to them prior to initiation of NIPPV, discussions need to be continued, particularly with increasing use of the ventilator. Coping with the changing situation is made easier when patients and carers have built up good relationships with both a respiratory and palliative care team. As the disease advances, patients are likely to be using the ventilator to treat breathlessness by day, as well as to improve sleep. Other treatments of dyspnoea such as opiates, benzodiazepines (e.g. lorazepam), or buspirone hydrochloride can be used to treat breathlessness and allow time off the ventilator. There are a number of practical difficulties in patients who are ventilator-dependent – in whom discontinuation of NIPPV will result in severe dyspnoea, if not respiratory arrest. A back-up ventilator must be available in case of malfunction. Interruption of electricity supply should be planned for. Patients and carers should be made aware that when the respiratory muscles are so weak that they cannot sustain spontaneous ventilation, sudden deterioration and death from ventilatory failure may occur. At this stage, symptomatic treatment of increasing breathlessness with pharmacological treatment in addition to NIPPV maybe the most appropriate course of action. This eventuality should be anticipated with patients and carers, and an acceptable management plan discussed and agreed. At this stage it may be appropriate for patients to be managed in the home or a hospice setting. As discussed above,[61] emergency intubation and ventilation has a very poor outcome, and should probably be avoided.

Patients should be aware that they can discontinue NIPPV at any time, and severe breathlessness and anxiety can be avoided in this event by premedication with opiates and anxiolytics.[53] This approach should not be regarded as unethical, nor does it amount to assisted suicide or euthanasia.

Although for the majority of ALS patients, NIPPV can successfully palliate symptoms, some cannot tolerate the therapy. In the UK, although at the present time home TV is difficult increasing numbers of patients will want to discuss this option. The following section will discuss tracheostomy ventilation in further detail.

Common complaints from ALS patients using NIPPV

Nasal discomfort

Patients frequently complain of nasal discomfort, particularly in the first few weeks of NIPPV use. Excessive nasal secretions (rhinorrhoea) can be treated by short-term use of an anticholinergic nasal spray (Rhinotec), although prolonged use may result in excessive drying. Occasionally, particularly if patients sleep in cool bedrooms, warming inspired air by entraining the ventilator tubing under the bedclothes may reduce rhinorrhoea. Nasal congestion responds to a steroid nasal spray, but frequently requires the addition of humidification. Humidifiers that can be inserted into the ventilator circuit are available, and room humidification may be helpful. Alternatively nebulized saline can be used.

Abdominal bloating

Patients may swallow excessive air during ventilation. This can be a particular problem if the patient is using a full-face mask, and may be solved by changing to a nasal interface. Drugs which increase gastric emptying, such as metoclopramide, may be useful. Relieving constipation is helpful.

Leaks

Air leaks can cause discomfort and may also reduce the efficiency of ventilation. Air leaks into the eye are particularly uncomfortable, and can cause conjunctivitis. A well-fitting mask is essential and should be changed regularly, as they can become stretched, and less fitting, with use.

Secretions

Good secretion management appears to be an important factor in acceptance of NIPPV. In our experience, patients with severe hypersiallorhoea find using NIPPV very difficult, and it is those patients who most frequently discontinue use (see Chapter 4b, p. 105, and Chapter 4d, p. 132 for further discussion of the management of secretions).

Increasing dyspnoea

Patients may notice that they are particularly dyspnoeic immediately after coming off the ventilator. This is likely due to the sudden increase in the work of breathing of the respiratory muscles. Patients should be advised to anticipate this, and reduce the load on the muscles by sitting up before removing the mask. The sensation will then generally abate. Patients may report dyspnoea whilst using the ventilator. In some cases, adjustment of the settings may be required to compensate for increasing respiratory muscle weakness. However, it is possible to overventilate patients and the resulting *hypo*capnia produces the sensation of dyspnoea. If increased ventilation does not reduce dyspnoea, then repeated increases should be avoided until ventilation-induced hypocapnia can be excluded by blood gas measurement.

Other aspects of respiratory care

Oxygen therapy

Oxygen can provide symptomatic relief of breathlessness in patients with hypoxia. However, it may decrease respiratory drive and make the symptoms of hypoventilation, such as headache worse. It may also lead to severe and unpleasant mouth dryness. The use of oxygen in ALS should be restricted to patients with a concomitant lung disorder such as COPD.

Prevention of infection

We advise patients to obtain influenza and pneumonia vaccinations.

Tracheostomy ventilation

Case history of an actual patient on TV

KL was a 55-year-old retired army sergeant major, a seven year-survivor of ALS. A leader in the ALS community, he was charismatic and optimistic about his role as a patient advocate, adviser and leader. After five years of NIV use, his time on ventilator reached 24 hours a day and he was having difficulty handling oral secretions. He had made the decision to undergo tracheostomy when he could no longer sustain life with NIV alone. After a prolonged winter of weight loss, increasing fatigue and eventually aspiration pneumonia, he underwent semi-elective tracheostomy and began TV. He remained several weeks in a Veteran's Administration hospital while his wife learned how to do endotracheal suction and valve change in order to permit vocalization through his tracheostomy as well as other nursing tasks required to safely bring him home. As he was already wheelchair-dependent, very few additional adaptations were needed to his home living situation. Within three months of TV, KL was again a major participant at ALS Association Fundraisers. Throughout his convalescence from TV, he continued to answer more than 50 e-mails a day from ALS patients all over the country. His message was consistent: 'Life can be good. Make it good.' He continued to hold family meetings although his wife joked that when the family was tired of his pontification she disconnected his speaking valve. They joked about the shared control they each maintained. Two years later he was actively mentoring young juvenile offenders at a local state penitentiary and getting involved in local government.

Treatment of ventilatory failure with invasive ventilation.

Although TV does offer the opportunity for prolonged survival for patients suffering from ALS,[33,39] its use remains highly controversial, even in those countries where it is most widely utilized. Long-term experience with TV in Japan has lead to the observation that, although postponing death, TV ventilation does not halt the progression of muscle weakness and therefore patients become progressively paralysed, dependent and eventually reduced to a locked-in state of existence. The quality of life for patients with ALS at this stage, although uncertain and untestable,[66] is regarded as not desirable by virtually all patients. Yet TV is a viable and desirable option for many ALS patients with bulbar dysfunction who have a desire to continue living and an inability to successfully use NIV. The majority of such patients report contentment and happiness with their choice of TV.[42,57,64]

Availability of TV

TV is not routinely available in most countries outside of the US and Japan due to the high financial burden it represents to individuals and society as a whole. In many countries with nationalized health care, long-term TV for chronic diseases like ALS is not a cost-effective option and therefore not offered. In contrast, in Japan where medical services have been available regardless of insurance coverage, the use of TV has been estimated to be as high as 24.5 per cent of those suffering with ALS.[67] In the US, where many different medical coverage plans exist and TV may or may not be feasible, the use of TV varies greatly. The total cost of TV, including home nursing needs, is so great that it routinely exceeds all insurance plan coverage and the individual out of pocket expense may be considerable.[57]

In addition to the limitation of availability of TV imposed by its expense, negative physician attitudes toward TV may contribute greatly to its relative unpopularity. One study evaluating the use of TV in various MDA centres in one US state found a wide variability from 1.6 to 14.3 per cent. This disparity in the use of TV correlated most closely with the personal attitudes of the physicians treating ALS patients at those centres. Physicians where the incidence of TV was greatest, when questioned, indicated they would use TV themselves if they developed ALS. In contrast, at those centres where TV was rarely used, physicians stated they would never use TV themselves and actively discouraged ALS patients from using it. In those centres with an intermediate incidence of TV use, physicans presented informed consent in a neutral fashion.[57] Physician predjudice against TV is based on concerns over quality of life, yet studies show that medical caregivers routinely under-report quality of life of patients on ventilator and that patients, when asked, rate their own QL higher than outside observers would predict. Ideally, additional information and assistance provided by other ALS patients using TV and their caregivers would provide prospective TV users and their families a more balanced informed consent process.[68]

The power of the clinician to influence the patient in the informed decision-making process has the potential to undermine patient autonomy. Some have even recommended a frank paternalistic approach to the choice of TV, stating that clinicians should assess quality of life of the patient 'independent of the patients' feelings' in determining whether or not to institute TV.[69] Paradoxically, the central ethical tenet agreed upon by clinicians, ethicists and most major religions is the tenet of patient autonomy.[14,62,70] Yet when the issue of TV is raised, opinions become polarized and it becomes difficult to truly share impartial medical information and allow patient autonomy.

Patient autonomy and competency in choosing TV

When ALS patients are asked who should make the decision regarding TV, they unanimously state they should make the decision for themselves. In an interview with 16 ALS patients contemplating the use of mechanical ventilation, nine discussed the decision in advance with family and friends, five with a physician and two reported that they did not discuss it with anybody.[71] Factors that patients considered most important in choosing a ventilator were: quality of life, severity of disability, ability to return home, ability to discontinue ventilation in the future if they so chose, and concern for their families' well-being.[71] In many cases the choice of TV is made knowing that it will entail a sacrifice of families' emotional, financial and physical well-being.

Historically, the competency of the ALS patient to make an informed decision regarding the use of TV has never been questioned as dementia was not believed to be a symptom of ALS. In fact, the predilection for involvement of the motor system with preservation of the intellectual functions was considered to be a hallmark of the disease and the presence of dementia would cast the diagnosis of ALS in doubt. Recently, it has been reported that there is cognitive involvement in as many as 60 per cent of patients with ALS[72] (see Chapter 4c). The pattern of dementia is a frontal executive dysfunction affecting the ability to plan for the future, make informed decisions and appreciate the consequences of those decisions (especially as those consequences affect others).[73] The cognitive deterioration, termed frontotemporal dementia, is higher in ALS patients with bulbar onset disease and is associated with decreased adherence to medical regimens and increased death rates.[74] Such bulbar onset ALS patients are poorly compliant with respiratory treatment regimens and would be expected to present to the emergency department in respiratory crisis. Perhaps this population of ALS patients with frontotemporal dysfunction at least in part explains the fact that the majority of ALS patients do not choose TV until they are in crisis. In a survey of ALS patients on mechanical ventilation in six states in the US, although 79 per cent said they had been informed by their physician about TV prior to their respiratory failure, only 21 per cent of them chose it in advance. Of those who were emergently intubated and ventilated when in crisis, another 21 per cent erroneously thought it would be only temporary.[57] In a prospective trial evaluating stated preferences regarding TV and actual choice of TV, 20 per cent of ALS patients who stated that they favoured TV had one in the 12 month follow-up period compared with 3.4 per cent of those who did not previously favour TV.[75]

Patient and family satisfaction with TV

Whether TV is chosen in advance or under the constraints of respiratory failure, 90 per cent of those cared for at home were glad of their choice and would choose so again,[41] whereas 72 per cent of those cared for in institutions were satisfied.[42] Interestingly, when their spouses were questioned regarding satisfaction with TV they answered enigmatically that they were glad the ALS patient had made the choice for TV but that they themselves would never choose TV because the decision made life too hard on the family. A study comparing QL of ALS patients with TV or NIPPV and their caregivers showed a comparable QL for the two patient groups, but a much higher burden for the TV caregivers.[76]

A neuropsychological assessment is an important part of the evaluation of an ALS patient. Extended counselling with both the ALS patient and family should then be instituted in order to facilitate informed decision-making. This would ideally be accomplished early in the course of ALS and at periodic follow-up intervals as patients with frontotemporal dementia would not only be expected to get into crisis earlier in the course of their illness, but they would be expected to display less sound judgement with regard to decision-making. In particular such patients may not be able to make sound decisions regarding TV as they may not be able to cognitively prioritize and consider the consequences of TV on the financial, physical and emotional well-being of not only themselves but their family. ALS patients with milder frontal executive dysfunction, able to make the decision to use TV, may progress and in time no longer appreciate the burden that continued TV presents to their family.

Factors predicting successful use of TV

When assessing patients for home-based TV, characteristics that most favour a positive outcome include:

1. a highly motivated ALS patient who is empathic to the needs of the family and engaged with the family and the community
2. a slowly progressive course of muscular paralysis
3. a thorough understanding of the alternatives to TV
4. a thorough understanding of the progression of ALS and the possible cognitive involvement
5. a well-informed family that is willing and able to take on the burdens of TV
6. the financial resources for equipment, caregiving needs and multidisciplinary support
7. an Advanced Directive for discontinuing TV[68]
8. capacity for both patient and family to remain flexible and adaptable to constantly changing caretakers, equipment and physical limitations.[77]

Hospitalization for TV

The length of hospitalization after TV varies but in the absence of critical illness, most patients will be moved from intensive care (ICU) to intermediate level care within 21 days of tracheostomy.[78] Patients and their families often begin TV training in the ICU and potentially continue in a longer-term rehabilitation setting until all the skills and knowledge required for safe home management of TV have been acquired. The development of a clinical pathway to ensure timely outcomes and focus on various aspects of family education and patient care can optimize the hospital effectiveness and shorten length of stay. A multidisciplinary approach includes input from pulmonology, neurology, gastroenterology, nursing, respiratory, occupational, physical and speech therapy, nutrition, social work and chaplaincy services. Communication must be re-established either with the patient's own voice and a passy-muir valve, or a ventilator assisted voice and fenestrated tracheostomy or lastly via augmentative communication device.[79] Re-establishing communication is essential in maintaining patient quality of life.

Preparation for discharge home on TV

Preparation for discharge begins with the initiation of TV and requires a designated case manager to coordinate and oversee all arrangements with community services and vendors. Assessment for home management of TV includes and assessment of the physical environment, technical support, nursing support and community support and resources.[80] O'Donohue[80] and the AARC Clinical Practice Guidelines[81] offer excellent checklists and guidelines for the management of the patient on TV in the home.

The physical environment is assessed by a home care team and equipment vendor to ensure the ability to meet the ALS patient's home equipment needs. The patient will need a room that allows easy egress in case of emergency and ideally the absence of stairs to facilitate frequent outings. The room will require four electrical outlets for equipment (ventilator, heated humidifier, suction machine, hospital bed) and the home will require enough electrical power to accommodate the equipment.

A physician must be available to coordinate total care. Ideally this is a pulmonary or rehabilitation specialist although in some centres, in the USA, the ALS neurologist functions in this capacity. Community support includes emergency personnel who is notified of and educated to the needs of a ventilator dependent person. Local social service agencies may be able to provide respite, financial and psychosocial support. Support from the respiratory equipment vendor must entail 24-hour availability with back-up equipment in the event of mechanical malfunction. Regular home visits must also be provided by respiratory therapists to service equipment and provide education to caregivers, as needed. Home care nurses must be trained in ventilator care and be identified prior to discharge from hospital. Due to nursing shortages, it is not uncommon for nursing agencies to be unable to provide full staffing needs even when there is guaranteed funding. A clear back-up plan must be in place with the family as well as a method to train and select future caregivers.

Finance issues should be clarified prior to discharge so that nursing coverage can be arranged and the amount of out-of-pocket expense clearly stipulated.

Many insurance plans in the USA cover only a fraction of home care nursing and durable medical equipment and therefore the ALS patient and/or family is responsible for the remainder.

The patient can then be discharged to home when there is clinical and physiological stability and a respiratory home care plan is in place. Anxiety levels of patient and caregiver are better managed by a clear written treatment plan which includes a comprehensive home respiratory care plan. Clear instructions and demonstration of necessary TV skills by the home caregiving team include:

1. cleaning and assembling the ventilator

2. an understanding the alarms, their importance and responses to them

3. care of artificial airway including suctioning and speech modalities

4. specific prescriptions for time off and on ventilator; settings, modes and measurements for ventilator while patient is in both resting and exercising states

5. other therapies including oxygen where necessary, medication and chest physical therapy.

During the first year, the tracheostomy site will require specialist follow-up and plans need to be in place for the patient to receive this care. Within a few months the stoma will have matured enough that the family may be trained in changing the tracheostomy tube and specialist follow-up may be less frequent.[82]

Day-to-day life for ALS patients on TV

Although the majority of ALS patients on TV rate their quality of life as good, a review of the daily activities of TV users reveals a very restricted lifestyle. TV users spend their days in simple activities: 21 per cent of ALS patients on TV never leave their homes, 95 per cent spend their days watching television or talking with family and friends.[41] More recently, with the popularity of home computers and the Internet, TV users are establishing a new social community built on technological support. ALS web sites are becoming an important source of medical information, emotional support and political power. Eventually, the ability to communicate in any fashion becomes threatened as patients become more limited, progressing from verbal communication to functional communication via an augmentative device to eye gaze systems, alphabet boards and ultimately to a complete locked-in state.[32] In such advanced cases, it becomes impossible to determine the desires or even state of cognitive awareness of the TV user.[66]

As TV users in such a locked-in state are unable to indicate pain, depression or the desire to terminate TV, an agreement should be reached before communication is lost as to an Advance Directive specifying the limits of TV. The physician and other caregivers involved in the management of ALS patients on TV again perform a role in the informed consent process at this juncture as most TV users will not specify limits of TV unless strongly advised to do so by their physicans.[82]

TV poses major challenges to family members: 58 per cent of caregivers when interviewed felt TV was a major burden and 47 per cent of caregivers reported that their own health had suffered as a result of caring for their ALS-affected family members.[41] In addition, caregivers reported a loss of privacy in their homes and decreased time for outside friendships, as well as increased tension, depression and anxiety.[64]

The medical relationship of ALS patients often change once TV is instituted as access to ALS care centres may be increasingly limited, especially if reliable transport and caregivers are not readily available. ALS patients may feel abandoned by the very centres that advised and encouraged TV initially. Patient care is often provided by home-based ventilatory teams headed by pulmonologists trained in invasive ventilatory management rather than the clinic-based multidisciplinary ALS team. This decreased access to the ALS community should be discussed in advance of the decision to use TV so that the new relationship may be anticipated and the impression of medical abandonment may be dealt with proactively.

Medical complications of TV

Medical complications of TV are frequent and can be serious. In a prospective study of 354 consecutive TV patients, a total of 400 complications occurred.[83] These included problems related to tracheostomy – pneumothorax, bleeding at the stoma site, subcutaneous emphysema, nosocomial infections, tracheomalacia, tracheoarterial fistula and tracheoesophageal fistula – as well as complications related to mechanical ventilation: pulmonary emphysema, pheumomediastinum, pneumopericardium, acute respiratory distress syndrome, venous air embolism, oxygen toxicity and systemic hemodynamic instability.[84] The medical course for ALS patients on TV is not smooth, but long-term survival is the rule, not the exception. In a study of 101 TV patients cared for at home, 87 per cent were alive one year later, 69 per cent at two years, 58 per cent at three year, 50 per cent at four years and 33 per cent at five years.[82] In another study of 52 ventilator dependent patients, survival ranged from 11 months to 14.5 years with a mean survival of 4.4 +/− 3.9 years.[33]

Death and discontinuation of TV

Deaths, when they occur, are predominantly due to medical complications and in particular ALS-associated circulatory collapse and sudden death.[85] Some TV users simply choose to discontinue life support.[53] In most countries the decision to discontinue life support is viewed ethically and legally equivalent to not choosing life support in the first place and therefore permitted upon the patient's request. Guidelines for the discontinuation of TV, including a step by step algorithm and medications to maintain the comfort of the patient have been published in the US.[14] Even where the ethical course is clear with regard to discontinuing TV, the practical course of how to do it is ambiguous. The family, although perhaps in principle in agreement with the decision, is always to some degree ambivalent about the role they play and certainly unable and unwilling to simply 'pull the plug', the patient cannot discontinue him or herself, and the clinician is not routinely accustomed to purposefully ending life. In some areas, hospice units may perform this service for the patient. The primary goal in withdrawing TV is to maintain patient comfort. In patients who are unable to communicate their comfort, tachycardia, tachypnea or restlessness may be indications of patient distress. Analgesia and sedation should be offered before, during and after the terminal weaning process.[53,86] Medications ideally should be given intravenously to bypass erratic gastrointestinal absorption due to poor tissue perfusion. Morphine is a preferred drug due to its wide therapeutic window, tendency to promote euphoria, dry airway secretions and dilate pulmonary vasculature. An initial bolus of 5–10 mg iv may be followed by a continuous infusion of 50 per cent of the bolus dose per hour. When the bolus dose must be repeated, the continuous infusion should be increased accordingly.[53] In addition, agitation may be managed by the addition of benzodiazepines. An initial bolus of 2–10 mg of midazolam, 2–4 mg of lorazepam or 5–10 mg of diazepam should be followed by the same dose as continuous hourly infusion. In this way, pain, fear and anxiety can be effectively relieved.[86] Supplemental oxygen and positive end expiratory pressure may be discontinued followed by conversion to a T-piece and spontaneous breathing.[87] Bedside nursing measures such as eliminating unnecessary procedures, removing unnecessary tubes, clearing secretions and administering antipyretics when indicated are also extremely helpful, especially to family members.

Additional support is sometimes needed for the medical team involved in terminal weaning and can be provided by reviewing the decision to discontinue TV in advance with an ethics panel comprising other colleagues, clergy and lay people in the community.

The physician's role in TV

In summary, the clinician's role in TV should be one of patient assessment, patient and family counselling, education and guidance, as well as safeguarding the patient's right to self-determination and human dignity. In helping to institute TV, the clinician must be cognizant of the possibility of cognitive involvement and diminished patient judgement, the relentless progression of ALS after TV, the burden imposed on family caregivers and the potential future responsibility of withdrawing TV support. Clinicians who believe themselves unable or unwilling to support the patient through the entire process of initiating, maintaining and ultimately withdrawing TV should refer patients on to another physician.[53] As the options for extending life become increasingly unlimited, we are all – clinicians, patients, family and community alike – searching for the ethical high ground.

References

1. Gay P. C., Westbrook P. R., Daube J. R., Litchy W. J., Windebank A. J., Iverson R. (1991) Effects of alterations in pulmonary function and sleep variables on survival in patients with amyotrophic lateral sclerosis. *Mayo Clinic Proceedings* 66: 686–94.

2. Ferguson K., Strong M., Ahmad D., George C. (1996) Sleep-disordered breathing in amyotrophic lateral sclerosis. *Chest* 110: 664–9.

3. Bye P. T. P., Ellis E. R., Issa F. G., Donnelly P. M., Sullivan C. E. (1990) Respiratory failure and sleep in neuromuscular disease. *Thorax* 45: 241–7.

4. Hetta J., Jansson I. (1997) Sleep in patients with amyotrophic lateral sclerosis. *Journal of Neurology* 244 (4 Suppl. 1): S7–9.

5. Brach B. (1979) Expiratory flow patterns in amyotrophic lateral sclerosis. *Chest* 75: 648–50.

6. Fallat R.J., Jewitt B., Bass M., Kamm B., Norris F.H. (1979) Spirometry in amyotrophic lateral sclerosis. *Archives of Neurology* 36: 74–80.

7. Vincken W., Elleker G., Cosio M. (1986) Detection of upper airway muscle involvement in neuromuscular disorders using the flow-volume loop. *Chest* 90: 52–7.

8. Garcia-Pachon E., Marti J., Mayos M., Casan P., Sanchis J. (1994) Clinical significance of upper airway dysfunction in motor neurone disease. *Thorax* 49: 896–900.

8. Zwillich C. W., Pierson D. J., Creagh C. E., Sutton F. D., Schatz E., Petty T. L. (1974) Complications of assisted ventilation. A prospective study of 354 consecutive episodes. *American Journal of Medicine* 57: 161–70.

9. Polkey M., Lyall R., Green M., Leigh P., Moxham J. (1998) Expiratory muscle function in amyotrophic lateral sclerosis. *American Journal of Respiratory and Critical Care Medicine* 158: 734–41.

10. Ertekin C., Aydogdu I., Yuceyar N., Kiylioglu N., Tarluci S., Uludag B. (2000) Pathophysiological mechanisms of oropharyngeal dysphagia in amyotrophic lateral sclerosis. *Brain* 123: 125–40.

11. Hadjikoutis S., Eccles R., Wiles C. (2000a) Coughing and choking in motor neurone disease. *Journal of Neurology, Neurosurgery and Psychiatry* 68: 601–604.

12. Hadjikoutis S., Pickersgill T., Dawson K., Wiles C. (2000b) Abnormal patterns of breathing during swallowing in neurological disorders. *Brain* 123: 1863–73.

13. Polkey M. I., Green M., Moxham J. (1995) Measurement of respiratory muscle strength. *Thorax* 50 (11): 1131–5.

14. Miller R., Rosenberg J., Gelinas D., Mitsumoto H., Newman D., Sufit R., Borasio G., Bradley W., Bromberg M., Brooks B., Kasarskis E., Munsat T., Oppenheimer E., and the ALS practice parameters task force (1999) Practice parameter; the care of the patient with amyotrophic lateral sclerosis (an evidence-based review). *Neurology* 52: 1311–23.

15. Allen S., Hunt B., Green M. (1985) Fall in vital capacity with posture. *British Journal of Diseases of the Chest* 79: 267–71.

16. Arnulf I., Similowski T., Salachas F., Garma L., Mehiri S., Attali V., Behin-Bellhesen V., Meininger V., Derenne J.-P. (2000) Sleep disorders and diaphragmatic function in patients with amyotrophic lateral sclerosis. *American Journal of Respiratory and Critical Care Medicine* 161: 849–56.

17. Varrato J., Siderowf A., Damiano P., Gregory S., Feinberg D., McCluskey L. (2001) Postural change of forced vital capacity predicts some respiratory symptoms in ALS. *Neurology* 57: 357–9.

18. Lechtzin N., Wiener C., Shade D., Clawson L., Diette G. (2002) Spirometry in the supine position improves the detection of diaphragmatic weakness in patients with amyotrophic lateral sclerosis. *Chest* 121: 436–42.

19. Lyall R. A., Donaldson N., Polkey M. I., Leigh P. N., Moxham J. (2001) Respiratory muscle strength and ventilatory failure in amyotrophic lateral sclerosis. *Brain* 124 (10): 2000–13.

20. Heritier F., Rahm F., Pasche P., Fitting J.-W. (1994) Sniff nasal pressure. A non-invasive assessment of inspiratory muscle strength. *American Journal of Respiratory and Critical Care Medicine* 150: 1678–83.

21. Fitting J., Paillex R., Hirt L., Aebischer P., Schluep M. (1999) Sniff nasal pressure, a sensitive respiratory test to assess progression of ALS. *Annals of Neurology* 46: 887–93.

22. Uldry C., Fitting J. W. (1995) Maximal values of sniff nasal inspiratory pressure in healthy subjects. *Thorax* 50: 371–5.

23. Bach J. (2002) Amyotrophic lateral sclerosis. Prolongation of life by non-invasive respiratory aids. *Chest* 122: 92–8.

24. Man W. D., Moxham J., Polkey M. I. (2004) Magnetic stimulation for the measurement of respiratory and skeletal muscle function. *European Respiratory Journal* 24 (5): 846–60.

25. Stambler N., Charatan M., Cedarbaum J. (1998) Prognostic indicators of survival in ALS *Neurology* 50: 66–72.

26. Hadjikoutis S., Wiles C. (2001b) Venous serum chloride and bicarbonate measurements in the evaluation of respiratory function in motor neuron disease. *Quarterly Journal of Medicine* 94: 491–5.

27. Velasco R., Salachas F., Munerati E., Le Forestier N., Pradat PF., Lacomblez L., Orvoen Frija E., Meininger V. (2002) Oxymetrie nocturne chez les patients atteints de sclerose laterale amyotrophique: analyse de son role predictif sur le survie. *Revue Neurologique (Paris)* 158: 575–8.

28. Bach J. R., Bianchi C., Aufiero E. (2004) Oximetry and indications for tracheotomy for amyotrophic lateral sclerosis. *Chest* **126**: 1502–7.

29. Elman L. B., Siderowf A. D., McCluskey L. F. (2003) Nocturnal oximetry: utility in the respiratory management of amyotrophic lateral sclerosis *American Journal of Physical Medicine and Rehabilitation* **82** (11): 866–70.

30. Sivasothy P., Brown L., Smith I., Shneerson J. (2001) Effect of manually assisted cough and mechanical insufflation on cough flow of normal subjects, patients with chronic obstructive pulmonary disease (COPD), and patients with respiratory muscle weakness *Thorax* **56**: 438–44.

31. Chatwin M., Ross E., Hart N., Nickol A., Polkey M., Simonds A. (2003) Cough augmentation with mechanical insufflation/exsufflation in patients with neuromuscular weakness. *European Respiratory Journal* **21**: 502–8.

32. Bach J. (1993a) Amyotrophic lateral sclerosis: communication status and survival with ventilatory support. *American Journal of Physical Medicine and Rehabilitation* **72**: 343–9.

32. Sancho J., Servera E., Diaz J., Marin J. (2004) Efficacy of mechanical insufflation–exsufflation in medically stable patients with amyotrophic lateral sclerosis. *Chest* **125** (4): 1400–5.

33. Bach J. (1993b) A comparison of long-term ventilatory support alternatives from the perspective of the patient and care-giver. *Chest* **104**: 1702–6.

34. Bach J. (1995a) Respiratory muscle aids for the prevention of pulmonary morbidity and mortality. *Seminars in Neurology* **15**: 72–4.

35. Bach J. (1995b) Amyotrophic lateral sclerosis: predictors for prolongation of life by non-invasive respiratory aids. *Archives of Physical Medicine and Rehabilitation* **76**: 828–32.

36. Bach J., Chaudhry S. (2000) Standards of care in MDA clinics. *American Journal of Physical Medicine and Rehabilitation* **79**: 193–6.

37. Bourke S., Williams T., Bullock R., Gibson G., Shaw P. (2002) Non-invasive ventilation in motor neurone disease: current UK practice. *ALS and Other Motor Neuron Disorders* **3**: 145–9.

38. Howard R. S., Wiles C. M., Loh L. (1989) Respiratory complications and their management in motor neuron disease. *Brain* **112**: 1155–70.

39. Annane D., Chevrolet J., Chevret S., Raphael J. (2000) Nocturnal mechanical ventilation for chronic hypoventilation in patients with neuromuscular and chest wall disorders. *Cochrane Database Systemic Reviews* CD001941.

40. David W., Bundlie S., Mahdavi Z. (1997) Polysomnographic studies in amyotrophic lateral sclerosis. *Journal of the Neurological Sciences* **152**, S29–S35.

41. Moss A. H., Casey P., Stocking C. B., Roos R. P., Brooks B. R., Seigler M. (1993) Home ventilation for amyotrophic lateral sclerosis patients : outcomes, costs and patient, family and physician attitudes. *Neurology* **43**: 438–43.

42. Cazzolli P. A., Oppenheimer E. A. (1996) Home mechanical ventilation for amyotrophic lateral sclerosis: nasal compared to tracheostomy-intermittent positive pressure ventilation. *Journal of the Neurological Sciences* **139**: 123–8.

43. Newsom-Davis I., Lyall R., Leigh P., Moxham J., Goldstein L. (2001) The effect of non-invasive positive pressure ventilation (NIPPV) on cognitive function in amyotrophic

lateral sclerosis (ALS): a prospective study. *Journal of Neurology, Neurosurgery and Psychiatry* **71**: 482–7.

44. Boitano L., Jordan T., Benditt J. (2001) Non-invasive ventilation allows gastrostomy tube placement in patients with advanced ALS. *Neurology* **56**: 413–14.

45. Thornton F., Fotheringham T., Alexander M., Hardiman O., McGrath F., Lee M. (2002) Amyotrophic lateral sclerosis : enteral nutrition provision – endoscopic or radiologic gastrostomy? *Radiology* **224**: 713–17.

46. Gregory S., Siderowf A., Golaszewski A., McCluskey L. (2002) Gastrostomy insertion in ALS patients with low vital capacity: respiratory support and survival. *Neurology* **58**: 485–7.

47. Pinto A., Evangelista T., Carvalho M., Alves M., Sales Luis M. (1995) Respiratory assistance with a non-invasive ventilator (Bipap) in MND/ALS patients: survival rates in a controlled trial. *Journal of the Neurological Sciences* **129**: 19–26.

48. Aboussouan L. S., Khan S. U., Meeker D. P., Stelmach K., Mitsumoto H. (1997) Effect of non-invasive positive pressure ventilation on survival in amyotrophic lateral sclerosis. *Annals of Internal Medicine* **127**: 450–3.

49. Kleopa K., Sherman M., Neal B., Romano G., Heiman-Patterson T. (1999) Bipap improves survival and rate of pulmonary function decline in patients with ALS. *Journal of the Neurological Sciences* **164**: 82–8.

50. Gruis K. L., Brown D. L., Schoennemann A., Zebarah V. A., Feldman E. L. (2005) Predictors of noninvasive ventilation tolerance in patients with amyotrophic lateral sclerosis. *Muscle Nerve* **32** (6): 808–11.

51. Farrero E. Prats E., Povedano M., Martinez-Matos J. A., Manresa F., Escarrabill J. (2005) Survival in amyotrophic lateral sclerosis with home mechanical ventilation: the impact of systematic respiratory assessment and bulbar involvement. *Chest* **127** (6): 2132–8.

52. Bourke S., Tomlinson T., Williams T., Bullock R., Shaw P., Gibson G. (2006) effects of non-invasive ventilation on survival and quality of life in patients with amyotrophic lateral sclerosis, a randomised controlled trial. *Lancet Neurol* **5**: 140–7.

53. Borasio G. D., Voltz R. (1998) Discontinuation of life support in patients with amyotrophic lateral sclerosis. *J Neurol* **245**: 717–22.

54. Melo J., Homma A., Iturriaga E., Frierson L., Amato A., Anzueto A., Jackson C. (1999) Pulmonary evaluation and prevalence of non-invasive ventilation in patients with amyotrophic lateral sclerosis: a multicenter survey and proposal of a pulmonary protocol. *Journal of the Neurological Sciences* **169**: 114–17.

55. Bradley W., Anderson F., Bromberg M., Gutmann L., Harati Y., Ross M., Miller R. (2001) Comparison of the ALS CARE database and the AAN practice parameter. *Neurology* **57**: 500–4.

56. McDonald E. R., Hillel A., Weidenfeld S. A. (1996) Evaluation of the psychological status of ventilatory-supported patients with ALS/MND. *Palliative Medicine* **10**: 35–41.

57. Moss A. H., Oppenheimer E. A., Casey P., Cazzolli P. A., Roos R. P., Stocking C. B., Siegler M. (1996) Patients with amyotrophic lateral sclerosis receiving long-term mechanical ventilation. Advance care planning and outcomes. *Chest* **110**: 249–55.

58. Jackson C., Rosenfeld J., Moore D., Bryan W., Barohn R., Wrench M., Myers D., Heberlin L., King R., Smith J., Gelinas D., Miller R. (2001) A preliminary

evaluation of a prospective study of pulmonary function studies and symptoms of hypoventilation in ALS/MND patients. *Journal of the Neurological Sciences* 191: 75–8.

59. Aboussouan L. S., Khan S. U., Banerjee M., Arroliga A. C., Mitsumoto H. (2001) Objective measures of the efficacy of non-invasive positive pressure ventilation in amyotrophic lateral sclerosis. *Muscle & Nerve* 24: 403–9.

60. Lyall R. A., Donaldson N., Fleming T., Wood C., Newsom-Davis I., Polkey M. I., Leigh P. N., Moxham J. (2001) A prospective study of quality of life in ALS patients treated with noninvasive ventilation. *Neurology* 57 (1): 153–6.

61. Bradley M., Orrell R., Clarke J., Davidson A., Williams A., Kullmann D., Hirsch N., Howard R. (2002) Outcome of ventilatory support for acute respiratory failure in motor neurone disease. *Journal of Neurology, Neurosurgery and Psychiatry* 72: 752–6.

62. Jackson D. J. (1979) Patient autonomy and 'death with dignity': some clinical caveats. *New England Journal of Medicine* 301: 404–8.

64. Gelinas D., O'Connor P., Miller R. (1998) Quality of life for ventilator-dependent ALS patients and their caregivers *Journal of the Neurological Sciences* 160, S134–6.

65. Mustafa N., Walsh E., Bryant V., Lyall R.A., Addington-Hall J., Goldstein L.H., Donaldson N., Polkey M.I., Moxham J., Leigh P.N. (2006) The effect of non-invasive ventilation on ALS patients and their caregivers. *Neurology* 66: 1211–7.

66. Bromberg M. B., Forshew D. A., Iaderosa S., McDonald E. R. (1996) Ventilator dependency in ALS: Management, disease progression, and issues of coping. *Journal of Neurological Rehabilitation* 10: 195–216.

67. Borasio G. D., Gelinas D. F., Yanagisawa N. (1998) Mechanical ventilation in amyotrophic lateral sclerosis: a cross-cultural perspective. *Journal of Neurology* 245 (Suppl. 2): S7–S12.

68. Oppenheimer E. A. (1993) Decision-making in the respiratory care of amyotrophic lateral sclerosis: should home mechanical ventilation be used? *Palliative Medicine* 7 (Suppl.): 49–64.

69. Dracup K., Raffin T. (1989) Withholding and withdrawing mechanical ventilation: assessing quality of life. *American Review of Respiratory Disease* 140: 544–6.

70. Goldblatt D., Greenlaw J. (1989) Starting and stopping the ventilator for patients with amyotrophic lateral sclerosis. *Neurologic Clinics* 7: 789–806.

71. Young J. M., Marshall C. L., Anderson E. J. (1994) Amyotrophic lateral sclerosis patients' perspectives on use of mechanical ventilation. *Health and Social Work* 19: 253–60.

72. Lomen-Hearth C. *et al.* (2003) Are ALS patients cognitively normal? *Neurology* 60: 1094–7.

73. Neary D. *et al.* (1998) Frontotemporal lobar degeneration: a consensus on clinical diagnostic criteria. *Neurology* 51: 1546–54.

74. Olney R. K., Murphy J., Forshew D., Garwood E., Miller B.L., Langmore S., Kohn A., Lomen-Hoerth C. (2005) The effect of executive and behavioral dysfunction the course of ALS. *Neurology* 65: 1774–7.

75. Albert S. M., Murphy P. L., DelBene M. L. and Rowland L. P. (1999) A prospective study of preferences and actual treatment choices in ALS. *Neurology* 53: 278–83.

76. Kaub-Wittemer D., von Steinbüchel N., Wasner M., Laier-Groeneveld G., Borasio G. D. (2003) Quality of life and psychosocial issues in ventilated patients with amyotrophic lateral sclerosis and their caregivers. *J Pain Symptom Manage* 26: 890–6.

77. **Make** B. J., **Gilmartin** M. E. (1990) Mechanical ventilation in the home. *Crit Care Clin* **6**: 785–796.

78. **Scheinhorn** D. J., **Stearn-Hassenpflug M.** (1998) Provision of long-term mechanical ventilation. *Critical Care Clinics* **14**: 819–32.

79. **Gracey** D. R. (1997) Options for long-term ventilatory support. *Clinics in Chest Medicine* **18**: 563–74.

80. **O'Donohue** W. J., Jr, **Giovannoni** R. M., **Goldberg** A. I., **Keens** T. G., **Make** B. J., **Plummer** A. L., **Prentice** W. S. (1986) Long-term mechanical ventilation. Guidelines for management in the home and at alternate community sites. Report of the Ad Hoc Committee, Respiratory Care Section, American College of Chest Physicians. *Chest* **90** (Suppl.): S1–S37.

81. **AARC Clinical Practice Guidelines** (1995) Long-term invasive mechanical ventilation in the home. *Respiratory Care* **40**: 1313–20.

82. **Oppenheimer** E. A. (1994). Respiratory management and home mechanical ventilation in amyotrophic lateral sclerosis. In Mitsumoto H., and Norris F. H. (eds) *Amyotrophic Lateral Sclerosis*, pp. 139–62. New York. Demos Publications.

84. **Sandur** S., **Stoller** J. K. (1999) Pulmonary complications of mechanical ventilation. *Clinical Chest Medicine* **20**: 223–47.

85. **Shimizu** T., **Hayashi** H., **Koto** S., **Hayashi** M., **Tanabe** H., **Oda** M. (1994). Circulatory collapse and sudden death in respirator-dependent amyotrophic lateral sclerosis. *Journal of the Neurological Sciences* **124**: 45–55.

86. **Campbell** M. L. (1993) Case studies in terminal weaning form mechanical ventilation. *American Journal of Critical Care* **2**: 354–7.

87. **Wilson** W. C., **Smedira** N. G., **Fink** C., **McDowell** J. A. and **Luce** J. M. (1992) Ordering and administration of sedatives and analgesics during the withholding and withdrawal of life support from critically ill patients. *Journal of the American Medical Association* **276**: 949–53.

Chapter 4b

Control of Symptoms:

dysphagia

Edith Wagner-Sonntag and Mario Prosiegel

Case history

Mr L, a 62-year-old active farmer, was admitted to our hospital with speech and swallowing problems of unknown etiology. Clinically he presented with rather unintelligible speech and a monotonous low voice. He reported difficulties with eating meat and bread, whereas drinking was quite normal. He had a weight loss of 5 kg within the last two months. The examination revealed a reduced tongue motility and tongue force with bilateral atrophy and fibrillations. Sometimes choking occurred on saliva with a markedly reduced reflexive cough. Mealtimes were very long and Mr. L. frequently stopped eating because of fatigue and loss of appetite. The diagnosis of ALS had been confirmed. Videofluoroscopy and fibreoptic endoscopy revealed a considerable risk of aspiration with reduced and uneffective cough on food as well as on thin liquids. Therefore, eating food of soft texture with caloric supplement and sipping or thickening liquids was recommended. The patient was informed about the advances of early insertion of a PEG-tube and the use of this type of nutrition as a supplement, especially when working. He decided to begin with a dietary modification. Three months later, after a weight loss of another 7 kg, he asked us to insert a PEG. Because his forced vital capacity was at that time below 50 per cent of predicted, a percutaneous radiological gastrostomy was inserted and some weeks later he reported a good experience with the new additional feeding.

Summary

Dysphagia is very common in ALS patients. The assessment comprises clinical examination and for specific questions instrumented methods such as videofluoroscopy and/or endoscopic evaluation of swallowing. Treatment of dysphagia in ALS patients includes an array of measures such as positioning, compensatory techniques, dietary modifications and safety strategies. In certain patients with severe dysphagia, augmented feeding techniques, i.e. nasogastric tube feeding or feeding via a percutaneous endoscopic gastrostomy or an jejunostomy, may be necessary. Many dysphagia-related symptoms like sialor-rhoea, thick mucous secretions and gastroesophageal reflux can be successfully treated pharmacologically. Palliative surgery, e.g. cricopharyngeal myotomy, is rarely indicated. Efficacy of palliative therapy can be assessed by measuring nutritional status, e.g. the body mass index, and by use of specific dysphagia-related scales as well as quality of life scales. Management of dysphagia in ALS requires a multidisciplinary team approach and ongoing assessment: physicians, nursing staff, speech and language therapists, dietitians, the patients and their relatives should thereby closely work together.

Eating and drinking are two of the most basic functions of life. Progressive loss of these abilities greatly impacts on both the patient and the family. The assessment of these swallowing problems and their management is crucial in the patient's care and requires a multidisciplinary approach.

Undernutrition and weight loss have functional consequences which may add to the disability of the underlying disease, causing both mental and physical deterioration, increased complications, and impaired quality of life. Starvation and weight loss are common in patients with ALS.[1] One study found that 21 per cent of patients were moderately to severely malnourished, including those with no apparent swallowing problems.[2]

Frequency of dysphagia in ALS

The site of significant neuronal loss and the duration of the disease will affect the development of dysphagia. The reported prevalence of dysphagia in ALS is highly variable, varying between 48–100 per cent.[3]

As far as disease duration is concerned, dysphagia appears on average four months after onset of the disease,[4] but during the course of the disease progression nearly 100 per cent of ALS patients have problems due to oral or pharyngeal involvement.[5] In the later stages of the disease dysphagia is a very common symptom and aspiration pneumonia, either on its own or in conjunction with respiratory insufficiency, may lead to death in ALS patients.[6]

A report from St Christopher's Hospice of 124 patients with ALS found that only 21 per cent of the patients were able to swallow all foods, 42 per cent semi-solids only, and 27 per cent liquidized or pureed foods; only 8 per cent of this series of patients required tube feeding. Moreover there were problems with patients' feeding and only 19 per cent of their patients were able to feed unaided, a further 24 per cent were only able to do so with specially prepared food of modified texture and the remaining patients all needed help with eating.[6] Another hospice study found that dysphagia was a problem for over 90 per cent of patients with ALS.[7]

Pathophysiology

The three anatomical levels which may be affected in ALS[8] are associated with the development of dysphagic symptoms:

1. Upper motor neuron (UMN) involvement causes supranuclear symptoms, also termed pseudobulbar palsy.

2. Lower motor neuron (LMN) involvement of the cranial nerve nuclei in the medulla oblongata and pons innervating the muscles of the jaw, face, tongue, pharynx and larynx affects chewing, swallowing, speech and voice with subsequent bulbar symptoms.

3. The motor neurons of the spinal cord can be affected and may lead to dysphagia as the result of progressive respiratory dysfunction. Regardless of the onset being bulbar or nonbulbar, dysphagia progresses as respiratory function declines.[9,10]

Dysphagic symptoms may develop as a result of neuronal loss at any of the three levels – supranuclear, bulbar and spinal – which are often affected in combination.

Since swallowing deals with two components – saliva and nutrition – patients have to manage both in order to avoid complications. At the onset of the disease there may be problems with coping with liquids or saliva. Many patients report that they produce too much saliva but it seems that there is no measurable increase in secretion, but rather a difficulty in handling the saliva, which creates the impression of too much secretion being produced.[11] Therefore, the term sialorrhoea should be preferred to hypersalivation. With increasing loss of muscle tone and muscle strength in lip closure the patients tend to drool. The inability to keep the lips closed leads to increased breathing through the mouth and this can tend to thicken the oral secretions, making them difficult to swallow.

As the disease progresses, a feeling of fatigue when eating arises as the motility and strength of the facial and oral/lingual musculature decreases. This leads to difficulties in the oral preparation, mastication and oral transport of food. Weak muscles make it difficult to manage thin liquids and dry and crumbly food. The swallowing reflex becomes difficult causing the subsequent problem of aspiration[12] and food spills downward before laryngeal closure can be initiated. With increasing weakness of laryngeal adduction the mechanism of compensating the late triggering of the swallowing reflex is no longer sufficient and laryngeal decompensation occurs with the ensuing risk of aspiration. Aspiration is defined as passage of material into the larynx below the level of the vocal cords, whereas penetration means passage of material into the larynx above the glottic level. At this stage it is crucial that the patient has a forceful cough reflex as the less effective the cough, the more dangerous oral intake becomes. Reduced tongue force, delayed triggering of the swallowing reflex and weak elevation of the hyoid and larynx result in reduced opening of the upper oesophageal sphincter. This leads to retention of saliva, food and liquids in the valleculae and piriform sinuses, also aggravating the risk of aspiration. A recent study showed that pressure profiles of the oesophageal sphincter are not disturbed in ALS patients.[13]

Laryngeal abduction and/or adduction may also be affected and worsen dyspnoea. In some cases, therefore, it will be necessary to discuss whether a patient could benefit from a tracheostomy (see Surgery below).

Assessment of dysphagia

A multidisciplinary approach is necessary for the assessment of dysphagia including in particular full assessment by a speech and language therapist, in collaboration with a dietitian. The clinical examination includes history taking, the evaluation of the body mass index, respiratory function (e.g. vital capacity) and the examination of swallowing abilities. During this assessment the speech and language therapist will examine the structures involved in swallowing, observe the patient's ability to manage food and drinks, define aspiration risks, plan therapeutic strategies to maintain a sufficient and secure oral intake and establish a current diet which the patient is able to manage. This assessment should be ongoing throughout the progression of the disease.

The following aspects of the oral phase of the swallowing process can be directly observed:

- Lip function: the ability to maintain a lip seal, which is important for the oral retention of food and fluid. Good lip seal also allows a positive pressure within the oral cavity allowing initiation of the swallowing and facilitating laryngeal elevation. The ability to take food from a utensil and to use a straw should be assessed.

- Tongue function: the strength, rate, coordination and range of tongue movement, from which inferences regarding the ability to collect and control a bolus within the mouth and to effectively push the bolus into the pharynx can be made. The efficacy of tongue function can also be observed by noting the presence of oral residue after a swallow.

- Pharyngeal function: while the pharyngeal phase cannot be directly observed, information can be inferred through observation of swallowing.

Coughing before, during and after swallowing may indicate that penetration or aspiration is occurring. It must however be remembered that some people do cough insufficiently or stop coughing because of weakness of the laryngeal closure and respiratory musculature. Penetration or aspiration without any subsequent cough is termed silent. Since there is usually no sensory pharyngolaryngeal deficit in ALS patients, silent penetration or aspiration is caused by the weakness of the laryngeal or respiratory muscles, as described above. The most effective way of ascertaining that aspirated material is cleared effectively through a cough is by videofluoroscopy or a fibreoptic endoscopic evaluation of swallowing. The timing and degree of laryngeal elevation during swallowing can be estimated by placing fingers on the suprahyoid muscles, the hyoid bone and larynx and noting the approximation of these structures during a swallow.

The assessment may be supported by the use of pulse oximetry (when a significant fall in oxygen saturation after oral intake suggests aspiration) or by observing respiration (when an increased respiration rate after oral intake suggests aspiration).

Videofluoroscopic and endoscopic swallowing evaluation

Videofluoroscopic swallowing study (VFSS) is an important technique in the evaluation of swallowing disorders for its ability to reveal insights into oro-pharyngeal, laryngeal and esophageal abnormalities. The assessment of an effective cough reflex or the presence of aspiration can be detected during the investigation. Based on these results, a treatment plan for swallowing therapy can be established and the decision made as to whether to provide dietary modification or alternative feeding methods.[14,15]

Because of the frequent finding of respiratory dysfunction and the high risk of aspiration in ALS patients with dysphagia, a modified barium swallow (MBS) may be dangerous with respect to aspiration pneumonia[16] and should, if at all, only be performed in patients with minor dysphagic symptoms. As hyperosmolar contrast media such as Gastrografin entail the risk of provoking life-threatening lung oedema if aspiration occurs[17] the isosmolar contrast agent Iotrolan,[18] which has no significant side-effects even in the case of aspiration, may be preferred.

Transnasal fibre–optic endoscopic evaluation of swallowing (FEES)[19] allows direct visualization of the pharynx and larynx and can be helpful in the assessment of swallowing.

VFSS and FEES are complementary methods and both have advantages and disadvantages.[20] FEES is generally well tolerated by the patients who can eat real food during the examination; it is more portable than VFSS and can even be performed in bedridden persons. VFSS provides an image of the entire duration of the swallow and allows viewing of the complete oropharyngeal tract including the upper oesophageal sphincter.

VFSS and FEES recordings are useful in the education of patients and carers as they reveal the process of swallowing very clearly and demonstrate the risks involved in swallowing and the benefits of modifications to the feeding process.[21]

Management of dysphagia

Positioning

The patient should be in a comfortable position while eating and drinking, usually in an upright position. Patients with ALS may require extra support as the effort may result in an unwanted increase in tone or fatigue. The involvement of a physiotherapist can be very helpful (see p. 194).

Compensatory techniques

There are several compensatory techniques that can aid the swallowing of patients and reduce the risk of aspiration:

- Supraglottic swallowing is a technique which helps to close the vocal cords during swallowing. The patient holds his breath while swallowing and exhales at full force immediately afterwards.[22] Food or secretion can be expelled from the laryngeal vestibulum by this technique in order to avoid aspiration. This technique is recommended when laryngeal closure becomes weak and triggering of the swallowing reflex is delayed and is appropriate for patients with minor oral, laryngeal and respiratory dysfunction.

- The Mendelsohn manoeuvre is a technique which helps to open the upper oesophageal sphincter and prolong its opening time. The patient has to hold the upward movement of the larynx during swallowing for about two seconds. This technique is especially appropriate for patients with deficient opening of the upper esophageal sphincter. In ALS patients where forceful movements become a problem, the Mendelsohn technique may be performed more moderately, since it should not distress the patient.

- Postural changes can be helpful. Patients with pseudobulbar symptoms, impaired tongue movements (and resulting difficulty initiating a swallow) but with intact pharyngeal phase of swallowing can tilt the head backwards to guide the bolus into the pharynx. Patients with bulbar symptoms, with difficulty in triggering the reflex and premature spilling of liquids can tilt the head forward, known as the "chin tuck". In order not to drool food or liquids patients should be encouraged to seal the lips with their hand.

Although neuropsychological disturbances may occur in ALS, they are in many cases only subtle and undetected without comprehensive neuropsychological testing[23] – see Chapter 4c. Therefore, for many ALS patients the cognitive prerequisites for adopting these strategies are good, even in late stages of the disease.

Exercises

There are no specific studies showing that the use of exercises to aid swallowing is of benefit to patients with ALS. It has not been shown that exercises improve swallowing function and they may merely exhaust the weakened muscles. For a small proportion of patients with very slowly progressing disease exercises may be of limited benefit in maintaining function. Exercises may be helpful in lip closure and tongue movements.

Patients may be encouraged to improve their swallowing rate by learning to swallow before trying to open the mouth or to speak. A simple timer can be used, which reminds them at an individually determined interval to swallow (for example every minute) following a 'beep' signal.

Since fatigue is a very common symptom which occurs frequently while performing exercises,[24] short therapy sessions several times a day with resting periods should be preferred.

Dietary modifications

As eating becomes more of a problem the patient should also be seen by a dietitian so that an assessment of the intake can be made and advice given on how to enrich the meals with calories, proteins and vitamins. Energy intake should correspond with the patients' changing requirements during the progression of the disease.[25] If the patient's eating is slowed it may be that they could adapt by taking longer over meals. In practice, they do not do this, possibly because slow eating induces earlier satiety, but also because they are embarrassed to take longer than others and curtail their meals accordingly. They increasing messiness with eating is also a source of embarrassment, and may cause them to avoid eating in company, or miss out items which cause them problems.

Dietary modification may be necessary with the aim of maintaining nutrition and preventing extensively long mealtimes, fatigue and dread of meals. Soft textures or puréed food can compensate for a poor oral preparation phase and ease oral and pharyngeal transport. Liquid supplements may be helpful, but beyond a certain stage there tends to be choking, especially with thin liquids, and patients find thickened drinks easier to manage. Food can be pureed or liquidized and mixed with commercial preparations such as Thick & Easy™ or Nutilis™, which make a semi-solid consistency that is easier to swallow. Puréed food can also be made much more attractive by reconstituting it into its original shape and appearance by using thickener and moulds. For example, meat, vegetables and potatoes can be given an almost normal appearance by liquidizing the different components, mixing them with thickener, and then moulding them on the plate in their original form, which retains the visual and hedonistic aspect of the food. Experience has shown that semi-solid food presented in this way is much more likely to be eaten than if it is presented in the form of a dull-coloured puree, like the weaning foods used for babies. It is also important to ensure food remains hot and palatable, using a heated tray or bowl.

Patients and relatives need instruction on how to prepare appropriate meals, like high-calorie food or specific textures that are easy to chew and swallow (including thickening of liquids to avoid dehydration). Another problem can be abdominal weakness and failure of glottic closure which can lead to constipation. In these cases dietary fibre has to be added. Triggering of the swallowing reflex can be enhanced by emphasizing taste or temperature. Cooled drinks are often easier to swallow.

A recent study showed that dietary modification is efficient in more than 90 per cent of patients with mild to moderate dysphagia.[26]

Rate of intake

Time must be allowed for the weakened muscles to coordinate their movements to complete swallowing and recover during meals. There is often a restriction in the size of bolus that can be tolerated by the patient. The task of feeding the patient can be tedious or cause trepidation and the speech and language therapist may need to spend time training carers, both family members and health care professionals, in the skills required to safely feed someone with dysphagia. It is also essential to ensure that food remains hot and palatable and retains the correct consistency during the entire meal.

Safety strategies

During mealtimes patients should avoid distractions such as conversation, television, radio or other noisy and stress-inducing situations. When patients show a significant level of fatigue, they are advised to eat several small meals a day.

When episodes of choking occur, the Heimlich manoeuvre can be applied by the carers.

Augmented feeding techniques

As dysphagia becomes more severe other feeding techniques may need to be considered. These decisions will need careful discussion with the patient and family and each patient will need an individual assessment and resulting management plan.

Nasogastric tube feeding

Fine-bore nasogastric tubes can be used for feeding, at least in the short term. There are problems of the tube becoming displaced and the tube is very obvious and uncomfortable for patient and family. Nasogastric feeding also appears to be associated with increased risks of ulceration and aspiration pneumonia[27] and there may be an increase in the amount of oropharyngeal secretions with the presence of a nasogastric tube.[28]

Gastrostomy and jejunostomy

The fine-bore percutaneous endoscopic gastrostomy (PEG) technique may be offered to patients with ALS quite early in their disease, since the risks associated with insertion are much less at this stage and the gastrostomy can be used just for supplementation. When respiratory muscle weakness has supervened, the procedure is much more hazardous, as mild sedation is necessary.[29] It is important to try and avoid putting the high-risk patient to unnecessary hazard, and also to be certain that the patients and their family really want it and understand its full implications. The decision to consider a PEG should only be made after careful discussion with the patient and family. It has been suggested that the discussion should be undertaken soon after the onset of dysphagia and when the patient's forced vital capacity is still over 50 per cent of predicted to reduce the risks of the procedure.[30]

The procedure is not without risk in patients earlier in the disease. The mortality of this procedure is less than 1 in 100, particularly from problems such as pneumonia. Clinical contraindications to this technique are abnormal coagulation, portal hypertension or ascites, gastric outflow obstruction, previous gastric surgery, major cardiorespiratory problems and *Clostridium difficile*-associated diarrhoea.

Although major complications such as peritonitis and cellulitis have been described, complications are usually minor and related to local skin infections, reflux, or mechanical problems with the tube, e.g. blocking or fracture of the hub. The technique of inserting a PEG is described widely.[31]

Jejunostomies have been used successfully in patients with neurological dysphagia. The advantage of this technique is that food is put directly into the jejunum, overcoming the problems associated with reflux of food into the pharynx. Unfortunately the insertion of a needle-catheter jejunostomy necessitates a general anaesthetic with a mini-laparotomy for its insertion. Alternatively, where reflux has been a problem, the PEG technique can be used, threading a fine-bore jejunal tube through the gastrostomy, round into the jejunum, under endoscopic guidance.

The insertion of a percutaneous radiological gastrostomy (PRG) does not require sedation.[32] It may be considered when the respiratory reserve of the patient is such that the insertion of a PEG may be considered to be very difficult and with increased risk of morbidity or mortality. Alternatively, non-invasive positive pressure ventilation with oxygen support and conscious sedation anesthesia can be administered during PEG or PRG insertion in patients with a forced vital capacity less than 50 per cent.[33]

Nourishment via a PEG has been shown to improve both the nutritional state of the patient and survival. A study of 35 ALS patients showed that there was an improvement of body mass index in patients with a PEG, whereas there was a reduction for controls. After six months the mortality of PEG patients was lower than the control group.[34] Other studies have shown a probable improvement in the quality of life and the majority of patients maintained or improved in weight. In addition there is increasing evidence that PEG insertion is better tolerated and associated with fewer side effects than nasogastric tube feeding.[28,31]

Ethical concerns have been raised about the use of augmented feeding techniques, as there is the risk of extending life, when the quality of the life is deteriorating and the patient does not wish to continue.[35] The patient and family need to be carefully involved in the decision about the insertion of a PEG and it is essential that there is adequate explanation of implications of the procedure, as well as the risks of not having the procedure, both on the quality and length of life. It is also important to ensure that the patient and family can cope with the procedures involved in feeding through the tube and that there are facilities and support for them in the community.[35]

Management of sialorrhoea and mucus secretions

Patients may experience problems with their oropharyngeal secretions. Although the total amount of saliva produced remains the same, sialorrhoea develops as swallowing is reduced. The patient should be reminded to swallow before trying to open the mouth or speak and to be aware of frequent swallowing to keep the mouth free of saliva.

Patients may complain of dryness, particularly on waking, but drooling may occur later in the day as fatigue increases or after meals. Depending on the nature of the problem different management approaches may be used. If the mucous secretions are thick and ropy, sipping fruit juices, especially dark grape juice, can be beneficial. Sipping water may be sufficient for dryness, but later in the disease artificial saliva may be required. Special, enzyme-containing dental care products like mouthwash and tooth paste, without alcohol and mint, or oral moistening gel may also be of benefit (see the section on Speech and language therapy, p. 218).

Pharmacological interventions

Reduction of salivary flow in ALS patients with drooling is possible with transdermal scopolamine lasting 24–72 hours[36] and other anticholinergic medication such as atropine, amitriptyline or doxepin.[25]

Botulinum toxin injection into the parotid glands has been proposed as a new treatment for sialorrhea in patients with ALS.[37]

If swallowing is disturbed because of thick mucous secretions, N-acetyl-cysteine may be helpful,[38] although of limited value for many ALS patients with a weak cough pressure.

Gastroesophageal reflux disease is frequent and may aggravate or even cause swallowing and respiratory problems.[39] Therefore, in ALS patients suffering from reflux, proton pump inhibitors such as omeprazole should be administered.

Surgery

Palliative surgery in ALS patients with dysphagia should be considered only in certain cases and then with caution, since surgical trauma may contribute to neuronal death and more progressive course of ALS.[40] Furthermore, in general anaesthesia the rate of perioperative mortality has been reported to be high.[41] Among surgical procedures the efficacy of cricopharyngeal myotomy remains controversial. There are four prerequisites for a cricopharyngeal myotomy:[42]

1. cricopharyngeal dysfunction,
2. normal elevation of hyoid and larynx,
3. swallowing therapy (e.g. by use of the Mendelsohn maneuver) not successful in achieving the opening of the upper esophageal sphincter,
4. pharyngeal pressure sufficient to propel a bolus through the open sphincter.

All these prerequisites occur rarely in ALS patients and a recent study showed that pressure profiles of the upper oesophageal sphincter are not disturbed in

ALS.[13] Therefore, for the majority of ALS patients treatment of dysphagia by cricopharyngeal myotomy may be inappropriate.

In order to avoid irreversible myotomy, botulinum toxin injections into the upper oesophageal sphincter are an alternative,[43] but share the same prerequisites as cricopharyngeal myotomy. Since a general weakness has been described in a patient with ALS after focal botulinum toxin injection,[44] this procedure cannot be generally recommended.

For ALS patients who cannot swallow their own secretions safely, the possibility of tracheostomy may be discussed with the patients and relatives[45] (see Chapter 4a).

Assessment of efficacy

Measurement of nutritional status plays a pivotal role. For this purpose, measures such as dietary histories and body mass index (BMI) can be recommended, in order to avoid malnutrition, i.e. BMI <18.5 kg/m^2. Dysphagia-specific scales such as the bulbar section of the Norris scale, the ALS Functional Rating Scale-R (ALS FRS-R) bulbar sections and the Dysphagia Outcome Severity Scale (DOSS) can also be used.[46] For assessment of dysphagia-specific quality of life, the recently developed and validated SWAL-QOL and SWAL-CARE are also suitable outcome tools.[47]

Conclusion

Attention to eating and drinking is part of the optimal care of all patients. When normal mechanisms begin to fail, the help of a speech and language therapist and dietitian should be sought to help the patient overcome mild to moderate degrees of activity limitation. The adoption of special techniques may aid swallowing, as may the provision of attractive food of semi-solid consistency. As dysphagia becomes more advanced, consideration should be given to the use of augmented means of feeding by gastrostomy, jejunostomy or nasogastric tube, but always with the full consent of the patient and the cooperation of family and carers. Nutrition is only one part of the overall management of patients with this distressing condition, which requires a multidisciplinary team approach.

Acknowledgements

The authors would like to acknowledge the contribution of the co-authors in the first edition, on which this chapter was based – Simon Allison, Consultant Physician, Department of Diabetics, Endocrinology and Nutrition, University of Nottingham; Jo Rawlings, Department of Diabetics, Endocrinology and Nutrition, University of Nottingham; Amanda Scott, Senior Clinician at Bethlehem Hospital and Lecturer at La Trobe University, Victoria, Australia; David Oliver, Consultant Physician, Wisdom Hospice, Rochester.

References

1. Kasarskis E. J., Beryyman S., Vanderleest J. G., Schneider A. R., McClain C. J. (1996) Nutritional status of patients with amyotrophic lateral sclerosis: relation to the proximity of death. *Am J Clin Nutr* **63**: 130–7.

2. Worwood A. M., Leigh P. N. (1998). Indicators and prevalence of malnutrition in motor neuron disease. *Eur Neurol* **40**: 159–63.

3. Kuhlemeier K. V. (1994). Epidemiology and dysphagia. *Dysphagia* **9**: 209–17.

4. McGuirt W. F., Blalock D. (1980). The otolaryngologist's role in the diagnosis and treatment of amyotrophic lateral sclerosis. *Laryngoscope* **90**: 1496–501.

5. Roller N. W., Garfunkel A., Nichols C., Ship I. I. (1974). Amyotrophic lateral sclerosis. *Oral Surg Oral Med Oral Pathol* **37**: 46–52.

6. O'Brien T., Kelly M., Saunders C. (1992). Motor neurone disease: a hospice perspective. *BMJ* **304**: 471–3.

7. Oliver D. (1996). The quality of care and symptom control – the effects on the terminal phase of ALS/MND. *J Neurol Sci* **139** (Suppl.): 134–6.

8. Lowe J. S., Leigh N. (2002). Disorders of movement and system degenerations. In Graham D. I., Lantos P. l. (eds) *Greenfield's Neuropathology*, Vol. 2, 7th edn, pp. 325–430. London: Arnold.

9. Hillel A. D., Miller R. (1989) Bulbar amyotrophic lateral sclerosis: patterns of progression and clinical management. *Head Neck* **11**: 51–5.

10. Strand E. A., Miller R. M., Yorkston K. M., Hillel A. D. (1996). Management of oral-pharyngeal dysphagia symptoms in amyotrophic lateral sclerosis. *Dysphagia* **11**: 129–39.

11. Newall A. R., Orser R., Hunt M. (1996). The control of oral secretions in bulbar ALS/MND. *J Neurol Sci* **139**: 43–4.

12. Robbins J. (1987). Swallowing in ALS and motor neuron disorders. *Neurol Clin* **5**: 213–29.

13. MacDougall G., Wilson J. A., Pryde A., Grant R. (1995). Analysis of the pharyngoesophageal pressure profile in amyotrophic lateral sclerosis. *Otolaryngol Head Neck Surg* **112**: 258–61.

14. Logemann J. A., Rademaker A. W., Pauloski B. R., Ohmae Y., Kahrilas P. J. (1998). Normal swallowing physiology as viewed by videofluoroscopy and videoendoscopy. *Folia Phoniatr Logop* **50**: 311–19.

15. Wright R. E. R., Jordan C. (1997). Videofluoroscopic evaluation of dysphagia in motor neurone disease with modified barium swallow. *Palliat Med* **11**: 44–8.

16. Tsokos M., Schulz F., Vogel H. (1998). Barium aspiration with fatal outcome. *Aktuelle Radiol* **8**: 201–3.

17. Trulzsch D. V., Penmetsa A., Karim A., Evans D. A. (1992). Gastrografin-induced aspiration pneumonia: a lethal complication of computed tomography. *South Med J* **85**: 1255–6.

18. Miyazawa T., Sho C., Nakagawa H., Oshino N. (1990). Effect of water-soluble contrast medium on the lung in rats. Comparison of iotrolan, iopamidol, and diatrizoate. *Invest Radiol* 25: 999–1003.

19. Langmore S. E. (ed.) (2001). *Endoscopic evaluation and treatment of swallowing disorders*. New York: Thieme.

20. Doggett D. L., Turkelson C. M., Coates V. (2002) Recent developments in diagnosis and intervention for aspiration and dysphagia in stroke and other neuromuscular disorders. *Curr Atheroscler Rep* 4: 311–18.

21. Leder S. B., Novella S., Patwa H. (2004). Use of fiberoptic endoscopic evaluation of swallowing (FEES) in patients with amyotrophic lateral sclerosis. Dysphagia 19: 177–81.

22. Ohmae Y., Logemann J. A., Hanson D. G., Kahrilas P. J. (1996). Effects of two breath-holding maneuvers on oropharyngeal swallow. *Ann Otol Rhinol Laryngol* 105: 123–31.

23. Abrahams S., Goldstein L. H., Al-Chalabi A., Pickering A., Morris R. G., Passingham R. E., Brooks D. J., Leigh P. N. (1997) Relation between cognitive dysfunction and pseudobulbar palsy in amyotrophic lateral sclerosis. *J Neurol Neurosurg Psychiatry* 62: 464–72.

24. Sharma K. R., Kent-Braun J. A., Majumdar S. *et al.* (1995). Physiology of fatigue in amyotrophic lateral sclerosis. *Neurology* 45: 733–40.

25. Hefferman C., Jenkinson C., Holmes T. *et al.* (2004) Nutritional management in MND/ALS patients: an evidence based review. *Amyotroph Lateral Scler Other Motor Neuron Disord* 5: 72–83.

26. Kuhlemeier K. V., Palmer J. B., Rosenberg D. (2001). Effect of liquid bolus consistency and delivery method on aspiration and pharyngeal retention in dysphagia patients. *Dysphagia* 16: 119–22.

27. Norton B., Holmer-Ward M., Donnelly M. T., Long R. G., Holmes G. K. T. (1996). A randomised prospective comparison of percutaneous endoscopic gastrostomy and nasogastric tube feeding after acute dysphagic stroke. *BMJ* 312: 13–16.

28. Scott A. G., Austin H. E. (1994). Nasogastric feeding in the management of severe dysphagia in motor neurone disease. *Palliat Med* 8: 45–9.

29. Mathus-Vliegen L. M. H., Louwerse L. S., Merkus M. P., Tytgat G. N. J., Vienney de Jong J. M. B. (1994). Percutaneous endoscopic gastrostomy in patients with amyotrophic lateral sclerosis and impaired pulmonary function. *Gastrointest Endosc* 40: 463–9.

30. Miller R. G., Rosenberg J. A., Gelinas D. F., Mitsumoto H., Newman D., Surit R. (1999). Practice parameter: The care of the patient with amyotrophic lateral sclerosis (an evidence-based review). *Neurology* 52: 1311–23.

31. Park R. H. R., Allison M. C., Lang J. *et al.* (1992). Randomised comparison of percutaneous endoscopic gastrostomy and nasogastric tube feeding in patients with persisting neurological dysphagia. *BMJ* 304: 1406–9.

32. Chiò A., Galletti R., Finocchiaro C. *et al.* (2004) Percutaneous radiological gastrostomy: a safe and effective method of nutritional tube placement in advanced ALS. *J Neurol Neurosurg Psychiatry* 75: 645–7.

33. Gregory S., Siderowf A., Golaszewski A. L., McCluskey L. (2002) Gastrostomy insertion in ALS patients with low vital capacity: Respiratory support and survival *Neurology* 58: 485–7.

34. Mazzini L., Corra T., Zaccala M., Mora G., Del Piano M., Galante M. (1995). Percutaneous endoscopic gastrostomy and enteral nutrition in amyotrophic lateral sclerosis. *J Neurol*, **242**: 695–8.

35. Lennard-Jones J. E. (1999). Giving or withholding fluid and nutrients: ethical and legal aspects. *J R Coll Physicians Lond* **33**: 39–45.

36. Talmi Y. P., Finkelstein Y., Zohar Y. (1989). Reduction of salivary flow in amyotrophic lateral sclerosis with Scopoderm TTS. *Head Neck* **11**: 565.

37. Bushara K. O. (1997) Sialorrhea in amyotrophic lateral sclerosis: a hypothesis of a new treatment – botulinum toxin A injections of the parotid glands. *Med Hypotheses* **48**: 337–9.

38. Kelly G. S. (1998). Clinical applications of N-acetylcysteine. *Altern Med Rev* **3**: 114–27.

39. Cote D. N., Miller R. H. (1995) The association of gastroesophageal reflux and otolaryngologic disorders. *Compr Ther* **21**: 80–4.

40. Sostarko M., Vranjes D., Brinar V., Brzovic Z. (1998). Severe progression of ALS/MND after intervertebral discectomy. *J Neurol Sci* **160** (Suppl. 1): 42–6.

41. Short S. O., Hillel A. D. (1989). Palliative surgery in patients with bulbar amyotrophic lateral sclerosis. *Head Neck* **11**: 364–9.

42. Kelly J. H. (2000). Management of upper esophageal sphincter disorders: indications and complications of myotomy. *Am J Med* **108** (Suppl. 4a): 43S–6S.

43. Schneider I., Thumfart W. F., Pototschnig C., Eckel H. E. (1994). Treatment of dysfunction of the cricopharyngeal muscle with botulinum A toxin: introduction of a new, noninvasive method. *Ann Otol Rhinol Laryngol* **103**: 31–5.

44. Mezaki T., Kaji R., Kohara N., Kimura J. (1996). Development of general weakness in a patient with amyotrophic lateral sclerosis after focal botulinum toxin injection. *Neurology* **46**: 845–6.

45. Borasio G. D., Sloan R., Pongratz D. E. (1998) Breaking the news in amyotrophic lateral sclerosis. *J Neurol Sci* **160** (Suppl. 1): 127–33.

46. Kidney D., Alexander M., Corr B., O'Toole O., Hardiman O. (2004). Oropharyngeal dysphagia in amyotrophic lateral sclerosis: neurological and dysphagia specific rating scales. *Amyotroph Lateral Scler Other Motor Neuron Disord* **5**: 150–3.

47. McHorney C. A., Robbins J., Lomax K. *et al.* (2002). The SWAL-QOL and SWAL-CARE outcomes tool for oropharyngeal dysphagia in adults: III. Documentation of reliability and validity. *Dysphagia* **17**: 97–114.

Chapter 4c

Control of symptoms:

cognitive dysfunction

Laura Goldstein

Case history

Explaining everyday difficulties: the value of a clinical neuropsychological assessment

Mr MK was a 55 year-old gentleman who had been diagnosed with ALS two years earlier. He was married with three children. He had recently become severely dysarthric but was now using a Lightwriter, although not particularly efficiently. His verbal output using this, and also through writing, was becoming increasingly limited, although he was able physically to write in a legible manner. His family was reporting that he appeared not to be remembering what they were telling him about recent events, appeared rather impulsive in his attempts to swallow food and was not able to follow the speech and language therapist's advice regarding safe feeding.

A clinical neuropsychology assessment suggested that Mr MK was experiencing impairments in a number of cognitive domains, which had implications for his everyday functioning. Thus his family's impression of his poor memory was borne out on testing, although assessment also highlighted his difficulty in understanding more complex grammar, which may have also led them to think that he was not remembering what they said to him, when he may simply not have understood them in the first place. He may also have had trouble trying to divide his attention between several people telling him different things which they expected him to remember. The perseveration observed during testing was also felt to contribute to his difficulties using his Lightwriter and, particularly importantly, also eating safely. His naming and word generation difficulties during testing also substantiated the everyday impression of his reduced verbal output when writing/using his Lightwriter.

The observations of cognitive deficits observed during testing were explained to Mr MK and his family so that they could improve how best to communicate with him, and were also relayed to the other members of the team working with Mr MK so that they could modify the complexity of the instructions given to Mr MK, reduce how much they expected him to remember without having written things down for him, and to address, in particular, the guidelines given to him regarding eating.

Summary

Although the traditional view of ALS was that it was not accompanied by cognitive change, a substantial body of evidence has now accumulated to show that, in addition to the relatively small percentage of patients in whom a frontotemporal-type dementia may occur, a substantial percentage of non-demented patents may nonetheless show mild to moderate cognitive change, predominantly of a dysexecutive nature. Memory deficits may also occur and, increasingly, language involvement has been noted. A number of disease-related factors (such as bulbar involvement, respiratory weakness) may compound cognitive impairment and need to be taken into account when assessing cognition. Affective disorder and medication may also impact on cognitive function. There is an absence of information concerning the effective use of psychological interventions for cognitive dysfunction in ALS, although more general cognitive neuropsychological rehabilitation techniques may be applicable. When developing interventions for dealing with behavioural changes that may occur in ALS-dementia, guidance needs to be taken from approaches used in other neurodegenerative diseases and frontotemporal dementias more generally. People with ALS should have access to clinical neuropsychologists who can assess the presence of cognitive dysfunction which may be present early on in the disease process and who can also, if necessary, undertake behavioural assessments, and work alongside other members of the clinical team to ensure the best provision of care for the person with ALS and also their carers.

Introduction

Despite the traditional view of ALS as a neurodegenerative disease that did not impact on cognitive functions, convincing evidence has now accumulated that, in at least some people, a detectable degree of cognitive involvement is present. This can vary in magnitude and at worst, there may be a frank dementia. The nature of the cognitive involvement will be documented below with comments on some of the practical implications of such compromised cognitive functions.

It is also important to note that many people with ALS and their carers are not aware of the potential for cognitive impairment. How professionals communicate such possible consequences of ALS may be particularly important, as people's own anticipation of being cognitively impaired has the potential to influence their future treatment choices.[1]

ALS and dementia

It is now well recognized that in at least approximately 3 per cent of sporadic cases and approximately 15 per cent of familial cases of ALS a frontotemporal dementia (FTD) may occur.[2,3] However more recent estimates suggest a higher prevalence of dementia in ALS[4,5] due to improved diagnostic criteria for FTD. In such cases a clear breakdown in behaviour, personality and cognition occur, reflecting frontal dysfunction.[2,6] Cognitive, personality and behavioural difficulties usually, but not always, precede the physical signs of ALS and approximately 10 per cent of people with FTD then develop ALS.

Where neuropsychological assessment is possible, impaired abstract reasoning, rigid thinking, reduced verbal fluency, poor response inhibition, impaired attention, reduced naming and a non-fluent dysphasia have been reported: memory is variably affected but more posterior functions are thought to remain unaffected.[2,7,8]

Although the practical implications of dementia for people with ALS have received little attention, the development of socially inappropriate and other problem behaviours, characterized in some cases as disinhibited, jocular, impatient, gluttonous and with stereotypical gestures[6] may produce disruption to everyday life and to the care provided. Schulz et al.[9] reported different subtypes of FTD in their sporadic ALS patients: the majority were characterized by dysexecutive behaviour typical of lateral frontal involvement, whilst small numbers demonstrated disinhibited behaviour, primary progressive aphasia, or semantic dementia. Others have suggested that whilst some ALS patients meet full criteria for FTD, others may only meet criteria intermittently.[10]

ALS-aphasia

Bak et al.[11] described six patients with ALS in whom communication problems developed at an early stage. They all developed a progressive non-fluent aphasia and five patients were also found to have deficits in syntactic comprehension. Interestingly, comprehension and production of verbs were consistently more affected than for nouns and this relative deficit persisted. The classical physical signs of ALS developed over the following 6–12 months. The behavioural symptoms ranged from mild anosognosia to personality change implicating frontal-lobe dementia, confirmed in three cases post mortem. Bak et al. support other views[12] that whilst the existence of ALS dementia has been well-recognized, the incidence of a possible ALS aphasia is possibly underestimated and can occur in the absence of the 'frontal' features characteristic of ALS dementia.

Cognitive impairment without dementia

The relatively recent emphasis on the potential compromise of cognitive functions in ALS has arisen out of, and in turn encouraged, a range of formal neuropsychological studies of people with ALS.[13–25] It is possible that for many people the deficits are sufficiently subtle and only revealed on formal neuropsychological testing, but in other cases aspects of changed everyday behaviour may suggest compromised cognitive ability. Whether such deficits are detected may be influenced by whether a clinic routinely refers all people with ALS for neuropsychological assessment (resources allowing) or only if cognitive deficits are suspected. From a practical viewpoint the physical care required by someone with ALS may detract from more subtle cognitive changes, which might otherwise be ascribed to mood changes or to other psychological reactions to the illness.

Executive functions

The most consistently reported cognitive difficulties for people with ALS have been in what are referred to as executive functions. These are functions typically defined as being involved in the organization and planning of behaviour, mental flexibly, the ability to switch between tasks and divide attention, to follow rules and inhibit responses when appropriate, think in abstract rather than only in concrete terms and also to be able to generate responses fluently.

A range of neuropsychological tests assess these abilities. Different studies have yielded a consistent pattern of results whereby people with ALS, as a group, appear impaired in their verbal fluency ability, i.e. their ability to generate rapidly written or spoken words. Although the most consistent findings have been for tasks requiring the generation of words beginning with predetermined letters,[13–16,19–21,26–30] the findings apply more variably to semantic categories.[13,15,28,31] Difficulties with fluent generation of responses may not just be limited to verbal material.[15,29] Taken together these findings indicate potential difficulties associated with the rapid generation of responses, and that these are associated with the thinking time involved in the generation of such responses and cannot simply be explained on the basis of slowed speech or impaired writing skills.

Deficits have also been found on a range of other executive function tests. Thus impairments have been found on a task of reasoning involving the logical sequencing of pictures to tell a story,[32] the ability to determine a rule in a task, follow it and then flexibly find new rules when the task changes,[14,18,30,33,34] and also to think sufficiently flexibly in order to generate random sequences.[14] In addition, evidence for rather poor planning and impulsive responding has been reported.[14] Verbal and visual attention tests may elicit deficits, and it is possible for people with ALS to have difficulties with focused and/or divided attention.[19,20,24,28,30,34,35] Deficits in reasoning, mental flexibility and attention, together with possible memory deficits (see below) may influence patients' ability to deal with changes to their lifestyle, and adhere to new treatment options, which may cause potential difficulties in care provision and uptake.

Memory

Deficits in memory in people with ALS have been reported, but generally these difficulties are found less consistently than those of executive function and the very wide range of memory tests employed in the different studies also limits comparisons between studies. Where deficits have been reported, they have included difficulties with word recognition, weak or impaired learning of lists or of pairs of words, recognition of visuospatial material, and impaired learning or reproduction of line drawings of objects.[14,16,18,19,21,22,24,26,28,30,34] In terms of remembering verbal material that is perhaps more similar to that in everyday life, some deficits have occasionally been reported in the recall of short stories.[24,36] It has been suggested that memory difficulties in people with ALS stem from weak encoding of the to-be-remembered material rather than its poor subsequent storage,[22] which may imply that care needs to be taken to ensure that the person has encoded the material sufficiently well in the first case to be able to recall it later on. Clearly this has implications for assessment of people's understanding of their treatment options and ultimately for determining their capacity to consent to treatment.

A new line of enquiry, relevant to the detection of memory changes in ALS, has begun to examine whether people with ALS show the typical profile of being better able to remember material that is emotional in nature than material that is neutral in valence. Papps et al.[37] have recently demonstrated that a group of people with ALS did not show this typical pattern when being asked to recognize previously seen words with either emotional or neutral valence and instead recognized a similar number of emotional words and more neutral words than control participants. It may be important to consider whether an alteration in the processing of emotionally salient material might influence people's reaction to their illness and what they remember of the information they are given about it, especially as other lines of work suggest that people with ALS may respond differently (more positively) from healthy controls to socio-emotional stimuli.[38]

Language

The potential for detecting a spoken language impairment in people with ALS is clearly more difficult where the person has pronounced bulbar impairment, but nonetheless a routine comprehensive language assessment for the person with ALS has been recommended.[39] This would seem particularly advisable if there is any doubt as to the person's ability to comprehend what is said to them. Accumulating evidence adds support for this view, although to date language impairments are found in a relatively small number of people with ALS.[32,40–42] No data exist concerning the relative difficulties in verb as opposed to noun processing seen in the ALS aphasia cases described earlier. In terms of spoken language, some evidence of deficits in confrontation naming (i.e. naming line drawings of objects) has been reported.[28,30,32,40–42] In our own recent studies, whilst object naming scores were lower than those for healthy controls, the patients' scores were not clinically impaired[16,43] and we have not always detected naming deficits.[15,21]

Visuoperceptual and visuospatial functions

Generally, although less emphasis has been placed on examining visuoperceptual functions, it would generally appear that a wide range of measures has elicited intact performance[21,28,32] but inconsistent findings have been reported for the Judgement of Line Orientation Test[16,28,30] and deficits have been found on the Motor Free Visual Perception Test.[42] The reported visuoconstructional deficits have not taken into account possibly confounding motor deficits.[28,31]

Summary of cognitive deficits in ALS

In terms of everyday manifestations of cognitive impairment, then, it is possible that the following may be apparent:

- Difficulty with generating thoughts/words – which may be manifest in limited conversation and poor word-finding – not to be confused with dysarthric speech
- Difficulty planning activities
- Difficulty switching from one idea to another and perseveration (i.e. continuing to do something even when it is no longer appropriate to the situation)
- Attentional/concentration difficulties, possibly leading to distractibility

+ Impulsivity
+ Forgetfulness/problems with learning new things
+ Language difficulties.

As the literature review illustrates, not all of these changes will necessarily be present in the same person, if at all, and they may be obscured by speech and other motor difficulties. It is also important to note that certain changes in cognition occur as a result of the normal ageing process and in relation to anxiety and depression, so a careful clinical evaluation will be necessary in order to determine the significance of any observed changes. In addition changes may be more prominent in the realm of behavioural difficulties rather than performance on specific cognitive tests. The everyday implications of identifying and characterizing cognitive dysfunction in someone with ALS are illustrated in the case example at the beginning of the chapter.

How common is cognitive impairment in ALS?

Ringholz et al.[24] note that previous studies have estimated the prevalence of cognitive impairment in people with ALS as falling between 1–75 per cent. However, the samples studied have varied in size and a range of cognitive measures has been employed. An earlier study of 146 patients from their centre indicated that around 35.6 per cent of patients were cognitively impaired (with impairment defined on the basis of performance at or below the fifth percentile on at least 2/8 neuropsychological tests administered).[30]

Ringholz et al.[24] obtained complete data sets on a wide range of neuropsychological tests and diagnostic rating scales on 252 patients with probable or definite ALS. They then used a range of statistical approaches to classify the extent to which patients were cognitively impaired. Depending on the classification measure used, 48.8–60.7 per cent of their ALS patients were classified as cognitively intact, 24.4–32.3 per cent as mildly cognitively impaired and 14.8–19.7 per cent as moderately–severely impaired. Excluding the intact group, the ALS group's cognitive profile was characterized by executive dysfunction and mild memory impairment; those with more severe cognitive impairment also had word-finding difficulties and produced sentences of shorter phrase length. Forty-three patients satisfied clinical diagnoses for dementia and of these 41 met criteria for FTD.

Ringholz et al.'s data suggest that approximately 40–50 per cent of ALS patients may show at least some degree of cognitive impairment. Confirming such prevalence figures has clear resource implications and suggests greater provision of neuropsychology services is needed for ALS patients. Whether similar prevalence figures would be obtained in a consecutive sample using other measures (for example our motor-speed adjusted measure of verbal fluency[14,15]) remains to be seen. It is certainly essential to avoid contaminating estimates of cognitive (dys)function by failing to take speech/motor ability into account[15] as some studies may have done.[5]

What factors might be associated with cognitive dysfunction in ALS?

It is important to be aware of a number of factors that may be associated with presence of cognitive impairment in ALS since some, but not all, are amenable to intervention.

Bulbar function

Early work[18] suggested that cognitive impairment was more prominent in patients with bulbar symptoms and advanced disease; however as most of that sample had bulbar impairment, clarification of this issue has required further investigation. Massman et al.[30] showed that cognitive impairment was present in 48.5 per cent of their patients with dysarthria – presumably reflecting bulbar dysfunction – although 27.4 per cent of their non-dysarthric patients were also cognitively impaired. It has been shown[14] that patients with evidence of pseudobulbar palsy (i.e. upper motor neuron involvement in the bulbar region) were more impaired than patients without pseudobulbar palsy on several neuropsychological tests of executive function, despite the group of ALS patients as a whole demonstrating deficits on measures of executive function and memory in comparison to healthy controls.

Inconsistent findings exist concerning the association between limb-or bulbar-onset forms of ALS and the extent of cognitive impairment detected in studies.[24,42] Certainly bulbar-onset ALS is not always associated with cognitive impairment[23] just as limb-onset may be associated with cognitive dysfunction.[42]

Respiratory weakness and nocturnal hypoventilation

Respiratory muscle weakness, producing sleep disruption (as a result of oxygen desaturation) accompanied by daytime sleepiness, headaches and loss of appetite may occur in as many as 44 per cent of ALS patients with bulbar symptoms.[44] It has been shown that ALS patients with evidence of hypoventilation, sleep disturbance and respiratory muscle weakness performed significantly worse on measures of memory and verbal fluency than did ALS patients without respiratory or sleep difficulties, and that improvements were seen in the former group following six weeks of nocturnal non-invasive positive pressure ventilation (NIPPV) on two of the memory measures, with a further trend towards improved verbal fluency.[45] Whilst it is unlikely that bulbar-associated respiratory weakness accounts for all the cognitive deficits reported to be associated with bulbar involvement, the role of potentially compromised respiratory muscle function should be borne in mind when considering the cognitive assessment of an individual and also whether any of the cognitive impairment is potentially reversible.

Mood and medication

Many of the cognitive studies of ALS patients have excluded the possibility that cognitive deficits might be accounted for by raised depression scores in ALS patients. Measures of mood may, however, vary over time independently of cognitive function.[17]

While we have been careful to exclude patients on psychotropic medication in our neuropsychological studies, most people do not comment on the medical regimens of their patients. However a range of psychotropic medications as well as other substances may affect cognitive functions,[46,47] and in different ways. Thus, for example, the use of benzodiazepines may affect new learning of material and the use of tricyclic antidepressants may cause sedation and impair memory.[46,47] In addition medication prescribed for ALS itself, such as riluzole, may have psychotropic effects and could potentially mask an otherwise measurable depression.[48]

Are cognitive deficits in ALS progressive?

Three studies have examined whether cognitive impairment in non-demented ALS patients is progressive. Whilst the sample sizes studied and the range of tests administered differ between studies, the findings are generally consistent.

Strong et al.[42] assessed 13 people with ALS and reassessed 8 of them after six months. The patients showed mild difficulties on tests of word generation, face recognition memory and motor-free visual perception. When reassessed, no major changes were noted for the ALS patients as a group, but those patients with bulbar as opposed to limb-onset ALS were impaired across more measures and showed deterioration over time. A similar finding in terms of greater deterioration in bulbar- as opposed to limb-onset ALS patients was recently reported.[49] Cognitive impairment may be present relatively early in the disease and may not increase significantly on follow-up, suggesting that cognitive decline does not occur in tandem with motor deterioration.[17, 49] Abrahams et al.'s[17] finding suggested that executive dysfunction (verbal fluency deficits) may occur relatively early in the disease with signs of language dysfunction developing as the disease progresses. This study did not, however, differentiate between those with bulbar- or limb-onset disease.

Primary lateral sclerosis and progressive muscular atrophy

Although the emphasis of this book is on people with ALS it is worth commenting briefly on what is known about cognitive deficits in patients with primary lateral sclerosis (PLS) and those with progressive muscular atrophy (PMA).

Such data as have been reported on neuropsychological functions in PLS seem to indicate the existence of executive dysfunction.[50] Although Le Forestier et al.'s[51] literature review indicated that PLS patients may be cognitively intact, in their own series of 20 patients they found evidence of disease involvement outside the motor system, and allude to executive dysfunction in nine of their patients but do not present any neuropsychological data. Certainly at this stage it would be difficult to estimate the prevalence of cognitive impairment in PLS, but the possibility must be considered in individual cases.

Scant attention has been paid to the possibility of cognitive dysfunction occuring in PMA patients. In two studies[19,20] there has been some indication that patients with only lower motor neuron involvement (presumed to be PMA) were impaired on fewer tests than people with ALS, although cognitive impairments, relative to controls, were noted on Raven's Coloured Progressive Matrices, and a measure of visual attention.[20] However, it is possible that the groups were poorly matched in terms of intelligence and that the other impairments reflected the lower motor neuron group's lower IQ scores. It is unclear, therefore, to what extent cognitive deficits should be realistically anticipated in PMA patients especially since neuroimaging studies have failed to detect significant changes between PMA patients and controls.[52]

Potential interventions

Very little has been written about the potential for alleviating the cognitive and behavioural changes that may occur in people with ALS, especially in the cases of full-blown dementia. The literature on managing cognitive and behavioural change in neurodegenerative diseases has largely focused on patients with Alzheimer's disease[53] and a number of techniques used in such patients have much in common with those who have suffered severe traumatic brain injuries.

Patients may have limited insight into their own cognitive/behavioural changes. When caregivers report changes to the clinician it is important for them to receive basic information about the types of changes that can occur in ALS, and for a full assessment to be arranged.[10] Lomen-Hoerth and Murphy[10] indicate that common complaints from caregivers, particularly in the context of a dementia, will include irritability and aggression, emotional withdrawal, suspiciousness, poor hygiene, refusal (or inability) to comply with treatment recommendations, or falls and choking incidents that might otherwise seem preventable. They also note that some families may refuse help from professionals to cope with these difficulties. This may be in part because such changes are seen as relatively insignificant in comparison to the person's physical difficulties.

Education for caregivers is at the centre of Lomen-Hoerth and Murphy's recommendations for intervening in cases where cognitive and behavioural changes occur.[10] They particularly recommend educating caregivers about the biological basis for many of these changes, and informing them that frontal lobe pathology is associated with symptoms such as aggression, impulsivity, and irritability and that there is also a biological basis for emotional lability, which carers may also find distressing. They also recommend informing caregivers that some reductions in certain behaviours (e.g. affection) may not be amenable to change whereas the development of disturbing behaviour (e.g. aggression, inappropriate language) may be addressed with, they suggest, a combination of psychotropic medication, particularly selective serotonin reuptake inhibitors (SSRIs) and behavioural interventions. They suggest that SSRIs may be particularly helpful for dealing with rigidity, agitation and compulsiveness, while severe agitation and aggression may be treated with atypical antipsychotics; however others clearly advise against the use of atypical antipsychotics in dementia cases.[54]

Interventions for cognitive and behavioural problems

Memory

Evans[55] has summarized a range of compensatory approaches that may be used when memory processes are failing. Since Münte et al.[22] consider encoding difficulties to be particularly relevant in ALS-related memory weakness, approaches that enhance learning may be particularly useful. For example encouraging and enabling the person to pay more attention to the material to be remembered, whilst also reducing possible distractions, may be helpful. Repetition of the to-be-remembered material, both initially and after increasing time intervals, may help the person recall the material better.

More elaborate techniques, such as that known as PQRST, may be helpful for people with mild–moderate memory difficulties who need to recall the contents of articles/documents, since this technique increases the meaningfulness and memorability of information.[55] Thus when someone wishes to recall the content of a letter detailing important changes, for example to financial arrangements/state benefits, they might be advised to:

- Preview the letter (ie read it through quickly first of all); then set themselves some

- Questions about what is contained in the letter (e.g. what are the main changes in my benefits? when do they come into force?); they would then

- Read the letter through again and would then

- State to themselves what the important information was. Finally they would Test themselves again by asking the relevant questions, and possibly repeating this testing after increasing time intervals.

Evans[55] suggests that for many memory-impaired people the use of mnemonics is too difficult, although many people do find 'mental retracing' (i.e. mentally retracing one's route to think about where one may have left something) may be helpful; he suggests that where the person is demonstrating a degree of impulsivity (reflective of executive dysfunction) a 'stop-think-retrace your steps' approach may be helpful. He notes however that the most commonly used memory aids tend to be 'external' aids, e.g. notebooks diaries, wall calendars, memo boards, alarms, pill reminders/dosette boxes, as well as signposts and labels on doors of cupboards etc.[55] As notebooks, diaries, calendars etc. are used by non-memory impaired individuals, they may be viewed as non-stigmatizing by the patient and may be particularly acceptable options.

Executive dysfunction

As noted above, a 'stop-think' approach may be of use when impulsivity is apparent in a person's behaviour. This may be of use, for example, when considering poor compliance with advice over swallowing food; thus a person with bulbar dysfunction who is tending to swallow food too quickly and without having chewed it sufficiently, could be encouraged, when eating, to count the number of times they have chewed their food, and then to stop before swallowing to ensure they have chewed it sufficiently, before concentrating on the advice regarding head position etc. that has been given to them by their speech and language therapist to enable them to swallow without choking.

Executive dysfunction is likely to result in a person having difficulty doing several things at once (multi-tasking) or dealing with a large amount of information at once. Reducing the 'cognitive load' placed on someone may help. Rather than asking the person complicated questions requiring the consideration of multiple sources of information, it is helpful to keep things simple and to try to get the person to restrict themselves to dealing with one problem at a time. Keeping questions phrased in simple terms may also be important should the person have any language comprehension difficulties. Spontaneous problem-solving skills may be reduced with executive dysfunction, so helping someone to talk through a problem, and providing the framework for them to consider their options may overcome their own limitations. This may be of particular value when the person needs to consider lifestyle choices and future treatment options.

If perseverative behaviour is present, then helping the person themselves to monitor how often they are doing/saying the same thing may be more effective in helping them to change their behaviour than simply telling them they are repeating themselves. Preventing sources of distraction may also help reduce potential distractibility.

Behavioural change

Gregory and Lough[56] provide some helpful illustrations of how challenging behaviours occurring in FTD may be dealt with using psychological interventions, and also indicate the value of adopting interventions designed for people who have had traumatic brain injuries when working with people with FTD. They describe a lady with whose mobility was restricted due to multiple sclerosis, but her case would be equally relevant if she were an ALS sufferer. This lady made repeated demands on her husband to give her medication for pain and to call the medical services, despite there being no obvious cause for her pain. Her calling out was perseverative and was also considered to be anxiety-driven. Gregory and Lough report that by distracting the lady when she began calling out (in this case by giving her a magazine and engaging her in conversation about it) it was possible to prevent her from engaging in this repetitive benaviour. They suggest that distraction can be used widely to address perseverative behaviour and that by removing articles from the environment that have become the focus of the perseverative behaviour, certain difficulties may be reduced.

Gregory and Lough[56] also illustrate the potential benefits of encouraging someone to use self-control statements when trying to reduce disinhibited behaviour. The presence of executive dysfunction might render it necessary for the person to have external prompts – e.g. flashcards with instructions – to encourage the person not to engage, for example, in verbal aggression or abuse in response to the presence of certain individuals, since spontaneously generating the self-control statements might be more difficult for the person, particularly when in a highly aroused state.

Conclusions

The potential for cognitive involvement, ranging from mild impairment to dementia in ALS cannot be ignored, even though not all patients will be affected. Specialist neuropsychological, and if necessary behavioural assessments should be available for people with ALS, irrespective of whether or not they have developed a full dementia. A clinical neuropsychologist should be available to work with other members of the clinical team to ensure the best provision of care for the person with ALS as well as their carers. Since cognitive involvement may occur very early in the disease process, their involvement should be an integral part of the service offered to people with ALS and their families.

Acknowledgements

Much of our group's research into the cognitive and broader psychological aspects of MND has been funded by the Medical Research Council, the Wellcome Trust and the Motor Neurone Disease Association, UK.

References

1. Silverstein M. D., Stocking C. B., Antel J. P., Beckwith J., Roos R. P., Siegler M. (1991) Amyotrophic lateral sclerosis and life-sustaining therapy: patients' desires for information, participation in decision making, and life-sustaining therapy. *Mayo Clinic Proceedings* **66**: 906–13.

2. Neary D., Snowden J. S., Mann D. M., Northen B., Goulding P. J., Macdermott N. (1990) Frontal lobe dementia and motor neuron disease. *J Neurol Neurosurg Psychiatry* **53**: 23–32.

3. Neary D., Snowden J. S., Mann D. M. (2000) Cognitive change in motor neurone disease/amyotrophic lateral sclerosis (MND/ALS). *J Neurol Sci* **180**: 15–20.

4. Barson F. P., Kinsella G. J., Ong B., Mathers S. E. (2000) A neuropsychological investigation of dementia in motor neurone disease (MND). *J Neurol Sci* **180**: 107–13.

5. Lomen-Hoerth C., Murphy J., Langmore S., Kramer J. H., Olney R. K., Miller B. (2003) Are amyotrophic lateral sclerosis patients cognitively normal? *Neurology* **60**: 1094–7.

6. Vercelletto M., Ronin M., Huvet M., Magne C, Feve J. R.(1999) Frontal type dementia preceding amyotrophic lateral sclerosis: a neuropsychological and SPECT study of five clinical cases. *Eur J Neurol* **6**: 295–9.

7. Peavy G. M., Herzog A. G., Rubin N. P., Mesulam M. M. (1992) Neuropsychological aspects of dementia of motor neuron disease: a report of two cases. *Neurology* **42**: 1004–8.

8. Vercelletto M., Delchoque C., Magne C., Huvet M., Lanier S., Feve J. R. (1999) Analysis of neuropsychological disorders coupled with 99m Tc-HMPAO Spect in amyotrophic lateral sclerosis. Prospective study of 16 cases. *Rev Neurol (Paris)* **155**: 141–7.

9. Schulz P. E., Ringholz G. M., Appel S. H. (2005) Spectrum of altered cognition in ALS. First International Research Workshop on Frontotemporal Dementia in ALS, May. London Ontario, Canada.

10. Lomen-Hoerth C, Murphy J. (2005) The neuropsychology of ALS. First International Research Workshop on Frontotemporal Dementia in ALS, May London Ontario, Canada.

11. Bak T. H., O'Donovan D. G., Xuereb J. H., Boniface S., Hodges J. R.(2001) Selective impairment of verb processing associated with pathological changes in Brodmann areas 44 and 45 in the motor neurone disease-dementia-aphasia syndrome. *Brain* 124: 1–20.

12. Doran M., Xuereb J., Hodges J. R.(1995) Rapidly progressive aphasia with bulbar motor neurone disease: A clinical and neuropsychological study. *Behav Neurol* 8: 169–80.

13. Abe K., Fujimura H., Toyooka K., Sakoda S., Yorifuji S., Yanagihara T. (1997) Cognitive function in amyotrophic lateral sclerosis. *J Neurol Sci* 148: 95–100.

14. Abrahams S., Goldstein L. H., Al Chalabi A., Pickering A., Morris R. G., Passingham R. E. *et al.* (1997) Relation between cognitive dysfunction and pseudobulbar palsy in amyotrophic lateral sclerosis. *J Neurol Neurosurg Psychiatry* 62: 464–72.

15. Abrahams S., Leigh P. N., Harvey A., Vythelingum G. N., Grise D., Goldstein L. H. (2000) Verbal fluency and executive dysfunction in amyotrophic lateral sclerosis (ALS). *Neuropsychologia* 38: 734–47.

16. Abrahams S., Goldstein L. H., Suckling J., Ng V., Simmons A., Chitnis X. *et al.* (2005) Frontotemporal white matter changes in amyotrophic lateral sclerosis. *J Neurol* 253: 321–31.

17. Abrahams S., Leigh P. N., Goldstein L. H. (2005) Cognitive change in ALS: A prospective study. *Neurology* 64: 1222–6.

18. David A. S., Gillham R. A.(1986) Neuropsychological study of motor neuron disease. *Psychosomatics* 27: 441–5.

19. Gallassi R., Montagna P., Ciardulli C., Lorusso S., Mussuto V., Stracciari A. (1985) Cognitive impairment in motor neuron disease. *Acta Neurol Scand* 71: 480–4.

20. Gallassi R., Montagna P., Morreale A., Lorusso S., Tinuper P., Daidone R. *et al.* (1989) Neuropsychological, electroencephalogram and brain computed tomography findings in motor neuron disease. *Eur Neurol* 29: 115–20.

21. Kew J. J., Goldstein L. H., Leigh P. N., Abrahams S., Cosgrave N., Passingham R. E. *et al.* (1993) The relationship between abnormalities of cognitive function and cerebral activation in amyotrophic lateral sclerosis. A neuropsychological and positron emission tomography study. *Brain* 116: 1399–23.

22. Munte T. F., Troger M., Nusser I., Wieringa B. M., Matzke M., Johannes S. *et al.* (1998) Recognition memory deficits in amyotrophic lateral sclerosis assessed with event-related brain potentials. *Acta Neurol Scand* 98: 110–15.

23. Portet F., Cadilhac C., Touchon J., Camu W.(2001) Cognitive impairment in motor neuron disease with bulbar onset. *ALS & Other Motor Neuron Disorders* 2: 23–9.

24. Ringholz G. M., Appel S. H., Bradshaw M., Cooke N. A., Mosnik D. M., Schulz P. E. (2005) Prevalence and patterns of cognitive impairment in sporadic ALS. *Neurology* 65: 586–90.

25. Wilson C. M., Grace G. M., Munoz D. G., He B. P., Strong M. J. (2001) Cognitive impairment in sporadic ALS: a pathologic continuum underlying a multisystem disorder. *Neurology* 57: 651–7.

26. Abrahams S., Goldstein L. H., Kew J. J., Brooks D. J., Lloyd C. M., Frith C. D. *et al.* (1996) Frontal lobe dysfunction in amyotrophic lateral sclerosis. A PET study. *Brain* 119: 2105–20.

27. Abrahams S., Goldstein L. H., Simmons A., Brammer M., Williams S. C., Giampietro V. *et al.* (2004) Word retrieval in amyotrophic lateral sclerosis: a functional magnetic resonance imaging study. *Brain* 127: 1507–17.

28. Hanagasi H. A., Gurvit I. H., Ermutlu N., Kaptanoglu G., Karamursel S., Idrisoglu H. A. *et al.* (2002) Cognitive impairment in amyotrophic lateral sclerosis: evidence from neuropsychological investigation and event-related potentials. *Cog Brain Res* 14, 234–44.

29. Ludolph A. C., Langen K. J., Regard M., Herzog H., Kemper B., Kuwert T. *et al.* (1992) Frontal lobe function in amyotrophic lateral sclerosis: a neuropsychologic and positron emission tomography study. *Acta Neurol Scand* 85: 81–9.

30. Massman P. J., Sims J., Cooke N., Haverkamp L. J., Appel V., Appel S. H. (1996) Prevalence and correlates of neuropsychological deficits in amyotrophic lateral sclerosis. *J Neurol Neurosurg Psychiatry* 61: 450–5.

31. Hartikainen P., Helkala E. L., Soininen H., Riekkinen P., Sr(1993) Cognitive and memory deficits in untreated Parkinson's disease and amyotrophic lateral sclerosis patients: a comparative study. *J Neural Trans-Parkinsons Disease & Dementia* 6: 127–37.

32. Talbot P. R., Goulding P. J., Lloyd J. J., Snowden J. S., Neary D., Testa H. J. (1995) Inter-relation between "classic" motor neuron disease and frontotemporal dementia: neuropsychological and single photon emission computed tomography study. *J Neurol Neurosurg Psychiatry* 58: 541–7.

33. Evdokimidis I., Constantinidis T. S., Gourtzelidis P., Smyrnis N., Zalonis I., Zis P. V. *et al.* (2002) Frontal lobe dysfunction in amyotrophic lateral sclerosis. *J Neurol Sci* 195: 25–33.

34. Frank B., Haas J., Heinze H. J., Stark E., Munte T. F. (1997) Relation of neuropsychological and magnetic resonance findings in amyotrophic lateral sclerosis: evidence for subgroups. *Clin Neurol Neurosurg* 99: 79–86.

35. Chari G., Shaw P. J., Sahgal A. (1996) Nonverbal visual attention, but not recognition memory or learning processes are impaired in motor neurone disease. *Neuropsychologia* 34: 377–85.

36. Iwasaki Y., Kinoshita M., Ikeda K., Takamiya K., Shiojima T. (1990) Cognitive impairment in amyotrophic lateral sclerosis and its relation to motor disabilities. *Acta Neurol Scand* 81: 141–3.

37. Papps B., Abrahams S., Wicks P., Leigh P. N., Goldstein L. H. (2005) Changes in memory for emotional material in amyotrophic lateral sclerosis (ALS). *Neuropsychologia* 43: 1107–14.

38. Lule D., Kurt A., Jurgens R., Kassubek J., Diekmann V., Kraft E. *et al.* (2005) Emotional responding in amyotrophic lateral sclerosis. *J Neurol* 252: 1517–24.

39. Strong M. J., Grace G. M., Orange J. B., Leeper H. A. (1996) Cognition, language, and speech in amyotrophic lateral sclerosis: A review. *J Clin Exp Neuropsychol* 18: 291–303.

40. Cobble M.(1998) Language impairment in motor neurone disease. *J Neurol Sci* 160 (Suppl.): 52.

41. Rakowicz W. P., Hodges J. R. (1998) Dementia and aphasia in motor neuron disease: an underrecognised association? *J Neurol Neurosurg Psychiatry* 65: 881–9.

42. Strong M. J., Grace G. M., Orange J. B., Leeper H. A., Menon R. S., Aere C. (1999) A prospective study of cognitive impairment in ALS. *Neurology* 53: 1665–70.

43. Abrahams S., Goldstein L. H., Simmons A., Brammer M., Williams S. C., Giampietro V. *et al.* (2004) Word retrieval in amyotrophic lateral sclerosis: a functional magnetic resonance imaging study. *Brain* 127: 1507–17.

44. Aboussouan L. S., Lewis R. A. (1999) Sleep, respiration and ALS. *J Neurol Sci* 164: 1–2.

45. Newsom-Davis I. C., Lyall R. A., Leigh P. N., Moxham J., Goldstein L. H. (2001) The effect of non-invasive positive pressure ventilation (NIPPV) on cognitive function in amyotrophic lateral sclerosis (ALS): a prospective study. *J Neurol Neurosurg Psychiatry* 71: 482–7.

46. Powell J. E. (2004) The effects of medication and other substances on cognitive functioning. In Goldstein L. H., McNeil J. E. (eds) *Clinical Neuropsychology. A Practical Guide to Assessment and Management for Clinicians*, pp. 99–119. Chichester, UK: John Wiley & Sons.

47. Stein R. A., Strickland T. L. (1998) A review of the neuropsychological effects of commonly used prescription medications. *Arch Clin Neuropsychology* 13: 259–84.

48. Ginsberg D. L. (2004) Riluzole for treatment-resistant depression. *Prim Psychiatry* 11: 16.

49. Schreiber H., Gaigalat T., Wiedemuth-Catrinescu U., Graf M., Uttner I., Muche R. *et al.* (2005) Cognitive function in bulbar- and spinal-onset amyotrophic lateral sclerosis: A longitudinal study in 52 patients. *J Neurology* 25: 772–81.

50. Caselli R. J., Smith B. E., Osborne D. (1995) Primary lateral sclerosis: a neuropsychological study. *Neurology* 45: 2005–9.

51. Le Forestier N., Maisonobe T., Piquard A., Rivaud S., Crevier-Buchman L., Salachas F. *et al.* (2001) Does primary lateral sclerosis exist? A study of 20 patients and a review of the literature. *Brain* 124: 1989–99.

52. Kew J. J., Brooks D. J., Passingham R. E., Rothwell J. C., Frackowiak R. S., Leigh P. N. (1994) Cortical function in progressive lower motor neuron disorders and amyotrophic lateral sclerosis: a comparative PET study. *Neurology* 44: 1101–10.

53. Moniz-Cook E., Rusted J. (2004) Neurorehabilitation strategies for people with neurodegenerative conditions. In Goldstein L. H., McNeil J. E. (eds) *Clinical Neuropsychology. A Practical Guide to Assessment and Management for Clinicians*, pp. 405–20. Chichester, UK: John Wiley & Sons.

54. Alzheimer's Society (2004) *Risperidone and olanzapine: restrictions on use for people with dementia. Information for care staff.* Information Sheet CSMinfo2. London: Alzheimer's Society.

55. Evans J. J. (2004) Disorders of memory. In Goldstein L. H., McNeil J. E. (eds) *Clinical Neuropsychology. A Practical Guide to Assessment and Management for Clinicians*, pp. 143–63. Chichester, UK: John Wiley & Sons.

56. Gregory C. A., Lough S. (2001) Practical issues in the management of early onset dementia. In Hodges J. R. (ed.) *Early-Onset Dementia. A Multidisciplinary Approach*, pp. 449–68. Oxford: Oxford University Press.

Control of symptoms:

other symptoms (including depression)

Gian Domenico Borasio and David Oliver

Symptoms of ALS can be divided in two groups (Table 4d.1): those deriving directly from the neurodegenerative process, and those which result indirectly from the primary symptoms. Treatment of dysarthria, dysphagia and dyspnoea is discussed in details in separate chapters. This chapter will focus on (mostly) pharmacological interventions for the other symptoms of ALS. Unfortunately, few of these recommendations are evidence-based, and more studies are required to establish the optimal pharmacological management of ALS symptoms.

Weakness and atrophy

These symptoms are the hallmark of ALS. The most effective way of helping patients is through the *timely* discussion and provision of adequate aids (from a walking stick to an AFO to a wheelchair etc.), which are reviewed in other chapters. Physiotherapy is very important to prevent contractures and maintain mobility, and is also discussed separately.

Pharmacologically, there are few ways to intervene. Acetylcholinesterase inhibitors may lead to a short-term improvement in muscle strength,

Table 4d.1 Symptoms due to ALS

Directly	Indirectly
Weakness and atrophy	Psychological disturbances
Fasciculations and muscle cramps	Sleep disturbances
Spasticity	Constipation
Dysarthria	Drooling
Dysphagia	Thick mucous secretions
Dyspnea	Symptoms of chronic hypoventilation
Pathological laughing/crying	Pain

Modified after Borasio and Voltz 1997.[1]

especially early during the disease. This seems more pronounced in bulbar patients. However, it is not seen in all, and it usually only lasts for day to a few weeks. Acetylcholinesterase inhibitors do not alter the course of ALS. The short-term use of pyridostigmine (up to 40 mg tid) can only be recommended for special situations, like a plane trip or a holiday. There is no rationale for long-term therapy with pyridostigmine in ALS, and more often than not, patients will have to be taken off this medication to avoid unnecessary side effects.

Clenbuterol has been advocated as a possible means of increasing muscle strength in ALS. It is a steroid with anabolic properties, and it is used in agriculture to increase the lean mass in meat animals, and by some professional athletes as a doping practice.[2] The use of anabolic drugs in ALS does not make sense from a pathophysiological point of view as the degenerative process involves the motor neurons, not the muscle cells. Offering an artificially increased muscle mass to a damaged motor neuron may very transiently increase force, but may also accelerate neurodegeneration in the long run.

Creatine monohydrate, which is also used by professional athletes, has shown interesting neuroprotective properties in the transgenic SOD1 mouse model.[3] Creatine has also been shown to increase force in a spectrum of muscular diseases. A recent study using creatine has shown no effect on muscle strength or survival in ALS patients.[4]

Muscle fasciculations, cramps and spasticity

Fasciculations (painless twitches of small numbers of muscle fibres, visible to the eye but with no movement effect on the joint) are often the first symptoms of the disease. They arise through degeneration of the intramuscular motor axons, and can lead to painful muscle cramps, which are not infrequently noticed by patients weeks to months before the onset of weakness. Cramps due to ALS may appear in unusual locations, such as the abdominal and paraspinal muscles, and may be the cause of significant discomfort. The drug of choice is quinine sulphate, followed by carbamazepine (Table 4d.2).

Spasticity of the extremities, which is due to degeneration of the upper motor neurons, can be clinically severe. In most, it can be effectively relieved by appropriate medication (Table 4d.3). With antispastic drugs, the patient has to titrate the dosage against the subjective clinical effect, since a moderate degree of spasticity is usually better for mobility than a fully flaccid paresis. Baclofen is the most widely used drug, although no specific study for ALS is available, as shown by a recent Cochrane review.[5]

Physiotherapy with passive movements, which can be continued very regularly several times a day by family or other carers, may be very helpful and it is

Table 4d.2 Medication for fasciculation and cramps*

Quinine sulphate	200 mg bid
Carbamazepine	200 mg bid
Phenytoin	100 mg qd tid
Magnesium	5 mmol qd tid
Vitamin E	400 IE bid
Verapamil	120 mg qd

* In all medication tables, the usual range of adult daily dosage is indicated; some patients may require higher dosages.
Modified after Borasio and Voltz 1997.[1]

Table 4d.3 Medication for spasticity

Baclofen	10–80 mg
Tizanidine	6–24 mg
Memantine	10–60 mg
Tetrazepam	100–200 mg

Modified after Borasio and Voltz 1997.[1]

essential to ensure that the patient is positioned carefully and comfortably. The physiotherapist may be able to assess the role of spasticity in the causation of pain, and assess the response to treatment.[6]

In severe instances, it may be necessary to deliver baclofen intrathecally via an implanted pump.[7] An alternative for such refractory cases, which are rather uncommon in ALS, may be intramuscular injections of botulinus toxin, which have been shown to be effective in multiple sclerosis.[8,9] Cannabis has been reported anecdotally to have a moderate effect on spasticity in ALS.[10] Dantrolene, which acts directly on the muscle, should not generally be used as first-line medication, because it enhances weakness. However, extreme spasticity in the terminal phase, which could only be relieved by high doses of intravenous dantrolene, has been reported.[11]

Pathologic laughing/crying (pseudobulbar affect)

A typical symptom, which needs to be differentiated from a depressed mood, is the development of uncontrollable bouts of laughter and/or tearfulness (the latter occurring more often), which is also referred to as "pseudobulbar affect". The pathophysiology is poorly understood.[12] It is not specific for ALS, but occurs also in other CNS diseases such as multiple sclerosis.[13]

Table 4d.4 Medication for pathologic laughing/crying

Amitriptyline	10–150 mg
Fluvoxamine	100–200 mg
Lithium carbonate	400–800 mg
L-Dopa	500–600 mg

Modified after Borasio and Voltz 1997.[1]

Pathologic laughing/crying occurs in up to 50%.[12,14] It is not a mood disorder, but rather an abnormal display of affect due to a dysregulation of the motoric components of emotional experience[15,16] and may be related to frontal cognitive dysfunction.[17] The symptom can be very disturbing for the patient in social situations.

Since pathologic laughing/crying is seldom volunteered by the patient, physicians should ask for it and point out that it is part of the disease and responds well to medication (Table 4d.4). The point must be made very clearly to patient and family that this symptom does not imply that the patient has some kind of psychiatric disturbance. The most widely used drug is amitriptyline,[13] but positive effects have also been reported for fluvoxamine,[18] dopamine[19,20] and lithium.[21] Since all these medications may also produce side effects, careful discussion with the patient is essential so that they are aware of the balance between a potential treatment and the possible side effects. Recently, a randomized study has shown good efficacy of a combination of 30 mg dextromethorphan hydrobromide and 30 mg quinidine sulfate twice daily in the palliation of pathologic laughing/crying.[22] The corresponding drug (Neurodex)® is currently under priority review by the FDA.

Symptoms indirectly due to ALS

Drooling

Drooling is a frequent complaint in ALS. It is due to a combination of facial muscle weakness and reduced swallowing ability. It is important to recognize and discuss the psychological problems associated with drooling, which often lead to a reduction in social activities. Therefore, adequate treatment of this clinically mild symptom may be of great importance for well-being.

Medications reducing salivary output are helpful (Table 4d.5), but anticholinergic side effects and contraindications must be kept in mind.[23,24] The most widely used drugs are glycopyrrolate[25,26] and amitriptyline, although no controlled trials are available for the latter. Transdermal hyoscine patches offer

Table 4d.5 Medication for drooling

Glycopyrrolate	0.1–0.2 mg sc/im tid
Amitriptyline	10–150 mg
Transdermal hyoscine patches	1–2 patches
Atropine/benztropine	0.25–0.75 mg /1–2 mg
Trihexyphenidyl	6–10 mg
Clonidine	0.15–0.3 mg

Modified after Borasio and Voltz 1997.[1]

the advantage of bypassing oral delivery, which may be very helpful in bulbar cases.[27,28]

Observational studies have found that botulinum toxin type A is safe and is beneficial at reducing refractory sialorrhea in some patients with ALS at doses ranging from 7.5 units to 20 units into each parotid gland[29] One placebo-controlled study found safety and efficacy in patients with ALS and other neurodegenerative disorders when using doses of up to 75 units into each parotid gland, with the highest doses producing the best results.[30] Submandibular gland injection should be considered if injection into the parotid glands alone is not beneficial.

Radiation therapy is another option for treating sialorrhea. It has been shown to be effective for patients with different neurologic diseases, including ALS, when directed at the parotid glands or the submandibular and sublingual glands.[31,32] Side effects include pain in the parotid area, dryness of the mouth, burning of the skin, sore throat, and nausea, and are usually transient, but on occasions they are more severe.

Thick mucous secretions

This is one of the most harrowing symptoms in ALS. Treatment options are insufficient so far. Late-stage ALS patients often suffer greatly because of thick mucous secretions blocking the upper airways, which result from a combination of diminished fluid intake and reduced coughing pressure, as well as chronic upper respiratory tract infections damaging the transporting ability of the mucosal hair cells.

Several attempts at treating thick mucous secretions in ALS have been tried, albeit none in a controlled fashion. N-acetylcysteine is helpful only in a minority of cases, because it requires a large fluid intake and basically dilutes the secretions, resulting in a higher secretion volume which does not necessarily ameliorate the problem if the coughing effort is insufficient. Since it is thought that thick secretions are produced by glands with beta adrenergic receptors, treatment with beta blockers such as propranolol or metoprolol might be considered in severe cases.[33]

Suction may become necessary, but is usually not fully effective unless performed via a tracheostomy. Both manually assisted coughing techniques and mechanical insufflation-exsufflation (In-Exsufflator, J.H. Emerson Co., 22 Cottage Park Av., Cambridge, MA 02140-1601; www.jhemerson.com) can assist in extracting excess mucus from the airway.[34,35] Physical therapy with vibration massage may also be helpful, especially in the initial stages (see Chapter 7a, pages 195–199).

Other treatments which have been shown benefit in an uncontrolled survey include dark grape juice, papaya enzymes, sugar free citrus lozenges grape seed oil and betablockers[36] (see Chapter 7c, Multidisciplinary care, speech and language therapy, p. 218). Reduction of alcohol and caffeine, substitution of dairy products, increased fluid intake, moistening of the air and steam inhalation may provide some benefit. A satisfactory therapy for thick mucous secretions in ALS is still not available and more research is needed in this area.

Psychological problems and depression

Most if not all patients with ALS undergo a phase of reactive depression after being told the diagnosis. Counselling is of paramount importance (see the Chapter 5, Psychosocial care, p. 144 for details). Clinically significant depression should be sought for and treated at all disease stages, particularly since psychological status strongly correlates with survival.[37] Amitriptyline is very useful, starting with 25 mg/d and slowly increase to 100–150mg/d as tolerated. If side effects such as dry mouth or constipation are a problem, serotonin reuptake inhibitors may be employed.

Suicidal thoughts are common at all stages in ALS, and particularly at the beginning, shortly after the diagnosis is communicated. Feelings of hopelessness and fear of becoming a burden to one's family are among the primary motivations. However, suicide attempts are rare. In a recent US survey[38] 57 out of 100 ALS patients said that they would ask for prescription of a lethal dose of medication if this were legal. However, only one patient said that he would actually make use of it in the next few weeks. The issue, therefore, seems to be more one of control than of acute suicidality. In our experience, the suicide rate among ALS patients lies below 1% (Neudert and Borasio, unpublished data). However, 20% of ALS patients in the Netherlands have been reported to die through active euthanasia or physician-assisted suicide.[39] In this context, it is important to remember that ALS patients may be hopeless without being depressed.[38] Assessing for hopelessness and instituting early nonpharmacologic interventions aimed at maintaining or restoring hope and a sense of meaning in life is likely to be the best way of preventing wishes for hastened death in ALS (see also Chapter 3b, Decision making, p. 43, Chapter 5, Psychosocial care, p. 143, and Chapter 6, Spiritual care, p. 169).

Sleep disturbances

These are usually secondary to other causes, the most common of which are:

* respiratory insufficiency with oxygen desaturation and dyspnea
* psychological disturbances, anxiety, depression, nightmares
* inability to change position during sleep due to weakness
* fasciculations and muscle cramps
* dysphagia with aspiration of saliva
* anxiety and/or depression.

The underlying reasons for sleep disturbances should be carefully sought for and treated accordingly. Sleep medication should be administered only after a careful search has excluded a treatable cause (Table 4d.6). It should be noted that frequent awakenings at night are amongst the earliest symptoms of nocturnal hypoventilation. However, most patients deny any subjective respiratory problems at this stage, since nocturnal oxygen desaturations in most cases do not give rise to a feeling of breathlessness after awakening. Assessment of nocturnal pO_2 is warranted in such cases — see Chapter 4a, Dyspnoea and respiratory symptoms, p. 64.

Table 4d.6 Sedatives dosage

Chloral hydrate	250–1000 mg
Diphenhydramine	50–100 mg
Zopiclone	7.5–15 mg
Flurazepam	15–30 mg
Diazepam	5–10 mg
(Beware of respiratory depression)	

Modified after Borasio and Voltz 1997.[1]

Constipation

Although the autonomic fibres innervating the intestine are not overtly affected by the disease, lack of exercise and reduced mobility can promote the development of constipation in ALS patients. The first step are dietary measures with food with high fibre content. Recipe books for ALS patients are available from several lay associations (see appendix for a list). Care should be taken to ensure adequate fluid intake, since dysphagia-induced dehydration may worsen constipation. The next step is a review of current medication, since muscle relaxants, sedatives and anticholinergics reduce bowel mobility. It should be kept in mind that constipation may become a major factor influencing quality of life, especially in the terminal stage. Mild laxative therapy should be prophylactically initiated in bed-ridden ALS patients and in all patients receiving opioids. If bowel pain arises, intestinal obstruction should be suspected and appropriate investigations performed.

Pain

Although there is no evidence that sensory nerves are affected other than subclinically by the disease process, pain does occur, primarily as the result of the changes imposed on the person as a result of the disease. The prevalence of pain in ALS is over 50% – 57% of patients on admission to a hospice were felt to have severe pain;[40] 64% of patients seen in a neurological service were found to have pain;[41] a survey of dying patients found a prevalence of 70% for patients dying at home and 70% for patients dying in the hospice;[42] 48% of patients had pain and 72% complained of "discomfort other than pain" in the last month of life.[43] The study of ALS patients attending a neurological clinic found that for men pain had been present for an average of 18 months[41] and at the hospice although 57% of the patients complained of pain only 12% had received a strong analgesic.[40] More recently in a group of over 1000 patients nearly 24% of patients reported pain and 75% had received medication to control pain.[44]

However, the pain is not always recognised by the professionals involved in the patient's care. A full multidisciplinary assessment is necessary to elucidate the cause of the pain. Careful examination and discussion with the patient and their carers, both family and professionals is essential. Families do seem to agree with the patient's assessments of pain and may be used in the assessment if communication is difficult.[45]

The pain may be due to:

- Muscle cramps, from muscle spasticity and fasciculations as a result of the degeneration of the neurones[1]
- Musculoskeletal pain – from the result of stress on bones and joints as the protective sheath of muscle has been lost due to muscle atrophy[1]
- Skin pressure pain, due to immobility. The patient may be unaware as to how severe the pain has become and talk only of 'discomfort'.[46]
- Other reasons (not ALS-related, e.g. concomitant diseases).

The treatment of the pain will depend on the causation. Cramps and spasticity are discussed above. For musculoskeletal pain, careful positioning and regular gentle movement may be helpful and support of flaccid arms, particularly in a car or wheelchair, should be considered.[6] Nonsteroidal anti-inflammatory medication can be useful, such as ibuprofen or naproxen. Intra-articular injections of local anaesthetic and/or steroids can be helpful if there is particular inflammatory pain in a single joint.[46]

As a patient becomes less mobile there is an increasing incidence of discomfort and pain. As the sensory nerves are unaffected the reduced movement leads to increasing skin pressure and this is perceived as pain. The treatment of this type of pain will need regular administration of analgesics, using the World Health Organization three step analgesic ladder[47] (Table 4d.7). The aim of the 'ladder' is to allow the progression from step to step, until pain control is achieved.

Initially patients may benefit from simple analgesics or weaker opioids, given on a regular basis and titrating to the patient's response. However many patients may require opioid analgesics to control the pain and discomfort. Many patients and their families fear the use of opioids, as do some medical and nursing practitioners, but the response to opioids can be dramatic and the quality of life can be greatly improved by their use. Experience in the care of cancer patients has shown that if analgesics are used correctly and carefully, titrating to the individual patient's pain, and given orally and regularly, pain can be controlled without appreciable side-effects,

Table 4d.7 WHO analgesic ladder

Step 1	Simple non-opioid analgesics, such as paracetamol, with/without adjuvants
Step 2	Step 1 drugs plus weak opioids, such as codeine based analgesics, with/without adjuvants
Step 3	Step 1 drugs plus strong opioids, such as morphine, with/without adjuvants

patients remaining lucid and alert.[48] The fear of shortening the patient's life through opioid medication is unfounded as shown by a recent meta-analysis.[49]

Morphine is the most widely used opioid – as morphine elixir or tablets every four hours, modified release tablets or capsules every 12 hours. Morphine can be used effectively and safely and a study within a hospice showed that the median maximum dose of morphine was 60 mg/24 hours and the mean duration of use was 95 days.[50] Other strong analgesics may be considered – such as oxycodone elixir, capsules or tablets or fentanyl trans-dermal patch, which can be particularly useful if swallowing is difficult and the pain syndrome is stable.

As well as the medication, it is important to consider the method of administration. If swallowing becomes difficult a liquid formulation may be necessary so that the medication can be given through the PEG. In the later stages of the disease process subcutaneous infusions, using a syringe driver, may be helpful, as this technique allows the administration of other medication, such as midazolam for stiffness or agitation and an anticholinergic, such as hyoscine, for secretions (see Chapter 9b, page 298).

The American Academy of Neurology Practice Parameters suggested that opioids be used and the WHO pain management recommendations should be the standard for the administration of analgesics.[51] However there has been little progress in the development of ALS specific protocols or further research into ALS related pain.[52] These are areas for further development.

Pain can come to dominate the patient's life, and that of the family and carers. The assessment and treatment of pain can have an enormous effect on the patient's quality of life and allow them to enjoy the company of their family and friends.

Less common symptoms

Gastroesophageal reflux disease (GERD) may occur in ALS due to diaphragmatic weakness involving the lower esophageal sphincter. Particular care is needed when starting a patient on PEG because of possible overfeeding which may lead to GERD and even aspiration. Treatment includes peristaltic agents (e.g., metoclopramide, cisapride) and antacids.

Dependent edema of the hands and feet occurs in weak limbs because of reduced muscle pump activity. Limb elevation, physiotherapy and compression hose are helpful. Diuretics may also be helpful, but may cause problems due to urinary frequency. If pain develops or swelling persists despite prolonged elevation, a deep venous thrombosis should be ruled out.

Urinary urgency and frequency in the absence of urinary tract infections can be due to spasticity of the bladder and responds favorably to oxybutinin (5 mg qd-tid).

Jaw quivering or clenching may develop in patients with pseudobulbar involvement in response to nox ious stimuli such as cold, anxiety or pain, and may be relieved by benzodiazepines (e.g., lorazepam sl or clonazepam).[53]

Laryngospasm (a sudden reflectory closure of the vocal chords) can cause panic due to a sensation of choking. Several types of stimuli (e.g., emotions, strong flavours or smells, cold air, fluid aspiration, gastroesophageal reflux) may provoke this symptom, which usually resolves spontaneously within a few seconds. Repeated swallowing while breathing through the nose can accelerate resolution.

Nasal congestion in bulbar patients with a weakening of the nasopharynx muscles can be helped by elevating the nasal bridge with nasal tape and application of topical decongestants.

Conclusion

Practice of symptomatic therapy in ALS varies widely between and even within countries. First attempts at setting standards have been made and are currently under revision,[51] but are still largely based on circumstantial evidence. Well-designed prospective studies are needed to provide an evidence-based foundation for the optimal palliation of symptoms in ALS.

References

1. **Borasio G. D., Voltz R.** (1997) Palliative care in amyotrophic lateral sclerosis. *Journal of Neurology* 244 (Suppl. 4): S11–S17.

2. **Prather I. D., Brown D. E., North P., Wilson J. R.** (1995) Clenbuterol: a substitute for anabolic steroids? *Medicine and Science in Sports and Exercise* 27: 1118–21.

3. **Klivenyi P., Ferrante R. J., Matthews R. T., Bogdanov M. B., Klein A. M., Andreassen O. A.** *et al.* (1999) Neuroprotective effects of creatine in a transgenic animal model of amyotrophic lateral sclerosis. *Nature Medicine* 5: 347–50.

4. **Shefner J. M., Cudkowicz M. E., Schoenfeld D.** *et al.* (2004) A clinical trial of creatine in ALS. *Neurology* 63: 1656–61.

5. **Ashworth N. L., Satkunam L. E., Deforge D.** (2006) Treatment for spasticity in amyotrophic lateral sclerosis/motor neuron disease. *Cochrane Database Syst Rev* (1): CD004156.

6. **O'Gorman B., Oliver D., Nottle C., Prisley S.** (2004) Disorders of nerve I: Motor neurone disease. In Stokes M. (ed) *Physical Management in Neurological Rehabilitation*, 2nd edn., pp. 233–251. Edinburgh: Elsevier Mosby.

7. **Marquardt G., Seifert V.** (2002) Use of intrathecal baclofen for treatment of spasticity in amyotrophic lateral sclerosis. *J Neurol Neurosurg Psychiatry* 72: 275–6.

8. Snow B. J., Tsui J. K., Bhatt M. H., Varelas M., Hashimoto S. A., Calne D. B. (1990) Treatment of spasticity with botulinum toxin: a double-blind study. *Annals of Neurology* 28: 512–15.

9. Restivo D. A., Lanza S., Marchese-Ragona R., Palmeri A. (2002) Improvement of masseter spasticity by botulinum toxin facilitates PEG placement in amyotrophic lateral sclerosis. *Gastroenterology* 123: 1749–50.

10. Amtmann D., Weydt P., Johnson K. L., Jensen M. P., Carter G. T. (2004) Survey of cannabis use in patients with amyotrophic lateral sclerosis. *Am J Hosp Palliat Care* 21: 95–104.

11. Raischl J., Hirsch B., Bausewein C., Borasio G. D. (1998) Hospice care for ALS patients in Germany: the Munich experience. Presentation at the 9th International Symposium on ALS/MND, Munich.

12. Gallagher J. P. (1989) Pathologic laughter and crying in ALS: A search for their origin. *Acta Neurologica Scandinavica* 80: 114–17.

13. Schiffer R. B., Herndon R. M., Rudick R. A. (1985) Treatment of pathologic laughing and weeping with amitriptyline. *New England Journal of Medicine* 312: 1480–2.

14. Caroscio J. T., Cohen J. A., Gudesblatt M. (1985) Amitriptyline in amyotrophic lateral sclerosis. *New England Journal of Medicine* 313: 1478.

15. Schiffer R. B., Cash J., Hernon R. M. (1983) Treatment of emotional lability with low-dosage tricyclic antidepressants. *Psychosomatics* 24: 1094–6.

16. Poeck K. (1996) Pathologisches Lachen und Weinen bei bulbärer myatrophischer Lateralsklerose. *Deutsche medizinische Wochenschrift* 94: 310–14.

17. McCullagh S., Moore M., Gawel M., Feinstein A. (1999) Pathological laughing and crying in amyotrophic lateral sclerosis: an association with prefrontal cognitive dysfunction. *J Neurol Sci* 169: 43–8.

18. Iannaccone S., Ferini-Strambi L. (1996) Pharmacologic treatment of emotional lability. *Clinical Neuropharmacology* 19: 532–5.

19. Udaka F., Yamao S., Nagata H., Nakamura S., Kameyama M. (1984) Pathologic laughing and crying treated with levodopa. *Archives of Neurology* 41: 1095–6.

20. Sieb J. P., Jerusalem F., Fresmann J. (1987) Symptomatische Therapie bei amyotrophischer Lateralsklerose. *Deutsche medizinische Wochenschrift* 112: 769–72.

21. Norris F. H., Smith R. A., Denis E. H. (1985) Motor neurone disease: towards better care. *BMJ* 291: 259–62.

22. Brooks B. R., Thisted R. A., Appel S. H. *et al.* (2004) Treatment of pseudobulbar affect in ALS with dextromethorphan/quinidine: a randomized trial. *Neurology* 63: 1364–70.

23. Camp-Bruno J. A., Winsberg B. G., Green-Parsons A. R., Abrams J. P. (1989) Efficacy of benztropine therapy for drooling. *Developmental Medicine and Child Neurology* 31: 309–19.

24. Reddihough D., Johnson H., Staples M., Hudson I., Exarchos H. (1990) Use of trihexyphenidyl hydrocholride to control drooling of children with cerebral palsy. *Developmental Medicine and Child Neurology* 32: 985–9.

25. Blasco P. A., Stansbury J. C. K. (1996) Glycopyrrolate treatment of chronic drooling. *Archives of Pediatrics and Adolescent Medicine* 150: 932–5.

26. Stern L. M. (1997) Preliminary study of glycopyrrolate in the management of drooling. *Journal of Paediatrics and Child Health* 33: 52–4.

27. Brodtkorb E., Wyzocka-Bakowska M. M., Lillevold P. E., Sandvik L., Saunte C., Hestnes A. (1988) Transdermal scopolamine in drooling. *Journal of Mental Deficiency Research* **32**: 233–7.

28. Lewis D. W., Fontana C., Mehallick L. K., Everett Y. (1994) Transdermal scopolamine for reductions in drooling in developmentally delayed children. *Developmental Medicine and Child Neurology* **36**: 484–6.

29. Simmons Z. (2005) Management strategies for patients with amyotrophic lateral sclerosis from diagnosis through death. *Neurologist* **11**: 257–70.

30. Lipp A., Trottenberg T., Schink T. *et al.* (2003) A randomized trial of botulinum toxin A for treatment of drooling. *Neurology* **61**: 1279–81.

31. Harriman M., Morrison M., Hay J. *et al.* (2001) Use of radiotherapy for control of sialorrhea in patients with amyotrophic lateral sclerosis. *J Otolaryngol* **30**: 242–5.

32. Stalpers L. J. A., Moser E. C. (2002) Results of radiotherapy for drooling in amyotrophic lateral sclerosis. *Neurology* **58**: 1308.

33. Newall A. R., Orser R., Hunt M. (1996) The control of oral secretions in bulbar ALS/MND. *Journal of Neurological Sciences* **139** (Suppl.): 43–4.

34. Bach J. R. (1993) Mechanical insufflation-exsufflation: Comparison of peak expiratory flows with manually assisted and unassisted coughing techniques. *Chest* **104**: 1553–62.

35. Bach J. R., Smith W. H., Michaels J., Saporito L. S., Alba A. S. *et al.* (1993) Airway secretion clearance by mechanical exsufflation for postpoliomyelitis ventilator assisted individuals. *Archives of Physical Medicine and Rehabilitation* **74**: 170–77.

36. Foulsom M. (1999) Secretion management in motor neurone disease. Tenth International Symposium on ALS/MND, Vancouver.

37. McDonald E. R., Wiedenfeld S. A., Hillel A., Carpenter C. L., Walter R. A. (1994) Survival in amyotrophic lateral sclerosis: the role of psychological factors. *Archives of Neurology* **51**: 17–23.

38. Ganzini L., JohnstonW. S., McFarland B. H., Tolle S. W., Lee M. A. (1998) Attitudes of patients with amyotrophic lateral sclerosis and their care givers toward assisted suicide. *New England Journal of Medicine* **339**: 967–73.

39. Veldink J. H., Wokke J. H., van der Wal G., Vianney de Jong J. M., van den Berg L. H. (2002) Euthanasia and physician-assisted suicide among patients with amyotrophic lateral sclerosis in the Netherlands. *New England Journal of Medicine* **346**: 1638–44.

40. O'Brien T., Kelly M., Saunders C. (1992) Motor neurone disease: a hospice perspective. *BMJ* **304**: 471–3.

41. Newrick P. G., Langton-Hewer R. (1985) Pain in motor neurone disease. *Journal of Neurology, Neurosurgery and Pyschiatry* **48**: 838–40.

42. Oliver D. (1996) The quality of care and symptom control – the effects on the terminal phase of ALS/MND. *Journal of Neurological Sciences* **139** (Suppl.): 134–6.

43. Ganzini L., Johnston W. S., Silveira M. J. (2002) The final month of life in patients with ALS. *Neurology* **59**: 428–31.

44. Mandler R. N., Anderson F. A., Miller R. G. *et al.* (2001) The ALS Patient Care database: insights into end-of-life care. *Amyotroph Lateral Scler Other Motor Neuron Disord* **2**: 203–8.

45. Adelman E. E., Albert S. M., Rabkin J. D. *et al.* (2004) Disparities in perceptions of distress and burden in ALS patients and family care givers. *Neurology* **62**: 1766–70.

46. **Oliver D.** (1994) *Motor Neurone Disease.* London: Royal College of General Practitioners.

47. **World Health Organization** (1990) *Cancer Pain Relief and Palliative Care.* Report of a WHO Expert Committee, Geneva: World Health Organization.

48. **Twycross R.** (1994) *Pain Relief in Advanced Cancer,* pp. 255–76 and pp. 333–47. Edinburgh: Churchill Livingstone.

49. **Sykes N., Thorns A.** (2003) The use of opioids and sedatives at the end of life. *Lancet Oncol* **4**: 312–18.

50. **Oliver D.** (1998) Opioid medication in the palliative care of motor neurone disease. *Palliative Medicine* **12**: 113–15.

51. **Miller R. G., Rosenberg J. A., Gelinas D. F., Mitsumoto H., Newman, D., Sufit R.** (1999) Practice Parameter: The care of the patient with amyotrophic lateral sclerosis (an evidence-based review): report of the Quality Standards Subcommittee of the American Academy of Neurology: ALS Practice Parameters Task Force. *Neurology* **52**: 1311–23.

52. **Mitsumoto H., Bromberg M., Johnston W.** *et al.* (2005) Promoting excellence in end-of-life care. *Amyotroph Lateral Scler Other Motor Neuron Disord* **6**: 145–54.

53. **Gelinas D., Miller R. G.** (2000) A treatable disease: a guide to the management of amyotrophic lateral sclerosis. In Brown R. H. Jr, Meininger V., Swash M. (eds) *Amyotrophic Lateral Sclerosis,* pp. 405–21. London: Martin Dunitz.

Chapter 5

Psychosocial care

Donal Gallagher and Barbara Monroe

Summary

Psychosocial care is the responsibility of everyone working with those affected by ALS. It includes the giving of bad news, respecting and developing coping strategies, acknowledging fears and maintaining hope. The assessment and continuing review of psychosocial concerns must recognize the particular issues faced by carers and children living with ALS. Good psychosocial care also recognizes the challenges for the professionals involved.

Case history

'On Christmas day I drove my car for the last time, the fingers of my left hand having become too weak to turn the ignition key. Ros had to cut up my Christmas meal although I fed myself. Eleanor and I pulled three crackers together; she insisted that I wore my blue paper hat and read aloud the old jokes from all the crackers.'

Christmas, a year later... 'I asked to be wheeled into the kitchen so that I could sit at the table with the family. Ros fed me and Eleanor pulled my cracker.'

Stephen Pegg's own words[1] provide a poignant example of how amyotrophic lateral sclerosis (ALS) affects everyday life and how its often relentless progression is vividly measurable. In addition, ALS impacts on the patient's roles and relationships with family and friends. For all concerned the experience is not just physical; the 'total pain' concept[2] which encompasses physical, emotional, social and spiritual elements, acknowledges the link between symptoms and psychological distress. A patient's experience of illness is a direct product of the interaction between all aspects of life. Worries about whether there will be enough money for shopping or how children are being affected have a bearing on total pain and the meaning of illness.[3]

Psychosocial care is a core component of good palliative care, and underpins the practice of all professionals and volunteers. At its heart is the principle of working with the patient, family and friends as the unit of care:

Psychosocial care is concerned with the psychological and emotional well-being of the patient and their family/carers, including issues of self-esteem, insight into and adaptation to the illness and its consequences, communication, social functioning and relationships.[4]

Working with the emotional, social and spiritual elements of an individual or family should not be apportioned to one professional.[5] A patient will choose who they talk to about these issues – so it may be with a speech therapist that they voice concerns about choking to death. A specialism of psychosocial care does exist and is most commonly provided by social workers, counsellors and psychologists. Each brings their expertise and ways of working, such as counselling (individuals, couples), family therapy, group work, direct interventions with children and bereavement care. Such professionals are a fundamental element of any palliative care team: where a team does not exist, access to a specialist in psychosocial care is important. Evidence supports the benefit of psychosocial interventions in cancer.[6–8] A diagnosis of ALS does not necessarily lead to depression. For those who do experience this Rabkin et al.[9] have shown these patients are more interested in life ending earlier, and whilst this does not manifest itself as increased interest in assisted suicide, depression predicts shorter survival time in ALS.[10] Responding to the psychosocial needs of patients, their families and carers influences their quality of life and may affect the quantity of life for some.

The practice of psychosocial care is founded on a secure base of knowledge, skills and values. These help in the initial assessment of the patient and family, which takes into account their experiences and capacity for change. Oliviere et al.[11] list the skills essential for carers, health professionals and volunteers (p. 7). Workers should respect the individuality of the patient and those connected with them: this is recognized by placing them at the centre of the care, offering realistic choices and being non-judgemental. Sheldon[12] discusses four key concepts in psychosocial palliative care: attachment, loss, meaning and equity. An understanding of these is essential to the practice of any palliative care professional: they are inextricably linked to much of this chapter. Some of the issues facing people affected by ALS will also be encountered in cancer or a chronic illness, such as Parkinson's disease, and distinguishing areas of emphasis specific to ALS psychosocial care is important. Naturally, the extent to which individuals and their families experience these will vary. Their inclusion here is intended to raise the awareness of professionals and volunteers and consequently improve the quality of psychosocial care.

Living with ALS

Breaking bad news

The difficulties in giving the diagnosis of ALS or other bad news, should not be minimized. Doctors may feel helpless where the role of healer is missing and feelings of sadness can be evoked in both the recipient and giver of the news. Dealing with other reactions, such as anger and despair, also cause concern. Faced with this there may be a tendency to give false reassurance, likened to a 'conspiracy of speech',[13] or use closed instead of open questions. There are techniques that can reduce the trauma for the patient, other supporters present and the doctor:

- Give the patient the choice of attending with someone. Ensure the location is private and quiet. Allow enough time for the appointment.

- Find out what the patient already knows about their condition to avoid incorrect assumptions. Do not assume the patient wants to know everything.

- Once the wish for further information is established, it can be given in a stepwise manner[14] with a 'warning shot' preparing the patient and those with them for the news. A clear diagnostic label can be helpful.[15]

- Provide clear honest information about the disease and its consequences, but beware of giving too much information at once. Write down information or have it taped if appropriate.[16]

- Check what has been understood.

- Communicate sensitively by being aware of your own body language. Allow pauses and silences in the discussion so information can sink in and emotions expressed.

- Establish what the concerns are and listen carefully to questions. Think about exploring the meaning behind a particular question.

- Further exploration of the emotional impact of the diagnosis can be done by a specialist member of staff, such as a social worker, either straight away or a few days later in the patient's home.[17] This approach acknowledges that the issue of breaking bad news is not a one-off affair.

◆ At the end of the meeting, clear direction should be provided about sources of further information and support. The patient should also understand what will happen next in their medical care, thus avoiding the impression that nothing can be done.

Assessing and responding to behaviour and feelings keeps the situation patient-focused and reinforces the importance of emotional care at an early stage. It gives a clear message that having and talking about feelings is normal and that all staff share the responsibility for this. This in turn has implications for professional training in communication skills.

Assessment

One of the challenges of psychosocial care is to recognize the interplay of the experience for the patient and those around them whilst also seeing each individual in the situation as just that – an individual. Each brings their own past, values, choices and feelings. No assumptions should be made about how each person will perceive or be affected by the illness based on visual clues, such as skin colour, age or gender. Comparisons should not be made between patients or families in apparently similar circumstances. As Earll et al.[18] conclude: 'it is important that professionals do not assume either that they can anticipate the patient's view of their condition, or that the medical perspective is the one adopted by patients'. The lack of clarity in attempts to determine a psychological profile of the ALS patient supports the individualized approach which is sensitive to the culture of the patient, family and community.[19–23] Consideration of the patient's competency is also required during assessment, given the prevalence of cognitive change in ALS.[24]

During assessment the practitioner creates a partnership with the patient and other individuals involved. It can touch on sensitive issues, which raise ethical concerns requiring careful moral scrutiny.[25] This demands that professionals explain the reasons for their inquiries, establish consent and check on it at intervals as the assessment progresses. Saying: 'If there is something you would rather not discuss, please let me know', is a clear way of 'handing back as much control as possible to the person whose body is out of control';[11] this is equally applicable to others being assessed. Establishing a partnership is also helped by discussing confidentiality and with whom information can be shared. This is crucial when working as part of a team.

Assessments vary in their formality. Whatever format is used, an initial assessment, which may not be completed in one visit, will identify those individuals and families at particular risk who will benefit from more support. Such an assessment will need to explore:

- An understanding of the individual patient.
- The effect of the illness on family roles and relationships.
- Personal histories of family members.
- Family life-cycle issues, e.g. births, children leaving home, marriages, retirement.
- Previous crises, how they were handled and additional concurrent crises.
- Other vulnerable individuals in the family, for example someone with learning difficulties
- The family's physical and social resources.

Numerous studies[26–29] stress the importance of not accepting patients or family members as proxies for one another's opinions and experiences.

Case history

Sally, aged 37, and her husband, Peter, described a stormy and sometimes physically aggressive relationship prior to her diagnosis with ALS. Sally only revealed the true extent of her distress when away from Peter and when directly asked about intimacy: 'Has your illness changed the ways you get close to your partner?' 'My husband is just raping me. Using my body for his needs, not mine.' She said that she felt increasingly frightened of him as she became more disabled. She eventually chose inpatient care.

Agreeing which problems can be changed and what the plan is to enable change keeps control firmly with the patient. Any plan must be based on realistic resources to support it and needs to be re-evaluated as the condition and circumstances alter. For example, Albert and colleagues[30] note the capacity of patients to express preferences for life-extending technologies, but caution that these may change over time and that education is required throughout the illness.

For some people with ALS who lose the ability to communicate verbally, alternative ways of gaining their thoughts and feelings must be considered. First, the patient and family should work with a system or aid with which they feel familiar and comfortable (e.g. Lightwriter). Discussing whether tiredness may affect the length of visits determines how focused assessments need to be and whether future visits should be planned. In these circumstances, a predominance of closed questions which draw on an awareness of the patient's situation can be helpful: 'Other people I have met with ALS have worried about becoming more dependent upon their family. Is this something you have thought about?' Whilst this type of question appears leading, the physical needs and limitations of the patient must be considered. If the assessor shows sensitivity to this issue, the patient is more likely to feel a partner in the process. If the patient wants to give a fuller answer, they must be allowed the time necessary, rather than the professional anticipating what the patient is trying to communicate after a few words on the Lightwriter.

Assessment is not just a means to an end. In work where time and contacts may be limited, the assessment is an intervention in its own right: 'building up a therapeutic relationship with the ill person and family, engaging them in a helping process, allowing them to feel safe and comfortable, communicating interest and respect, carving out time to allow their anxieties to surface'.[11]

Hope

Attempts have been made at defining hope: Buckley and Herth[31] summarize it as 'an inner power or strength that can enrich lives and enable individuals to look beyond their pain, suffering and turmoil'. What is the relevance of such a concept to someone given a diagnosis of ALS with a limited life expectancy? The presence and experience of hope will depend in part upon the way in which information about the diagnosis, prognosis and treatment is given. If it is understood that the future will be dramatically different from that envisaged before the diagnosis, then the way hope is viewed will also be affected. For many with ALS the shock of the diagnosis is compounded by the relentless progression of the condition with one loss following another: this can easily leave them feeling helpless and hopeless. Maintaining hope even under these conditions is evident, but may be different from, for example, someone undergoing chemotherapy. Hope is often attached to treatment, whether curative or palliative . Even now, with treatment regimes for MND in their infancy, individuals will readily agree to new medication or take part in trials, some in the hope of a better future for themselves but others selflessly to promote a better future for those diagnosed later.

Kim[32] suggests that 'an individual's level of hope determines whether human beings live or die'. Identifying what hope means to them, what helps maintain their hope, what causes them to lose hope and how it changes during an illness is important in psychosocial care. Palliative care professionals and volunteers can play their part alongside the patient's family and friends in fostering hope through categories identified by Buckley and Herth.[31] Maintaining relationships with children, considering spiritual issues – see Chapter 6 – and supporting independence for as long as possible are some areas to focus on, even as death approaches. Working on a life review with the patient[33] not only gives the opportunity to recall the highlights of their life but may also be done with fun and humour, the benefit of which others have commented on.[34] Others may describe their experience in terms of suffering: there are parallels between this multidimensional concept[35] and the loss of hope for people with ALS.[36] Attempts to understand how terminally ill people suffer presents challenges and opportunities. Whilst suffering is more complex than purely physical pain, good symptom management is essential in combating suffering.[36,37] It is equally clear that the wider understanding of and engagement with suffering lies beyond medicalization.[38] This is essential if the extent and language of suffering and hope is to be fully comprehended. Only then will professionals develop the competencies to work with them effectively.[39,40]

Case history

Mary was diagnosed with ALS and later asked how she saw hope in her situation. She said she had been told she would live between three and five years. Her hope was in the belief that she would live five rather than three years.

Loss

Psychosocial interventions may assist the person with ALS to deal with the many losses they encounter. Such losses occur at different levels of visibility and different stages of the disease. At diagnosis, the patient and family may grieve for the future they had planned and expected. It will be difficult to grieve for subsequent losses, as they overlap. We often have the human capacity to adapt to loss and cope with the concomitant stress. This usual adaptive model, however, does not allow for a spiralling scenario in which a period of adjustment and equilibrium is interrupted by the next loss. ALS seems set apart from other chronic illnesses in this respect.[41] The reformation of self for a burns survivor[42] following enormous losses is possible during rehabilitation. Those with ALS, who experience irreversible and unremitting physical losses, including breathing difficulties, will not necessarily view this as affecting their quality of life[43,44] though there is an apparent association with depression.[45] The meaning of an apparent loss may have other underlying and devaluing implications; losing a job can affect status, role in the family and self-esteem. The full implications will probably emerge only later, by which time the patient may have had to face loss of mobility or communication. If willing, they may find it helpful to talk about the numerous losses with an outsider, given permission to mourn the changes and express powerful emotions.

Control and choice

Issues of loss and control are linked. Feelings of being out of control may predate the diagnosis: testing, misdiagnosis and increasing problems may produce lack of faith in medical professionals. Hearing about the history of the illness at the initial assessment acknowledges that the way a patient feels today may stem from an unresolved or unspoken past event. Unobtrusive questioning, precise summarizing along with genuine interest in the feelings about the events, demonstrate tangible concern. Returning a sense of control to the patient and family is a hallmark of good psychosocial care. Though ALS patients are no more or less likely to feel an internal sense of control,[20] those who do believe in chance or the power of others over their health are more likely to feel hopeless.[46] The extent to which they feel in control of their life will vary from person to person and probably from day to day. ALS does not deprive patients of their ability to convert their early treatment preferences into real choices.[30] Similarly, professional involvement need not leave the patient, family and carers feeling disempowered if it includes those willing to partici-pate in decision-making. Working with issues of the patient's and family's choosing maximizes their strengths, and shifts the locus of control from external to internal. A patient-held record is a positive and visible way of creating this shift and enhancing communication between professionals.[47]

Providing adequate and timely information, suggesting separate means for patients and their families to become knowledgeable (e.g. helplines, books/ leaflets, self-help groups) means realistic and informed choices can be made. Making a decision to enter a hospice or another establishment either for respite care, symptom control or terminal care will often evoke powerful conflicting feelings in an individual whilst simultaneously creating differences of opinion between the patient and family. Planning ahead wherever possible and giving families and individuals the support (alone and together) and time they need to make a mutually agreeable decision is vital. A visit before admission may help dispel myths or fantasies about an institution and the care it offers. Utilizing those parts of the home care regime that can be transferred whilst acknowledging the distinct difference between the two locations (e.g. ward routines, health and safety requirements) will establish a care contract after admission based on mutual knowledge and agreement. Individuality is preserved when patients can continue to inform and review their care plan. Staff must make efforts to preserve patient dignity and be flexible in their practice so that individual identity and needs are not sub-merged in standardized protocols. Those family members who want to be involved in care during the stay should be included in discussions; this will facilitate a transfer of skills and ways of working between the two locations and help alleviate any guilt feelings the relative or carer may have.

Fears of death and dying

At all stages, but especially as death approaches, the person with ALS may wish to discuss both the process of dying and death itself. It is important to indicate a willingness to discuss difficult topics, but not to press the point with those who are reluctant. Appropriate questions may both offer prompts and legitimize discussion: 'Do you ever find yourself thinking about the future and how things will go?' Anticipation of future losses can be as worrying for patients and carers as current ones.[48,49] Breathlessness, pain, incontinence and dying by choking may be some concerns. Many will welcome information about how deterioration will be recognized and what symptoms mean in terms of illness progression and survival. They will value information about physical aids and adaptations, help in the home and medications for symptoms. Written information[50,51] may be helpful, but reassurance is vital as fears are often greater than reality: for example, only one patient out of over 200 at St Christopher's Hospice died in a choking attack.[52]

Case history

As 47-year-old Susan's condition deteriorated, she became more panicky, spending long periods sobbing uncontrollably. She was helped by discussing her fears. She wanted to die but was frightened by the manner and timing of her death. She was relieved to know that 'it probably won't be much longer now', to be told that death usually followed the weakening of the respiratory system and that she would probably gradually lapse into unconsciousness and peacefully stop breathing. She was also told what medication would help if things should be more difficult.

Fears about the future may lead some to conclude their new world is unbearable and judge an early death to be preferable.[53] Cues can be provided: 'Does your situation ever make you feel like it's not worth going on?' A positive response requires serious exploration of the issue and any fear, such as dependency.[54] Drawing up an advance directive (whether legally enforceable or not) may help with a sense of control. Whatever the legal position about euthanasia, good palliative care will inform and expand patients' options. However, Sheldon reminds us, it is important

[that] assurances are given that despite any disagreements about this issue, the team will continue to offer their skill and experience and will strive to respect the patient's wish to remain in control in all other areas, provided these do not infringe the autonomy of others.[12]

Careful risk assessment, incorporating multidisciplinary working, must differentiate between those whose wish to die is rational and those suffering from mental ill health. The extent to which clinical depression exists in ALS is disputed (see Goldstein and Leigh[45] for summary). Talking about the future is a sensitive matter, but a brave professional can provide patients and their families with the opportunity to discuss issues such as preparing a will, future care of children and options about the desired place of death.

Coping strategies

The complexity of losses, including plans, privacy, skills and changed relationships, all place great stress on someone with ALS and those close to them. It is more surprising that 'in the face of an incurable disabling disease...the majority of people' are 'neither depressed nor even in serious psychological difficulty'.[18] To cope with the demands patients, family members and carers adopt, often unconsciously, strategies to make the situation bearable. These will change depending on the difficulties encountered and their current perception of their illness and disability.[55] A patient may use different coping strategies from his family or carers.[56] The way individuals deal with stressful events will partly be determined by their past and the extent to which threats have been successfully combated before. Horta[57] remarks that 'neither the initial nor the ongoing emotional reaction of patients to ALS is merely a "here and now" response' and professionals can use the assessment in part at least to discover an individual's past coping abilities. This process may help them and the worker to recognize their strengths or alternatively their need for support.

The use of denial is common in situations in which a person's known world and integrity are threatened. It replaces the reality of the diagnosis and its implications with an alternative reality. It is a valid and perhaps necessary coping mechanism when adjusting to loss (see Task 1 in Worden[58]); Horta summarizes that 'denial is a protective and primarily unconscious method of retaining psychological equilibrium'.[57] One daughter of a person with ALS remarked that 'denial...is a rather convenient and tidy way to control the amount of reality to be dealt with at any one time'.[59] Putting pressure on someone resistant to a different perception of the illness may reinforce the denial, although Hogg et al.[60] showed it to be predictive of psychological ill health. Having regard for the patient's family and carers is essential in detecting clashes of coping styles and needs.[61] Scenarios in which a patient talks of getting better and going back to work whilst his partner wants to plan for a different future, can cause tremendous tension and resentment. There may be limits to an outsider establishing consensus between the two; equal respect for each individual's position is the starting point. Thereafter, providing opportunities for the individuals, alone and together, to discuss the other's views may help maintain a relationship when they need one another most.

People who use denial present dilemmas for everyone (non-professional and professional alike), particularly as those who rely upon it may be more physically impaired.[60] Many use it as a short or medium-term measure along with a need to take one day at a time to reframe their world and future. This allows a patient to control their life and emotions by no longer defining it in terms of pre-ALS life but rather finding meaning and purpose in the present.[34] One patient talked of feeling more positive as a result of a support group for ALS patients. He realized that he was not 'as bad off' as other patients. Peer group support may also afford exchange of helpful ideas between patients and families.

People with ALS can be helped by active problem-solving for themselves, for instance by alternative or complementary therapies.[18] 'Intellectual stimulation'[34] can be positively affected by professionals who enable patients to access information. As a patient's condition deteriorates, page-turners or access to the Internet can maintain a knowledge base and contact with other ALS patients through online discussion groups. In contrast to the earlier example, one woman with ALS was horrified at the prospect of being in a room with other people with ALS whose greater degree of disability and dependence would cruelly predict her future. This different perception of the usefulness of a particular activity underlines the point that individuals will select, often unwittingly, ways that help them to carry on living with stability. O'Brien[62] revealed how this control over information can be sabotaged by unsolicited sources such as the media. Psychosocial care can involve expanding an individual's coping repertoire[63] by suggesting ways that have helped others cope. Recognizing the value of normality, and taking time off from the disease, has parallels with Stroebe's Dual Process Model of Coping.[64] It can be reflected in a practitioner's intervention by not just concentrating on the disease and its consequences but also showing genuine interest in whatever else the person wants to talk about. The sensitive use of humour with patients not only conveys warmth and humanity but mirrors how some people with ALS maintain personal relationships and reframe terrifying prospects.[34]

Family, carers and friends

All patients have a family, whether they live alone, are a sole survivor or part of a large intergenerational group. The family is a complex system that changes over time, and has a past and a future that exerts pressures on the present. Patients will also connect to other networks containing significant relationships, some of which may be more important than biological links. The entire patient network exists within a social and cultural context that helps define the possibilities for the individual and their family.[68] Cultural expectations about the roles, rights and responsibilities of individual family members also have an impact.[12,41,65]

Help for the family can get lost in anxiety for the patient. Family life will deteriorate along with that of the patient, but patient and family members have different needs at different times, require different supports and may have conflicting agendas.[45,59] Care for the family has an important preventive health component. Family members will live on into a future shaped by their experience of the patient's illness and death. With help they can emerge strengthened into a changed but safe family future. Kissane and Bloch's[66] research on families affected by cancer emphasizes the importance of family functioning during the illness to adaptive grief outcome and the pivotal importance of psychosocial care.

Carers' needs

Carers face conflicting demands, for example, juggling employment and children with the demands of physical caregiving. They also receive bewildering advice from friends, family and professionals and may pay a price for support received in invasion of privacy and potential criticism.[67,68] Changes in family structure may also add to the burden; e.g. divorce, split and reconstituted families, geographic distance. Practical support is a priority.[69] Many families strugglie with rapid frightening changes in the physical needs and capacities of the ill person and physical caring tasks. They need knowledge of what is available, how to obtain it and advocacy to obtain it in time. Sykes et al.'s[70] study sadly demonstrated how often practical supports arrived too late.

Carers require:

- ◆ Adequate nursing support.
- ◆ Confident, committed family doctors.
- ◆ Good symptom control for the patient.
- ◆ Coordinated care that is individual and flexibly delivered.
- ◆ Access to specialist care.
- ◆ Practical help: household tasks, personal care, equipment.
- ◆ Respite care as an inpatient or a home sitting service.
- ◆ Knowledge about the illness and training in skills to enhance patient comfort.

- Financial support.
- Advice and information on services available and help to secure them.
- Emotional support directed specifically at the carer.[71–73]

Individual time for carers needs to be negotiated at the start of the relationship so that it is part of the contract rather than offered when difficulties arise, when it may be harder for the carer or patient to accept separate meetings without suspicion and guilt. Rabkin and colleagues[9] demonstrated high concordance between patient and caregiver distress and suggested that attention to the mental health needs of caregivers may alleviate patient distress. As Payne[74] notes, it is important to balance accounts of carer burden[44] with the positive aspects and rewards of caring.

What helps patients and their families?

- Ensuring clear adequate information and an opportunity for questions.
- Acknowledging emotional pain and anxieties and facilitating their expression.
- Permission to grieve the person who was.
- Reassurance about powerful unfamiliar feelings.
- Timely interventions that anticipate fears and problems. Generalization can help here: 'Many families tell us . . . What is it like for you?'
- Offering acceptable frameworks for why people are behaving as they are.
- Confirming coping and acknowledging positive aspects of caring.
- Helping the family decide what is important and giving them the confidence and/or resource to act upon it.
- Addressing uncertainty and the distress it causes. Simple open questions that acknowledge feelings help: 'What is the worst thing at the moment? Who are you most worried about?'
- Affirming individual needs and offering help in ways acceptable to the individual.

Case history

Gill had ALS and showed evidence of cognitive impairment. Her husband found it difficult to accept her deterioration. He was angry about her diminished quality of life. 'I don't believe in God. How can this be allowed?' He needed to control his contact with professionals and expressed himself best in casual meetings with staff on the stairs or at meal times, preferring this to formal talking time. 'I must keep the shreds of my dignity. I don't want to break down and expose myself.'

Special pressures occur in families where the patient has lived with ALS for over five years (McDonald 1994).[28] The preliminary findings by the Northern Regional Care Advisers of the MND Association UK in 1999 indicate that most carers had been told the prognosis was relatively short. This led to them giving up everything. When the illness stretched into five or more years they felt enormous guilt about being unable to cope. Equally the patient felt in some cases that they had wasted the life of their partner.

Family meetings can anticipate and address difficult decisions and conflict.[75] Some guidelines are:

- Effective preparation: who should attend, where should it be held, potential objectives.

- Decide what should be said to begin. Explain the rules, for example the right to speak for yourself and give some idea of the time frame.

- Speak in language that all can understand and check this frequently.

- Be neutral and find out how everyone defines the problem. All need to feel that the professional understands their viewpoint.

- Define problems in a positive form. 'You love your children and you want to protect them.'

- Anticipate and acknowledge differences and conflicts. Try to find similarities: 'You are both feeling lonely and resentful.' Help people negotiate and compromise, which may mean helping them retreat from fixed positions.

- Be realistic and encourage focus on concrete, specific, achievable goals.

- Check agreements, rehearse potential difficulties and summarize clearly.

- End the interview in a safe place; refer to a lighter topic, use humour etc.

- Do not do all the work. Remember the aim is to help the family solve the problem in a way they feel comfortable with, not to sort it all out for them.

Intimacy and sexuality

Individuals within a relationship experience ALS very differently. In McDonald's survey,[28] spouses were more lonely than patients and often experienced psychological or spiritual distress at different stages of the illness. Ginsberg[76] discusses how anger and frustration at loss of independence causes demanding and regressed behaviour on the part of the patient, provoking resentment in family members. Marital boundaries and roles blur and change. Old issues of power and control re-emerge in the anger and frustration engendered by the illness.[72,77] It is important that professionals help couples retain a sense of intimacy and enjoyment in previous shared activities, even if this requires paid carers to take over some physical provider roles. Carers will need encouragement to take a break from caring and pursue individual activities.

Case history

Laura had been living with Martin for three years prior to his diagnosis with ALS. She now felt trapped by a commitment to him that seemed to be destroying her own life. She could not bear to spend time in the same room as him unless actively engaged in his physical care. Martin shouted and screamed at her, sometimes spitting food in her face. In individual conversations with staff he said he felt he was turning into a 'monster'. He said that he was afraid to tell her he loved her in case she did not want to hear it. Alone, Laura admitted that she wished he were dead. With help they were able to acknowledge how hard it had become to talk together, how much they had both lost and how different their reactions to coping with stress were. A barrier was broken when Martin cried in front of Laura.

Intimate relationships and body image may be deeply affected by ALS yet are largely neglected in the literature.[78] Issues of intimacy and sexuality are about much more than intercourse. They concern fundamental needs to communicate and receive love, to feel at ease with their bodies and physical closeness. The combination of sex, disability and death is a powerful inhibitor. Professionals' anxieties about their own sexuality may lead to defensive designation of the whole area as one that requires a particular specialism. Yet if professionals remove sex from the agenda they can isolate people further from the help they need to gain the love and acceptance that will support them in losses in so many other areas. In reality the communication skills required are the same as any other sensitive topic. Indeed a recent palliative care study[79] found that patients with all types of cancer were willing to discuss the impact on their sexual lives. The research of Kaub-Wittemer and colleagues[44] confirms that sexuality is important for many ventilated ALS patients, although less so for their caregivers.

Although most professionals cannot be expected to become specialist psychosexual counsellors, all have a responsibility to become comfortable with offering and responding to cues about sexuality, offering first line help and referring for specialist support[80]. In Vincent et al.'s[81] study of women with cancer of the cervix, 80 per cent of those receiving treatment wanted more information about the impact on their sexuality, but 75 per cent said they would not raise the question first. Vulnerable individuals often give the professional a cue to test out whether he is safe enough to receive their confidences. An example would be the man who said of his wife: 'She just doesn't seem to love me any more.' Bland reassurances may confirm that this subject is indeed too difficult and painful to discuss. Graded, open questions may help: 'How has your illness changed your work life, home life, life as a couple, ability to get close to one another physically?' It also helps to generalize to give permission: 'People often have questions they'd like to ask about the sexual side of life.' Monroe (p. 106) offers a useful set of history taking questions.[11]

Concerns may be expressed about body image, sexual function or both. In some relationships the physical dependency created by the illness can disturb a well-established pattern of lack of intimacy. Some partners find that their change of role to carer alters their feelings and sexual desires, or that the physical deterioration in a partner creates similar changes. Many patients feel anxious about the changes in the way their body looks and behaves. Anxiety about rejection can lead to retreat and a wall of silence which may be eased by a facilitated discussion. Some couples appreciate advice about alternative positions or alternative methods of love-making such as mutual caressing. Professionals should avoid assumptions based on age, gender, culture, marital status, apparent relationship or experience. Those without a partner may discuss the relationships they had in the past or those they now fear they will never have. Sadly, a young couple may be offered a double bed and an individual room in a hospice where the same facilities are thought less important for an older couple.

Children and their needs

When someone in the family is ill everyone is affected, including children. However, adult desire to protect children may leave them alone and confused, at the mercy of their fears and fantasies which may be worse than reality. Children are always aware when something is happening in the family. They sense adult anxiety, overhear conversations, are aware of practical changes and often hear adult gossip from school friends. Many research studies show the cost of inadequate support and involvement for children facing bereavement.[82–85]

Children need:

◆ Respect and acknowledgement.

◆ Information about what is happening, and why, and what might happen next. Information needs to be clear, simple, truthful and to be repeated as children struggle to come to terms with what is happening.

◆ Reassurance. Children become frightened as they watch a parent or relative becoming dependent or emotionally labile or irrationally angry. They need an explanation, to know that they did not cause the illness and cannot catch it.

◆ Children will want reassurance about practical issues such as what is going to happen to the family and their own care after the person has died.

- Appropriate involvement in helping the patient.
- A chance to talk about feelings and know facts with adults who are prepared to share theirs.
- A variety of mediums for self expression, e.g. drawing, writing, playing games.
- Opportunities to reflect and remember, to know that life will go on and it is all right to have fun.

Many studies confirm the importance of pre-death experiences in mediating and influencing the course and outcome of bereavement.[85,86] Significant factors include the relationship of the child with the ill person before the death, the openness of family communication, the availability of community support, and the extent to which the child's parenting needs have continued to be met.[87]

Caring adults are often struggling with seemingly impossible and conflicting demands and may need help to negotiate compromises. For example, a parent struggling with the impending death of a partner may lose sight of their child's fear they are losing not one parent but two.

Helping parents

Parents know their children best and children need their families, who will be around long after the professionals. The professional task is to support parents to help their children. Professionals should work with what parents can manage and help them to develop a sense of confidence and competence.[88] What and how children are told about the situation is the responsibility of their parent(s) or guardian. Parents will need encouragement and support to understand how best to communicate with and involve their children. They may have good reasons for their reluctance to share information about illness and death with their children. They are often struggling to maintain control in the midst of uncertainty and may feel both physically and emotionally overwhelmed. They may be avoiding the truth and wonder if they can cope with the child's grief when anxious about managing their own. They may underestimate what a child understands and worry about saying the wrong thing or making matters worse. Research indicates that children as young as three years old begin to understand what the word death means.[89,90] Children informed about their parent's impending death are less anxious (Rosenheim and Richter 1985 cited in[83]). It is important to support parents with their own emotional needs before they contemplate those of their children.

Parents often welcome the opportunity to think about what their children might ask and how they might respond. Christ's[91] meticulous study confirms the value of helping parents to understand and respond to their children's developmental needs. Parents will need advice on how to anticipate and understand altered behaviour in their children; why they are more clingy, do not want friends to come home, seem to be frightened or embarrassed by the person who is ill. For many parents rehearsal of the issues with a professional will be sufficient and they will want to speak to their children alone, perhaps with a later opportunity to review the conversation and concerns raised. Others will welcome sharing the task with a professional and may gain confidence from the presence of a doctor, nurse or social worker as they try to answer their children's questions. Parents can be helped by being offered appropriate resources, such as suggestions of books to read to their children, or for their children to read.[92]

Parents may need encouragement to widen their children's support network by involving other adults close to them: a relative, another adult friend, a youth club leader and, most importantly, the school. They may need support with strategies to manage other friends or family members resistant to involving the children. Everyone will need reassurance about children's resilience. The aim should be to help parents talk to their own children themselves. Rarely when this is impossible and the professional undertakes direct work with the child, care must be taken to work within family values and culture. The professional must discover what knowledge is permissible in the family and what words have already been used, and should negotiate an agreement with the child and parent about how and what to tell the parent about the content of the session.

Case history

Luke was eight. He stayed overnight with his grandparents every weekend. His grandfather was diagnosed with ALS and over a period of a few months found it more difficult to get about. Luke had always played football with his grandfather but this became impossible. Luke became angry and upset about this, saying his grandfather did not love him any more. Luke's grandfather used this opportunity to tell Luke more about his illness, using the MND Association (UK) booklet for children. He also made sure that Luke's mother was involved in what Luke had been told. The social worker provided Luke's mother with a workbook in which Luke could write and draw to explore further with his mother any unresolved questions and worries.

Young people

Adolescents face a particular struggle between balancing independence and attempts to find a new identity, with an event that draws them back into a changed family and additional unwelcome demands.[93] They often value a separate opportunity to talk to a professional about the illness and may also want to discuss difficulties in relationships with their friends. A serious illness is frightening and embarrassing for their peers, making them different just when they most want to be the same. In separate work with adolescents it is important to have clear agreements about confidentiality with them and their parents. Parents need help to understand that a young person's withdrawal is not just careless or selfish. Information about feelings can help young people feel more in control, especially when in written form so that they read it when they choose. The MND Association (UK) has a good example: *When your parent has MND.*[94] It is important to remember that talking is not the only solution to helping young people;[95] keeping a diary, watching films, reading books, playing sport as a release, or practising relaxation techniques all help adolescents express their feelings. Above all young people need affirmation wherever possible. Professionals must also be aware of the needs of young people and children who are acting as carers, often in single parent families. Frank[96] offers useful principles and guidelines for this.

Working with ALS

Many professionals and volunteers have commented on the emotionally taxing nature of caring for ALS.[28,76,97] ALS may confront professionals with fears about their own mortality[98] and their own death. Carroll-Thomas[99] reminds us that how we intervene in and react to a family will be based upon our own values, psychological make up and professional culture. She asserts: 'The more challenging the problem, including feelings of helplessness, the more likely that cultural values will emerge in clinician and patient interactions.' Professional attitudes and values can affect the allocation of resources and choice of language may affect the quality of information given. Multiprofessional teams extends the services and options for the patient and family, optimizing coordinated care and an effective response to complex needs.[45,100] Research demonstrates the impact of teamwork in better care outcomes.[101,102] Working in teams also offers the chance to share dilemmas, ethical questions and stresses of caring for ALS. Even someone who works alone can create a team by thinking flexibly and imaginatively about those involved. Teams must respect the autonomy of the individual and the family's own style. Professional views on safety may need to be balanced against patient and family wishes and the importance of allowing families to do the things in the way they choose.

Case history

Patricia was married with two children aged four and ten. She had ALS. Her ten-year-old daughter undertook the bulk of her physical care while Patricia's husband busying himself with his job and his four-year-old son. Patricia's daughter stayed off school to look after her for the last fortnight of her life, despite professional anxieties. A year later the family was coping well and Patricia's daughter and her father often talked proudly of their joint achievements.

A multiprofessional team should include someone specializing in psychosocial care, not only for the needs of the patient and family and sometimes to advocate for them in team discussions, but also to take a lead in the care of the professionals; for example, encouraging appropriate personal disclosure and team review of complex pieces of work. Papadatou[103] explores the grief experiences of health care professionals and emphasises the importance of team-based meaning-making.

Individual professionals have a duty of care for themselves. They need to acknowledge their feelings and when necessary find support for them.[104] Carmack[105] has some helpful insights on balancing engagement and detachment in caregiving. She comments that the longer and more intense the caregiver's involvement, the more important to learn this balance.

Caregivers can be taught how to do what they can, while letting go of the need to control the outcome ... Caregivers may need instruction in setting and maintaining clear limits and boundaries. Many caregivers have never learned either the legitimacy of setting limits or the means to do so.[105]

Conclusion

For now ALS remains incurable. Psychosocial care plays a particularly important role in determining how patients and families respond to the impact of illness. It can help them cope with experiences of loss and change and expand their sense of what is possible. McDonald states:

In many cases quality of life had little to do with physical disability. Many patients and families maintain high quality lives at all stages of physical disability and all lengths of illness. The key lies in their psychosocial and spiritual well-being. [28]

The psychosocial care described is not a luxury, but essential in the kind of effective palliative care that can help the patients and those close to them move into a changed future with a sufficient sense of confidence.

References

1. **Mann I.** (1991) Never 'eard of it. Northampton: MND Association (UK).
2. **Saunders C.** (1993) Introduction – history and challenge. In Saunders C., Sykes N. (eds) *The Management of Terminal Malignant Disease*, 3rd edn, pp. 1–14. London: Hodder and Stoughton.

3. **Barkwell D. P.** (1991) Ascribed meaning: a critical factor in coping and pain attenuation in patients with cancer-related pain. *Journal of Palliative Care* 7 (3): 5–14.

4. **National Council for Hospice and Specialist Palliative Care Services** (1997) *Feeling Better: Psychosocial Care in Specialist Palliative Care. A Discussion Paper.* Occasional paper 13, August 1997. London: National Council.

5. **Monroe B.** (2004) Social work in palliative medicine. In Doyle D., Hanks G., Cherny N. I., Calman K. (eds) *Oxford Textbook of Palliative Medicine*, 3rd edn, pp. 1005–17. Oxford: Oxford University Press.

6. **Spiegel D., Bloom J., Kraemer H. C. Gotheil E.** (1989) Effect of psychosocial treatment on survival of patients with metastatic cancer. *Lancet* 2 (668): 888–91.

7. **Fallowfield L.** (1995) Psychosocial interventions in cancer. *BMJ* 311: 1316–17.

8. **Fawzy F. I., Fawzy N. W., Canada A. L.** (1998) Psychosocial treatment of cancer: an update. *Current Opinion in Psychiatry* 11 (4): 601–5.

9. **Rabkin J. G., Wagner G. J., Del Bene M.** (2000) Resilience and distress among amyotrophic lateral sclerosis patients and caregivers. *Psychosomatic Medicine* 62 (2): 271–9.

10. **Johnston M., Earll L., Giles M., McClenahan R., Stevens D., Morrison V.** (1999) Mood as predictor of disability and survival in patients newly diagnosed with ALS/MND. *British Journal of Health Psychology* 4: 127–36.

11. **Oliviere D., Hargreaves R., Monroe B.** (1998) *Good Practices in Palliative Care: A Psychosocial Perspective.* Aldershot: Ashgate.

12. **Sheldon F.** (1997) *Psychosocial Palliative Care: Good Practice in the Care of the Dying and Bereaved.* Cheltenham: Stanley Thornes.

13. **Carey J. S.** (1986) Motor neuron disease – a challenge to medical ethics: a discussion paper. *Journal of the Royal Society of Medicine* 79: 216–20.

14. **Borasio G. D., Sloan R., Pongratz D. E.** (1998). Breaking the news in amyotrophic lateral sclerosis. *Journal of the Neurological Sciences* 160 (Suppl. 1): S127–S133.

15. **Johnston M., Earll L., Mitchell E., Morrison V., Wright S.** (1996) Communicating the diagnosis of motor neurone disease. *Palliative Medicine* 10 (1): 23–34.

16. **McClement S. E., Hack T. F.** (1999) Audio-taping the oncology treatment consultation: a literature review. *Patient Education and Counselling* 36 (3): 229–38.

17. **Ackerman G., Oliver D. J.** (1997) **Psychosocial support in an outpatient clinic.** *Palliative Medicine* 11 (2): 167–8.

18. **Earll L., Johnston M., Mitchell E.** (1993) Coping with motor neurone disease – an analysis using self-regulation theory. *Palliative Medicine* 7 (Suppl. 2): 21–30.

19. **Brown W. A., Mueller P. S.** (1970) Psychological function in individuals with amyotrophic lateral sclerosis. *Psychosomatic Medicine* 32: 141–52.

20. **Houpt J. L., Gould B. S., Norris F. H.** (1977) Psychological characteristics of patients with amyotrophic lateral sclerosis (ALS). *Psychosomatic Medicine* 39 (5): 299–303.

21. **Peters P. K., Swenson W. M., Mulder D. W.** (1978) Is there a characteristic personality profile in amyotrophic lateral sclerosis? *Archives of Neurology* 35: 321–2.

22. **Montgomery G. K., Erikson L. M.** (1987) Neuropsychological perspectives in amyotrophic lateral sclerosis. *Neurologic Clinics* 5: 61–81.

23. **Armon C., Kurland L. T., Beard C. M., O'Brien P. C., Mulder D. W.** (1991) Psychological and adaptational difficulties anteceding amyotrophic lateral sclerosis: Rochester, Minnesota, 1925–1987. *Neuroepidemiology* 10: 132–7.

24. **Strong M. J., Lomen-Hoerth C., Caselli R. J., Bigio E. H., Yang W.** (2003) Cognitive impairment, frontotemporal dementia, and the motor neuron diseases. *Annals of Neurology* **54** (Suppl. 5): S20–23.

25. **Randall F., Downie R. S.** (1999) *Palliative Care Ethics: A Companion for all Specialities,* 2nd edn. Oxford: Oxford University Press.

26. **Hinton J.** (1994) Can home care maintain an acceptable quality of life for patients with terminal cancer and their relatives? *Palliative Medicine* **8** (3): 183–96.

27. **Hinton J.** (1996) Services given and help perceived during home care for terminal cancer. *Palliative Medicine* **10** (2): 125–35.

28. **McDonald E. R.** (1994) Psychosocial-spiritual overview. In Mitsumoto H., Norris F. H. (eds) *Amyotrophic Lateral Sclerosis: A Comprehensive Guide to Management,* pp. 205–27. New York: Demos.

29. **Maguire P., Walsh S., Jeacock J., Kingston R.** (1999) Physical and psychological needs of patients dying from colo-rectal cancer. *Palliative Medicine* **13** (1): 45–50.

30. **Albert S. M., Murphy P. L., Del Bene M. L., Rowland L. P.** (1999) A prospective study of preferences and actual treatment choices in ALS. *Neurology* **53** (3): 278–83.

31. **Buckley J., Herth K.** (2004) Fostering hope in terminally ill patients. *Nursing Standard* **19** (10): 33–41.

32. **Kim T-S.** (1990) Hoping strategies for the amyotrophic lateral sclerosis patient. *Loss, Grief and Care* **4** (3–4): 239–49.

33. **Lester J.** (2005) Life review with the terminally ill – narrative therapies. In Firth P., Luff G. , Oliviere D. (eds) *Loss, Change and Bereavement in Palliative Care,* pp. 66–79. Buckingham: Open University Press.

34. **Young J. M., McNicoll P.** (1998) Against all odds: positive life experiences of people with advanced amyotrophic lateral sclerosis. *Health and Social Work* **23** (1): 35–43.

35. **Salt S.** (1997) Towards a definition of suffering. *European Journal of Palliative Care* **4** (2): 58–60.

36. **Ganzini L., Johnston W., Hoffman W.** (1999) Correlates of suffering in amyotrophic lateral sclerosis. *Neurology* **52** (7): 1434–40.

37. **Chapman C. R., Gavrin J.** (1993) Suffering and its relationship to pain. *Journal of Palliative Care* **9** (2): 5–13.

38. **Kissane D. W.** (1998) Models of psychological response to suffering. *Progress in Palliative Care* **6** (6): 197–204.

39. **Öhlén J.** (2002) Practical wisdom: competencies required in alleviating suffering in palliative care. *Journal of Palliative Care* **18** (4): 293–9.

40. **Deneault S., Lussier V., Mongeau S., Paillé P., Hudon E.** *et al.* (2004) The nature of suffering and its relief in the terminally ill: a qualitative study. *Journal of Palliative Care* **20** (1): 7–11.

41. **Cobb A. K.** (1994) The effect of cultural expectations on progression responses in ALS. In Mitsumoto H., Norris, F. H, (eds) *Amyotrophic Lateral Sclerosis: A Comprehensive Guide to Management,* pp. 229–40. New York: Demos.

42. **Morse J. M., Carter B. J.** (1995) Strategies of enduring and the suffering of loss: modes of comfort used by a resilient survivor. *Holistic Nursing Practice* **9** (3): 38–52.

43. **Robbins R. A., Simmons Z., Bremner B. A., Walsh S. M., Fischer S.** (2001) Quality of life in ALS is maintained as physical function declines. *Neurology* **56**: 442–4.

44. Kaub-Wittemer D., von Steinbüchel N., Wasner M., Laier-Groeneveld G., Borasio G. D. (2003) Quality of life and psychosocial issues in ventilated patients with amyotrophic lateral sclerosis and their caregivers. *Journal of Pain and Symptom Management* 26 (4): 890–6.

45. Goldstein L., Leigh N. (1999) Motor neurone disease: a review of its emotional and cognitive consequences for patients and its impact on carers. *British Journal of Health Psychology* 4: 193–208.

46. Plahuta J. M., McCulloch B. J., Kasarkis E. J., Ross M. A. Walter, R. A. *et al.* (2002) Amyotrophic lateral sclerosis and hopelessness: psychosocial factors. *Social Science and Medicine* 55: 2131–40.

47. McCann C. (1998) Communication in cancer care: introducing patient-held records. *International Journal of Palliative Nursing* 4 (5): 222–9.

48. Hunter M. D., Robinson I. C., Neilson S. (1993) The functional and psychological status of patients with amyotrophic lateral sclerosis: some implications for rehabilitation. *Disability and Rehabilitation* 15 (3): 119–26.

49. Leach C. F., Delfiner J. S. (1989) Approaches to loss and bereavement in amyotrophic lateral sclerosis (ALS). In Klagsbrun S. C., Kliman G. W., Clark E. J. Kutscher, A. H. DeBellis R., Lambert C. A. (eds) *Preventive Psychiatry: Early Intervention and Situational Crisis Management,* pp. 201–11. Philadelphia, PA: The Charles Press.

50. MND Association [UK] (2003) *Death and Dying.* Leaflet, obtainable from MND Association [UK]. www.mndassociation.org.

51. MND Association [UK] (2003) *How Will I Die?* Obtainable from MND Association [UK]. www.mndassociation.org.

52. O'Brien T., Kelly M., Saunders C. (1992) Motor neurone disease: a hospice perspective. *BMJ* 304: 471–3.

53. Ganzini L., Johnston W. S., McFarland B. H., Tolle S. W., Lee M. A. (1998) Attitudes of patients with amyotrophic lateral sclerosis and their care givers toward assisted suicide. *The New England Journal of Medicine* 339 (14): 967–73.

54. Seale C., Addington-Hall J. (1994) Euthanasia: why people want to die earlier. *Social Science and Medicine* 39 (5): 647–54.

55. Johnston M., Marteau T., Partridge C., Gilbert P. (1993) Changes in patient perceptions of chronic disease and disability with time. In Schmidt L. R., Schwenkmezgar P., Weinman J., Maes S. (eds) *Theoretical and applied aspects of health psychology,* pp. 361–71. Pennsylvania Harwood Academic Chur.

56. Goldstein L. H., Adamson M., Jeffrey L., Down K., Barby T., Wilson C. *et al.* (1998) The psychological impact of MND on patients and carers. *Journal of the Neurological Sciences* 160 (Suppl. 1): S114–S121.

57. Horta E. (1986) Emotional response to ALS and its impact on management of patient care. In Caroscio J. T. (ed.) *Amyotrophic Lateral Sclerosis – A Guide to Patient Care,* pp. 282–9. New York: Thieme Medical Publishers Inc.

58. Worden J. W. (1991) *Grief Counselling and Grief Therapy,* 2nd edn. London: Routledge.

59. Centers L. C. (2001) Beyond denial and despair: ALS and our heroic potential for hope. *Journal of Palliative Care* 17 (4): 259–64.

60. Hogg K. E., Goldstein L. H., Leigh P. N. (1994) The psychological impact of motor neurone disease. *Psychological Medicine* 24: 625–32.

61. **Bolmsjö I., Hermerén G.** (2001) Interviews with patients, family, and caregivers in amyotrophic lateral sclerosis: comparing needs. *Journal of Palliative Care* 17 (4): 236–40.

62. **O'Brien M. R.** (2004) Information-seeking behaviour among people with motor neurone disease. *British Journal of Nursing* 13 (16): 964–8.

63. **Hoffman R. L., Decker T. W.** (1993) Amyotrophic lateral sclerosis: an introduction to psychosocial and behavioural adaptations. *Journal of Mental Health Counselling* 15 (4): 394–402.

64. **Stroebe M., Schut H.** (1999) The dual process model of coping with bereavement: rationale and description. *Death Studies* 23: 197–224.

65. **Oliviere D.** (2004) Cultural issues in palliative care. In Sykes N., Edmonds P., Wiles J. (eds) *Management of Advanced Disease*, 4th edn, pp. 438–49. London: Arnold.

66. **Kissane D. W., Bloch S.** (2002) *Family Focused Grief Therapy*. Buckingham: Open University Press.

67. **Hull M.** (1990) Sources of stress for hospice care – grieving families. *The Hospice Journal* 6 (2): 29–54.

68. **Kirschling J., Trilden V. P., Butterfield P. G.** (1990) Social support: the experience of hospice family caregivers. *The Hospice Journal* 6 (2): 75–93.

69. **Aoun S. M., Kristjanson L. J., Currow D. C., Hudson P. L.** (2005) Caregiving for the terminally ill: at what cost? *Palliative Medicine* 19 (7): 551–5.

70. **Sykes N. P., Pearson S. E., Chell S.** (1992) Quality of care of the terminally ill: the carer's perspective. *Palliative Medicine* 6 (3): 227–36.

71. **Neale B.** (1991) *Informal Palliative Care: A Review of Research on Needs, Standards and Service Evaluations*. Occasional Paper No. 3. Sheffield: Trent Palliative Care Centre.

72. **Sebring D. L., Moglia P.** (1987) Amyotrophic lateral sclerosis: psychosocial interventions for patients and their families. *Health and Social Work* Spring: 113–20.

73. **Thorpe G.** (1993) Enabling more dying people to remain at home. *BMJ* 307 (9): 915–18.

74. **Payne S.** (2004) Carers and caregivers. In Oliviere D., Monroe B. (eds) *Death, Dying and Social Differences*, 181–98. Oxford: Oxford University Press.

75. **Monroe B., Sheldon F.** (2004). Psychosocial dimensions of care. In Sykes N., Edmonds P., Wiles J. (eds) *Management of Advanced Disease*, 4th edn, pp. 405–37. London: Edward Arnold.

76. **Ginsberg N.** (1986) Living and coping with amyotrophic lateral sclerosis: the psychosocial impact. In Caroscio J. T. (ed.) *Amyotrophic Lateral Sclerosis – A Guide to Patient Care*, pp. 273–80. New York: Thieme Medical Publishers.

77. **Luloff P. B.** (1986) Reactions of patients, family, and staff in dealing with amyotrophic lateral sclerosis. In Caroscio J. T. (ed.) *Amyotrophic Lateral Sclerosis – A Guide to Patient Care*, pp. 267–71. New York: Thieme Medical Publishers.

78. **Gilley J.** (1988) Intimacy and terminal care. *Journal of the Royal College of General Practitioners* 38: 121–2.

79. **Anath H., Jones L., King M., Tookman A.** (2003) The impact of cancer on sexual function: a controlled study. *Palliative Medicine* 17 (2): 202–5.

80. **Stausmire J. M.** (2004) Sexuality at the end of life. *American Journal of Hospice and Palliative Care* 21 (1): 33–39.

81. **Vincent C. E., Vincent B., Greiss F. C., Linton E. B.** (1975) Some marital concomitants of carcinoma of the cervix. *Southern Medical Journal* **68**: 552–8.

82. **Rutter M.** (1966) *Children of Sick Parents.* Oxford: Oxford University Press.

83. **Black D., Wood D.** (1989) Family therapy and life-threatening illness in children or parents. *Palliative Medicine* 3 (2): 113–18.

84 **Black D., Young B.** (1995) Bereaved children: risk and preventive intervention. In Raphael B., Burrows G. (eds) *Handbook of Studies on Preventive Psychiatry*, pp. 225–44. Amsterdam: Elsevier.

85. **Worden J. W.** (1996) *Children and Grief: When a Parent Dies.* New York: Guilford Press.

86. **Silverman P. R., Worden W. J.** (1993) Children's reactions to the death of a parent. In Stroebe, M. Stroebe, W. Hansson R. (eds) *Handbook of Bereavement*, pp. 300–16. Cambridge: Cambridge University Press.

87. **Harris T., Brown G., Bifulo A.** (1986) Loss of parent in childhood and adult psychiatric disorder: the role of lack of adequate parental care. *Psychological Medicine* 16: 641–59.

88. **Monroe B.** (1995) It is impossible not to communicate – helping the grieving family. In Smith S. C., Pennells M. (eds) *Interventions with Bereaved Children*, pp. 87–106. London: Jessica Kingsley.

89. **Kane B.** (1979) Children's concepts of death. *Journal of Genetic Psychology* 4: 15–7.

90. **Lansdown R., Benjamin G.** (1985) The development of the concept of death in children aged 5–9. *Child Care Health Department* 11: 13–20.

91. **Christ G. H.** (2000) *Healing Children's Grief. Surviving a Parent's Death from Cancer.* Oxford: Oxford University Press.

92. **MND Association [UK]** (1996) *When Someone Special has Motor Neurone Disease.* Obtainable from MND Association [UK]. www.mndassociation.org.

93. **Fleming, S. J., Adolph R.** (1986) Helping bereaved adolescents: needs and responses. In Corr C. A., McNeil J. N (eds) *Adolescence and Death*, pp. 97–118. New York: Springer.

94. **MND Association [UK]** (2004) *When Your Parent has Motor Neurone Disease.* A booklet for young people. Obtainable from MND Association [UK]. www. mndassociation.org.

95. **Ribbens-McCarthy J., with Jessop J.** (2005) *Young People, Bereavement and Loss: Disruptive Transitions?* London: National Children's Bureau.

96. **Frank J.** (1995) *Couldn't Care More: A Study of Young Carers and Their Needs.* London: The Children's Society.

97. **Meininger V.** (1993) Breaking bad news in amyotrophic lateral sclerosis. *Palliative Medicine* 7 (Suppl. 2): 37–40.

98. **O'Brien T.** (1993) Palliative care and taboos within motor neurone disease. *Palliative Medicine* 7 (Suppl. 2): 69–72.

99. **Carroll-Thomas S.** (1993) Ethics and the clinician: the daily experience with MND. *Palliative Medicine* 7 (suppl. 2): 11–3.

100. **Traynor B., Alexander M., Corr B., Frost E., Hardiman O.** (2003) Effect of a multidisciplinary amyotrophic lateral sclerosis (ALS) clinic on ALS survival: a population based study : 1996–2000. *Journal of Neurology, Neurosurgery and Psychiatry* 74: 1258–61.

101. **Findley L. J.** (1991) *Can Care be Organised in the Management of Motor Neurone Disease?* A report of Ciba Foundation discussion meeting, 5 February 1991. London: Ciba, St Christopher's Hospice, MND Assoc (UK).

102. **Jones R. V. H.** (1993) Teams and terminal cancer at home: do patients and carers benefit? *Journal of Interprofessional Care* 7 (3): 239–44.

103. **Papadatou D.** (2000) A proposed model of health professionals' grieving process. *Omega* 41 (1): 59–77.

104. **Monroe B.** (2004) Emotional impact of palliative care on staff. In Sykes N., Edmonds P., Wiles J. (eds) *Management of Advanced Disease*, 4th edn, pp. 450–60. London: Edward Arnold.

105. **Carmack B.** (1997) Balancing engagement and detatchment in caregiving. *Image: Journal of Nursing Scholarship* 29 (2): 139–43.

Chapter 6

Spiritual care

Robert Lambert

Summary

Spiritual care is of great importance in the treatment of ALS. It is essential to consider the importance of spiritual issues, within both the illness and its treatment, to the whole person, rather than in the physical aspects alone. Spirituality is defined to include both religious and non-religious elements. Spirituality can be considered as a resource for coping, as a potential source of conflict and suffering, and as an arena to explore in finding meaning. There are many different universal spiritual themes which may be expressed in ALS: faith, hope, a sense of the sacred, meaning, gratitude, forgiveness, vocation and acceptance of death. We need clinically based, non-denominational spiritual care and it is important for all clinicians to be aware of their patients' spiritual values.

Paradox

People with ALS live with paradox. Paul the Apostle wrote some 2000 years ago that 'In the midst of life, we are in death,' expressing this universal human dilemma. Knowing that we shall die, how do we make sense of life? We manage to keep the thoughts of our own death out of conscious awareness most of the time. We may be reminded of it while watching a film, attending a relative's funeral, or waiting outside the office on a visit to the doctor, but we manage to push it aside and carry on with life. A diagnosis of ALS forces this sudden awareness through the compression of time, the daily reminders of physical decline, consecutive losses and the reactions of loved ones. A second paradox is expressed in ALS. Not only are we more than our bodies, it is sometimes in the absence of physical capacities that people are most profoundly alive. This was put simply by a friend a few years ago as he approached his own death due to a brain tumour: 'It's odd, but I feel just as alive now that I am near death as I was years ago when it was still far off... maybe even more so.' Here we are in the realm of the spiritual – that aspect of life that has little to do with physical quality or capacities – that which is at once most dynamic and enduring about a person.

What do we mean by spiritual?

In an earlier age the terms spiritual and religious were synonymous, and everyone knew what they meant. It is no longer so simple. The advance of the sciences, secularism and critical scholarship in religious studies have separated these terms in the west. Now religion is more often associated with public practices, such as membership in an institution, participation in rituals and adherence to the teachings of a tradition. Spiritual has become associated with the private realm of one's personal experiences, beliefs, and values.[1] Both refer to the inner life of a person, but religion is more likely to be shared with others and to bind one to a culturally defined group. 'Religion is organized, institutionalized spirituality.'[2]

Spirituality seeks meaning in lived experience. It uncovers and tries to understand truth, not as fact, but as meaning. Spirituality encompasses religious beliefs and practices but is not limited by them. We might say then that all people are spiritual; some people are also religious. Robert Fuller notes that we are spiritual whenever we wonder why we are here or what happens when we die. We are spiritual when we are 'moved by values of beauty, love, or creativity that seem to reveal a meaning or power beyond our visible world.'[1]

The crisis of terminal illness heightens one's awareness of the spiritual. With patients, I find that the spiritual surfaces in three different ways. First, spirituality may be a resource for coping with illness. People turn within to find spiritual resources: beliefs, values, trusted experiences or images, which give them strength, encouragement or comfort. Some may seek strength in the practice of their faith, through the support of their community and in the guidance of religious leaders.

Second, spiritual conflicts may emerge. One person's spiritual life can be a source of strength and joy: another's can be a source of pain and suffering. The spiritual may even be a dark place filled with punitive gods, failure to live up to ideals, memories of rejection or judgement by religious figures, or frightening images of the afterlife. Some associate illness with judgement, punishment, or the injustice of a capricious god.

Third, the spiritual emerges in the searching questions which arise from within. Reflecting on their past and future, people may engage in a search for meaning. Why am I here? Why is this happening to me? What should I do with my remaining time? The questions are not only about the meaning of this event but about life itself. Illness becomes an occasion for going deeper, for reinterpreting the meaning of one's life, and for understanding how this new chapter connects to all the rest. Fleischman states that this is what religion (spirituality) is about.

It differs from our philosophical self in that it seeks to discover meanings, not to create them; and it differs from our scientific self in that it seeks to discover meanings, not causal forces. Seen from the standpoint of psychology, religion refers to those overt and covert aspects of personality in which there is a questioning drive, a quest, to relate meaningfully the particular to the whole.[3]

As one finds meaning in the present, it is possible for life to be experienced as deeper, richer, and more rewarding even while one is living with physical decline.

Spiritual themes

People with ALS do not face different spiritual issues from everyone else, but a terminal illness intensifies spiritual needs and questions. The spiritual issues I will discuss below are universal ones. All religions have their ways of addressing these issues and each person, religious or not, seems to confront them sooner or later. The field of pastoral care, in its evolution into a clinical discipline, recognized the advantage of seeing these themes through a clinical lens rather than a partisan one. Hiltner's suggestion of a pastoral diagnosis,[4] and Pruyser's proposal of 'diagnostic variables,'[5] were great steps forward toward viewing spiritual themes through clinical eyes. This list of spiritual themes is neither unique nor exhaustive, but it describes the themes that I have heard repeated while accompanying patients with ALS.

Does life make sense? The existential question

Why is this happening to me? What will become of me? The lack of a scientific explanation for the cause of ALS is not at the root of these questions – people with other illnesses ask the same questions. The question is one of meaning and not of causality. When someone hears the diagnosis of a terminal illness there is a sense of shock, of being knocked off balance. What one had expected from life has been taken away and replaced by another scenario, difficult to believe and even more difficult to accept. As the news sinks in questions about meaning emerge, and behind these questions are the greater questions about life itself: What is life all about? If this thing that makes no sense is happening to me now, does anything else make sense?

Religious people may speak of God's will, God's plan, or a divine purpose. The monotheistic religions speak about the goodness of God, the created order of the universe and natural laws. Although it is mysterious, somehow illness can and must be accounted for within those thoughts. Ancient writings like the book of Job are attempts to make sense of illness within this frame. Other religions have their way of describing the order of things. Buddhism's fourfold noble truth begins by stating that to live is to suffer. The nature religions fit illness and death into the natural cycles of the earth. Religions speak of a world in which there is a meaningful connection between people and events.

The spiritually inclined may look for a benevolent goodness, an intelligent design, or at least a natural order. Inherent in all of these approaches is the idea of providence, of the goodness of the created order, despite all possible appearances to the contrary. Fleischman refers to this as the need for lawful order.[3] If there is an order to things, then even our crises and hardships fit into this purpose in some way that we can discover.

But without some sense of goodness and order what can we trust, what is worth doing, what is good and what is not? The seemingly random nature of ALS is difficult to fit into such an order. The age-old questions are raised, as they are when people are hit with tsunami or a hurricane. But ALS does not happen to a region, it happens to one person. How could God allow this to happen to me? Some find a way to make sense and others do not.

Jean-Yves Leloup suggests that this process is more difficult in our era. He writes that the predominance of atheistic humanism as a world view in our time makes death a scandal, an offence, an absurdity, and therefore much more difficult to face. 'This attitude about death is at the source, at one and the same time, of various attitudes of denial, avoidance, prolonging life through unnecessary treatments, and support for assisted suicide.'[6]

On the other hand, if illness and eventual death are part of a natural or a God-created order, then one can, in accepting death, participate in that order. One patient, a woman of 45, was diagnosed with ALS five years ago. Raised in a strict Christian family, she had a mostly negative experience of a severe religion and no longer practised it. But in her mid-30s a friend invited her to a lecture on Buddhism, which piqued her interest. She was drawn to the accepting environment and to the ordered thinking of Buddhist teachings. She began practising meditation, attending lectures, until eventually she identified herself as a Buddhist. Here is how she makes sense of her illness:

I am fortunate that I was already practising when I got ALS. Where I grew up they would have told me that this was a punishment from God. But it's not. This is not from God. In Buddhism, life itself is suffering. And this is my suffering. It will transform me. Everyone has to live with suffering but this is just life. My life won't end with this suffering, only this life. I must finish this life with the right attitude and in peace so my soul will continue in a higher life later. I am suffering now, but I'm not attached to this suffering. I can see beyond it. That is why I meditate, to detach and be at peace.

We can hear how these teachings make sense of what she lives by finding order and goodness in spite of the illness. But even for someone who is not religious there is a way to make sense. A man who was diagnosed at age 66 said this:

I am sad to be nearing the end. I love life. It's good and it has been good to me. But it has to be my turn sometime, and my turn is now. That is the way life is made. It's my turn to go, and someone else will be next. I look around and think, what can I expect? Sixty years seems young, but when you look around the world, you know I've lived longer than I would have in most places! So this is the way things are designed and I have to accept it.

Both of these patients are coming to terms with this illness through belief in an ordered world and by finding how they fit within it.

Is anything sacred?

The wife of an ALS patient told me that her husband's illness was so distressing for her that she could find comfort only when she attended the service at the Anglican Church. She and her husband had attended there for more than 30 years. He could no longer come with her and she missed him beside her there. She described how she would lose herself in the music of the organ and the choir and find a refuge in the familiar sights and symbols of the liturgy. At the moment of receiving communion she felt God was present and she would be all right. I asked her husband if he missed the services. He said he had gone mostly to support his wife, but it was not there that he felt the divine presence. What he missed were the late summer evenings at their cottage on the lake. There surrounded by his family and watching the sunset he felt a sense of awe and reverence that gave him peace inside. 'The church is fine,' he said, 'but it's there at that lake that I know we are not alone.'

These two halves of a couple demonstrate very different ways of experiencing something unifying and similar: the sense of the sacred. Pruyser[5] noted that nearly everyone has some sense of the sacred, the awareness that there is something holy, beyond the human realm, if asked the question: does anything give you a sense of awe and reverence? Some will describe overtly religious experiences. Others speak of nature, music, art, or of some aspect of human relationships such as love, fidelity or trust.

A cardiologist told me that as a young man he became so fascinated with the intricate functioning of the cardiopulmonary system that he had no choice but to become a heart specialist. He said he could only imagine a divine nature at work to create such a marvellous system to support life. Another patient told me in great detail, with awe and gratitude, about his visit to Israel. It was his lifelong dream to visit the holy sites of his religion but he had put it off until his neurologist advised him to do what was important while he was still able. Another patient described a new interest in listening to birds on his deck in the mornings. Before he had ALS he had neither the time nor the interest to notice the life of nature around him. Now each morning he felt accompanied by all of life.

In experiences of awe, reverence and transcendence people touch what is sacred to them and feel a connection beyond that of the body. Such experiences are not merely a resource to help someone to live with illness, but a way of living more deeply with more satisfaction than before.

Faith

The word faith is often used to describe something static, an intellectual idea, a doctrine, or an allegiance to a particular set of beliefs. We say, 'I have faith (believe) in God' or 'She is of the Moslem faith.' But faith also describes something much more dynamic. Faith is a person's stance toward life. It refers to the motivating force within a person, to what drives them and nourishes them to continue. The theologian Paul Tillich spoke of faith as 'the courage to be'.[7] Faith is also related to trust and confidence. I asked a patient about her faith:

I have faith in God that he will take care of me. God always takes care of us and it's always through others and their kindness. In my life I have tried to do the same for others because I know that God works through me for their sake. So now it's important to trust. I have to trust that my husband and daughter will continue to be there for me. The aides who come to help us each morning and night, I have to trust them. There is a lesson here for me somewhere and I will have to learn it. My faith gets stronger every time I see someone reaching out to me.

Another patient described how he looked within himself for the courage to continue. His children and his wife wanted him to live as long as possible. Despite his discouragement and fatigue he tried to continue for them. He said he was not religious but felt perfectly natural praying for courage. I asked to whom he prayed.

To whatever force there is beyond us. I don't think we have to know all about it in order to pray. After all, we got here without asking to be born, so there's a force somewhere that carries us along.

Thankfulness and grace

Religions describe life as something received which points to a transcendent other from which we come. There is an unmerited quality to life, reflected in celebrations of thanksgiving, prayers of gratitude, requests for divine help, or rituals, which enact the receiving of goodness from beyond ourselves. Religions cultivate gratitude and underpin the experience of grace. Grace is the experience of receiving what one did not earn or could not merit only because of the generosity of another. One may experience grace when receiving a gift, when granted a reprieve, or even when waking up, taking the next breath, or moving forward to the next moment.

Illness can make it difficult for one to experience thankfulness or grace. ALS appears to strike in a random and unmerited way: there is nothing one could have done to have caused it and one may feel unfairly singled out for mistreatment. Grace is challenged by such an illness and can easily be replaced by resentment. Yet some patients maintain and express a sense of thankfulness about life in spite of their illness. A dignified orthodox Jewish man demonstrates how gratitude can be a spiritual strength.

When I come here I really am reminded that life is a gift. I have had 70 very good years. I am not happy to be sick but I am 70 and I look around me and see others of 30 or 40 with this disease, and I cannot help but think I blessed I am to have had 70 years of health and happiness! Some people have said to me that this is not fair. You know, in fact, it's more than fair to me. I did nothing to deserve a longer life than some of these others around me, and I can only be grateful that I have lived so well.

He was not always positive, becoming sad and withdrawn for long periods and expressing frustration at his declining abilities. But at his core he remained thankful, expressing this to God in his daily prayers and in more concrete ways to the people around him. The smallest act of kindness from his wife, his children, his friends and colleagues, or professionals in the hospital received a word of thanks, a nod of appreciation, or sometimes a written note. This thankfulness was a spiritual resource that helped him to cope until the end and sometimes compensated for his other moods.

Another patient, age 60, had lived a life of illness and hardship even before being diagnosed with ALS. He struggled with the question of fairness: 'Why me?' He asked, 'When will I get a break?' He complained often about health services and seemed unappreciative of the efforts of others. This was not new on his part, but it added to his isolation and loneliness.

Then a strange thing happened after the first few years of a slowly progressing illness. As he became increasingly dependent he also came into frequent contact with other patients, some more debilitated than he was. Two of the patients that he befriended were very kind to him. But their illness progressed more quickly than his and they both died. He began to ask: 'Why am I still here when they are not?' 'How could they be so kind to me when they were going faster?' He had a kind of subtle transformation over time and began to be more at peace. One day he said:

I was pretty angry about being sick. But this is not the worst illness I have lived with in my life. I've been sick many times with more pain and difficulty than this. I guess I'm one of the lucky ones if you could call it that. Five years and I'm still here. I never thought I'd be around to get acquainted with my grandchildren. And now that I'm retired I've got time to spend with them.

Gratitude can take curious twists and turns and we are wise to seize a moment of grace, however it arrives.

Guilt, forgiveness and change

When one is suddenly faced with a foreshortened future, time becomes precious and the past looms large. Coming to terms with the past sometimes feels urgent. In the literature about dying it is common to speak about 'life review'. As people review what was good about their lives they inevitably uncover regrets. It is important that these regrets find some expression and relief, but people may also wish to make changes and live differently in the time that remains.

Repentance, literally to turn again, is a basic spiritual need of human beings. This capacity to regret is fundamental to making sense of one's life. Without it there is no sense of agency, of responsibility for one's actions and choices. Viktor Frankl wrote in his book[8] about life in a concentration camp, how important it is to choose one's actions, even when the range of one's possible choices are extremely limited. The ultimate choice even if facing death, he wrote, is to choose how to think about it.

Religious traditions take the freedom and responsibility of being human seriously. Even if ultimate powers are attributed to God or to higher beings, human beings bear responsibility for their actions and choices. Through rituals of confession, acts of atonement, or prayers for forgiveness, religions create mechanisms to acknowledge guilt, regrets and remorse, and provide avenues to be freed of one's past errors.

To be sure, religion is not always at its best when dealing with guilt, forgiveness and repentance and many people have turned from religion precisely because of an overemphasis on these themes. But if religions have not handled these themes well, secular culture has not done much better.

We live in a time when the shifting of blame and responsibility away from oneself is considered normal. From the highest political leaders down through every level of society we have developed the skill of pointing away from oneself and denying responsibility. At a spiritual level we pay a high price by feeling less than fully alive and connected on one hand, or by living under the burden of regret on the other.

As one nears the end of life with a diminished capacity for independent action, this issue often surfaces as a powerful spiritual need. One patient had spent his entire life at the office and made a mountain of money. It is a classic story. When his two daughters were young he was rarely home. As young adults they were angry and distant coming to him only to ask for money. Now at 55 he had been diagnosed with ALS. A moment of repentance arrived, not because of a revelation from above nor out of religious conviction, but because his 27-year-old daughter, who had just given birth to her second child, confronted him in anger.

You have another chance. You were never there for us; you can be there for your grandchildren. They need to know you and you have no more excuse because you're home all the time! Don't blow it!

The patient told me this story with tears in his eyes and a shy smile on his face as his daughter sat beaming beside him. She visits him three times a week with both of her children. 'You know what?' he said, 'My grandchildren don't even care that I can't walk!' Facing the past led to peace in the present and three generations were healed in this one moment. Most stories are less dramatic and many do not end with such resolution, but it is important that people have a chance to express their regrets in words or in actions.

Belonging

Belonging is less about which religious group someone is part of it than it is about the sense of connectedness one feels to others, to the world, to life itself. Fleischman suggests that to understand a person one must ask the question, 'Of what whole is this person a part?' Though the answer will vary widely the importance of that question is the same.

Human beings need 'a place inside of, and an orientation to, history. This need to overcome one's individual skin, one's isolation and fragmentariness, to have a group, an affiliation, a community, can be called a need for membership'.[3]

This need may be met through participation in a religion, membership in a political party, identification with culture, language, an ethnic group, or it may be through bonds of family, neighborhood, or colleagues.

One of the most disturbing aspects of ALS is that it separates the patient from the community, the group, the whole to which he or she belongs. Isolation as a result of progressive paralysis and immobility, loss of communicative abilities, and increasing dependence lead to isolation from former groups. When one loses the sense of belonging and 'membership' one's inner integrity and wholeness is challenged. Who am I when stripped of my relational and role identities, my participation with others and the mutuality of giving and receiving? An elderly patient described the inability to eat and the loss of speech as the two worst losses he had endured because of ALS. They were more difficult than the loss of his mobility and more upsetting than the thought of dying. He had been an intensely social man, involved in business, community groups, volunteering in several associations and as a leader in his congregation. His extended family was accustomed to long, happy hours around the table each week. Though adequately nourished through a PEG, he now found it too painful to be present while others ate and drank. He found it unbearable to be present in his former community groups since he could no longer respond to people verbally. The loss of belonging was an attack on his self-esteem and identity. He maintained his sense of belonging as well as he could by seeing a few of his former colleagues individually in his home, but it was a sad compromise.

It is important to notice what aspects of belonging are lost for a patient and to look for ways to maintain or replace them when possible. One ventilated patient developed complications and was hospitalized for an extended period of time while awaiting placement for long-term care. Though able to communicate only through eye blinking, small hand movements, and a letter board, she developed a remarkable circle around her, of nurses, volunteers, housekeeping staff and others. The staff became so attached to her that they held a party when she was finally transferred some months later. Every staff member who had cared for her signed the goodbye gift, hand made by one of the nurses. One wonders if it was only her own needs that were being met, or if she was also touching the need for belonging in the staff.

Hope

In medicine hope is often linked to prognosis, which is to say, hope for survival and a longer life. By contrast, religions speak of hope beyond this life: salvation, heaven, or nirvana. What do patients hope for when they know that they will eventually die of ALS? Some continue to hope for a cure or a miracle, but most let go of this fairly soon. Others hope for salvation beyond this life. Surprisingly, even religious people are less focused on this hope than one might expect. As the disease progresses and people begin to adjust a diminished physical state, we hear them hope more in the immediate sense: for comfort, dignity, intimacy, or for daily satisfactions. Some hope for the completion of projects or to live long enough to participate in a particular event.

One of our patients was 33 at the time of diagnosis. Warm and personable, he talked openly with the staff about his losses and his hopes. His life's hope was to be a father and raise children. He had been married only a year at the time he entered the clinic and his wife was pregnant with their first child. Shattered by the diagnosis, it was especially difficult when he realized that the disease was progressing rapidly. But within a few months he regained his determination to live. His sights were focused entirely on the pregnancy and the coming birth of their first child. 'I will be there for my wife when this baby is born' he told me. 'I must be there. Pray that I will live until this child knows me.' He did live for nearly nine months after his child's birth. Though he could no longer speak, his whole face lit up as his wife showed photos to the clinic staff and talked about their baby.

Some hopes look further into the future. The Buddhist patient mentioned earlier found hope in the teachings about reincarnation and the practice of mediation. They have helped her to adapt to illness and to be less afraid of dying. She believes she will be reincarnated and continue her development in another form.

At the beginning you just hope that they are wrong about the diagnosis and that you will discover that you don't have ALS after all. Gradually, after enough symptoms come and they don't go away, you start to realize that its true and you will have to deal with it. Then you start hoping they will find a cure. In time you realize that it will be too late, and that this is going to be your life until the end. Then you can hope in something more after this life and that is the real hope.

She explained how meditation, cultivating peace, showing compassion and living without inner conflict would help her be peaceful at the time of dying. This peacefulness will allow her next life to be at a higher plane. She meditates several times a day to achieve this peace. In spite of her losses, the difficulties of daily life with ALS, and a shortened future, there is a genuine joyfulness about her. She faces physical changes with a certain calm acceptance. Hope based on her spiritual life is a strength for living in the here and now.

Near the end hope can take a different form. It is sometimes heard in the longing for death as release from dependency, discomfort, or from the trials of life in a body that no longer moves or breathes on its own. People express hopefulness related to how they will die. 'I don't want to be alone at the end,' one says. 'I want to go before my family is exhausted from caring for me,' another. Those who have religious or spiritual ideas about an afterlife often turn to them near the end. A Roman Catholic patient hospitalized with pneumonia expressed this simply: 'I'm tired and I've had enough. Can you ask the priest to come?' In his way he was looking forward with hope.

Vocation

The young father to be was determined to live long enough to know his child. This sense of purpose motivated him not only to survive but also to be involved with his wife in the preparations for their new arrival. It gave him hope and a new identity to replace the one he was losing.

When a person becomes a patient and is faced with the loss of work, social role and parental responsibilities, there is a deep crisis of identity. It is a spiritual crisis as well as a psychological one, touching not only identity but the very meaning of life. People ask, 'Why am I here?' 'Who needs me?' and 'What must I do?' In traditional religious terms these questions defined one's vocation or calling. There is something one is meant to do. Doing so fulfils both an inward need and an outward one: the needs of someone else. Without this sense of vocation there is an emptiness and a loss of connection (belonging) with others.

A physician who was diagnosed with ALS continued to practice until the last moment possible. Near the end of his practice he could no longer use his hands. Attached to a teaching hospital, he counted on the residents in his charge to conduct physical exams, to take blood pressures and to carry out treatments, while he looked on as supervisor. His patients appreciated his continued presence, trusting in his experience and knowledge of their cases and feeling that he cared about them. The crowd at his funeral was a sea of former patients, their families, former students and colleagues who spoke proudly of how he had touched their lives.

Another patient, a college instructor for 20 years, found the most difficult loss to be ending his career on disability. He could no longer function at the university because of his lack of strength but he found the days at home interminable. He was depressed and withdrawn until a neighbour, an elementary school teacher, convinced him to accept two of her students as a tutor. He met those two, then more until his schedule was full, meeting one or two students every afternoon to help with their reading, maths and history lessons. His depression lifted and he spoke with satisfaction about his renewed vocation.

Acceptance of death

One of our basic needs is to make sense of our own end. Related to the need for belonging, one strives to see how their arrival and their passing fits into the order of things. Related to vocation, one looks to know if their mission is complete. I have saved this issue for the end, not because of the obvious chronology of things, but because there is a tendency to think of religion and spirituality as concerned primarily with death. While religions do have ways of addressing death, neither religion nor spirituality is focused there. Religion seeks to structure common meanings for the life of a people. Within religion the reality of death is lifted up to underscore the precious and sacred nature of life itself. Because we die, life is limited and must be valued. Spirituality, whether separate from or part of religion, is involved in deepening one's awareness and connection to daily life. It is about living more fully, more deeply until the end. Realizing one's finitude, the present time becomes precious.

Many people have observed that paradoxically, in coming to terms with death, they are then free to live more fully. The wise old professor with ALS says to his student in the book *Tuesdays with Morrie*: 'Learn how to die, and you learn how to live.'[9] He explains how knowing that he might die any day leads one to paying attention to the spiritual: loving relationships, the universe, the things we take for granted. He continues to explain how, being confined to his room, he appreciates the window more than his student, who can get up and go outside at will.

Patients describe this paradoxical truth again and again. The man who earlier described his new-found appreciation for the singing of the birds also spoke of being a better father since becoming ill. Previously he had little patience for the concerns of his three teenaged children. Now less distracted by his worries about work and money, and finding himself at home with enormous amounts of free time, he took an interest in his children's days and in their preoccupations. Realizing he was slowly losing them, none of the small matters that had previously irritated him were important. 'I can listen to them for hours!' he said. 'I'm just so happy to have them around and that they will sit and talk with me!'

Not all patients come to an acceptance of death and not all learn from its approach, but many do. In the process some need to discuss how the end will arrive for them. Some are fearful of suffocation, of choking to death, or of dying alone. They need to be reassured of how their care will be provided and of their power to make choices at the end. In my experience, concerns about assisted suicide or about having life artificially prolonged often point to a need to communicate about how death will come and what it will mean. Patients need to know that their rights and wishes will be respected and they may need to find some reassurance that they are still valuable as human beings.

Some simply need to talk about dying with someone who does not turn away from the subject. To listen patiently and without reaction communicates to the patient that we are not fearful about what is happening to them and that we believe they are capable of living all the way into that mystery which is death. Listening demonstrates that we believe in the strength that lies within them to face their own end. 'In the end, to accept the spiritual dimension of the other is to have confidence in what the other is becoming.'[6] Conversations about dying nearly always open a door to the spiritual. When facing death, Fleischman writes:

The least religious or superstitious persons will still feel themselves to be in the presence of an unknown. A door opens. Both the dying and those with them, who do not close off in fear, feel deepening love, and life itself never feels more ephemeral and indomitable.[3]

Indeed, as witnesses to the final days, we are put in touch with just how 'ephemeral and indomitable' life is. I was particularly moved and instructed by one patient whom I had followed for several years. A few weeks before his death he related to me what had happened at their synagogue the week prior. The rabbi had invited him to come forward to read from the Torah in honor of the couple's fiftieth wedding anniversary. He was surprised and embarrassed at first, knowing that he could no longer speak and could barely walk with assistance. But he dutifully went to the front with the help of his son and his grandson. He was surprised again as his grandson lifted the Torah and announced, 'Today I will read from the Torah in honor of my grandfather who taught me his faith.' His grandson had completed his bar mitzvah just a few weeks earlier, symbolizing his entrance into the faith as an adult.

In these few moments were captured the fulfilment of vocation, belonging, an encounter with the sacred and a sense of order. It was also a moment of preparation for his death. As he repeated the story he wrote at the bottom of his pad, 'Something is finished. I can go in peace.' A few weeks later he died.

Spiritual care as accompaniment

Spirituality is to 'take one more step.' Take one more step in accepting my fatigue, in accepting my limits, the limit of my intelligence, of my lack of understanding in the face of suffering ... to take one more step with or without belonging to a religion. . . . To be spiritual is simply, wherever one is, to take another step. To accompany then is to help the other person to do just that, in the midst of their suffering, at the heart of who they are...

One who offers spiritual accompaniment is therefore someone who can accompany this 'restarting' and encourage that opening, while helping the other to avoid stopping at their symptoms and identifying with them.[6]

I met the patients mentioned above in the ALS outpatient clinic of a neurological hospital in Canada. My role there is pastoral counsellor, chaplain (the traditional terms) or spiritual care provider. The field of pastoral care is evolving as the population continues to diversify and become more secular and as needs are increasingly identified as spiritual rather than religious. In our context the spiritual care provider is a non-denominational, clinical member of the multidisciplinary health care team.

This necessitates a clinical approach by those providing spiritual care. A clinical approach means that contacts with patients are interventions whose goals are therapeutic and supportive. It assumes that these interventions are not partisan or biased toward the religious or spiritual point of view of the clinician. It assumes that one has adequate clinical training in addition to a background in theological or religious studies. To take a clinical approach means to respect the patient's beliefs and values and to view them with certain objectivity. The clinician must consider how a particular aspect of the patient's spiritual life might contribute to health or to illness and how it might be a factor in treatment decisions.

Participation on the team also encourages all members of the multidisciplinary team to be aware of the patient's spiritual values. In the same way that the contributions of the social worker encourage the team's awareness of social needs, conversations about the spiritual beliefs and practices of the patient brings them into focus. The whole team is invited to view the patient somewhat differently. Marie de Hennezel writes about the importance of health care professionals 'welcoming' the spiritual needs of the patient.

The 'spiritual request' is rarely formulated as such, but it is nearly always present, because it is actually the request to be recognized as a person, with all his mystery and his depth. This request is not addressed to 'spiritual specialists'; it is addressed to every human encountered:
You who cares for me or who accompanies me, how do you see me? Am I reduced to a broken body wasting away? What value or what meaning do you place on the time that remains for me to live?[6]

The patient examples discussed above illustrate some of the ways that spiritual issues emerge during treatment of ALS and the important impact that they can have on the quality of life. We noted that spiritual issues can emerge in three ways: as a resource to the patient; as an area of conflict or suffering; or in the search for meaning while nearing the end of life. These three suggest the kinds of intervention to be offered by the spiritual care provider in the relationship of accompaniment.

When spirituality is a resource, the clinician's goal is to strengthen and support what is already present. The Buddhist patient described earlier finds support and encouragement in discussing her practices of meditation and how they offer her inner peace. In addition, it is important that the team understand this as a core value for her, which impacts on both her decisions and how she feels about dying.

When spiritual beliefs create conflict for the patient, the spiritual care specialist seeks to play a therapeutic role. The goal of the intervention is the resolution of conflict, to the degree that it is possible, so the patient will not have the burden of spiritual pain added to their physical problems. The orthodox Jewish man mentioned above had previously never missed a day of saying the traditional prayers aloud morning and evening. This gave him peace, comfort, purpose and a sense of belonging. But when his voice became too weak to pray aloud he was in a spiritual crisis. His family, his rabbi, and the clinic staff all minimized the importance of this (it seemed obvious he could simply pray in silence) but he remained troubled. As we talked (through writing) about how this affected him I discovered that it was a deep source of shame. His own father had always said the prayers aloud, even on the day of his death. Not only did this connect him to his father and ancestors, but it also fulfilled a duty, praying aloud as a daily witness to his children and grandchildren. The importance of this loss had to be fully understood and recognized before he could move beyond this particular grief and be at peace with silent prayers.

In other situations the spiritual care specialist is engaged in an exploration of the meaning of what is happening to the patient. This is not to find the cause, but to deepen the experience of life, even in the midst of serious illness, by finding meaning and connecting this moment to the rest of life. The man who talked of listening to the birds on his deck each morning also observed that he had a new interest in his children. 'I'd rather have come to this without getting sick' he said, 'but maybe it took getting sick for me to become a real father. It sounds strange but actually I'm happier than I was a few years ago.' This was a spiritual discovery. However long or short his life, each day has more meaning than before.

This brief review of spiritual issues present in patients with ALS illustrates the importance of spiritual care as an integrated part of the multidisciplinary team. Of course there is a role for clinically trained spiritual care specialists. More importantly there is a need for all who are involved with treatment to be attentive to the spiritual meanings expressed by our patients: to be present, to listen, to respect and recognize the inner importance of what each one is living until the last moment.

Notes

The names and identifying data of all persons described have been altered to protect their anonymity. Most are composites of several patients who expressed similar experiences.

References

1. Fuller R. C. (2005) Spiritual but not religious. Accessed 27 August 2005. Available at http://www.beliefnet.com/story/109/story_10958_1.html.
2. Smith H., Lesser E. (2001) Letters from the heart. Accessed 27 August 2005. Available at http://www.spiritualityhealth.com/Nmagazine/issue.php?id=36.
3. Fleischman P. (1989) *The Healing Zone*. New York: Paragon House.
4. Hiltner S. (1958) Preface to *Pastoral Theology*, pp. 98–113. Nashville: Abingdon.
5. Pruyser P. M. (1976) *Guidelines for Pastoral diagnosis. The Minister as Diagnostician*, pp. 60-79. Philadelphia, PA: Westminster Press.
6. de Hennezel M., Leloup J-Y. (1997) *L'art de mourir*, p. 40. Paris: Editions Robert Laffont. English translation of this and subsequent texts cited here are by Robert Lambert.
7. Tillich P. (1952) *The Courage to Be*. New Haven, CT: Yale University Press.
8. Frankl V. (1984) *Man's Search for Meaning: An Introduction to Logotherapy*. New York: Simon and Schuster.
9. Albom M. (1997) *Tuesdays with Morrie*. New York: Doubleday.

Chapter 7a

Multidisciplinary care:

physiotherapy

Ulrike Hammerbeck and Alison Garrett

Summary

The physiotherapist has an important role within the multidisciplinary team in the assessment and management of mobility issues, spasticity, pain, the provision of aids, such as collars and splints, and in respiratory care. The aim of this intervention is to facilitate the provision of person-centred care, allowing the quality of life to be as good as possible. 'The rehabilitation of these patients can be as rewarding as any other difficult mission in medicine if health care providers will regard these patients as individuals living with, rather than dying from, their disease.'[1]

Introduction

The physiotherapist, as part of the multidisciplinary team, plays an important role in the care of the patient with amyotrophic lateral sclerosis (ALS). Progressive weakness can be one of the major causes of discomfort for patients with the disease and as the individual's exercise tolerance gradually decreases localized weakness becomes apparent.[2] The presentation and progression of ALS varies significantly according to the site and extent of motor neuron damage in the nervous system: therefore management has to be tailored to the specific needs of every individual.

The initial physiotherapy assessment will establish the individual's need by demonstrating their current impairments as well as any restrictions in activity and participation, and will highlight all treatable aspects of the disease.[1] The findings will provide important information to assist the multidisciplinary team in coordinating care and can be used to predict and monitor progression at the re-assessment stage and throughout the course of the disease. The assessment will focus on the musculoskeletal system with regards to muscle length, power and tone and joint range of movement (ROM) as well as respiratory function, activity levels and fatigue. It will highlight any difficulties an individual experiences with mobility and activities of daily living as well as their perceived limitations.

The findings from the initial assessment enable the therapist to assist the patient in setting treatment goals. This ensures a person-centred approach, promotes autonomy and should give the patient a sense of control.[3,4,5] The goals will enable the physiotherapist to plan an appropriate, comprehensive and meaningful rehabilitation programme.[1] In the initial stages of the disease, therapy goals may be aimed at optimizing function and independence: with further disease progression the goals may change to focus on maintaining functional mobility, muscle length and ultimately, maximization of quality of life.[4]

Physiotherapy intervention in conjunction with the multidisciplinary team is aimed at:

+ Maintaining independence and maximizing quality of life
+ Advice and provision of an exercise programme to increase exercise tolerance and fitness
+ Maintenance of the musculoskeletal system in terms of ROM and muscle strength
+ Fatigue management
+ Maintaining mobility
+ Comfort and positioning
+ Prevention and treatment of respiratory complications
+ Pain relief.

A crucial role for the multidisciplinary team is to ensure that the individual with ALS is in contact with their appropriate local agencies. Liaison within the team and a thorough assessment will ensure this. Well coordinated, multidisciplinary care will enhance the health of the individual, increase lifespan and improve their quality of life.[1,3,6]

Throughout the course of the disease different physiotherapy settings will be more appropriate depending on the individual's levels of mobility and function. Consideration should be given to what setting is most beneficial to the patient and may be determined by factors such as ease of access, available expertise and multidisciplinary input. The patient's intervention path could therefore lead from treatment in the outpatient physiotherapy department into the community or hospice. Consistent and close collaboration with the wheelchair service is of great importance as the positioning needs of clients with ALS can change quite rapidly and they will need to be reviewed regularly.

Exercise in ALS

The general benefits of exercise are well recognized.[7] These include:

+ Increased efficiency of muscles
+ Increased endurance
+ Reduced fatigue levels
+ Improvement in aerobic capacity
+ Improved psychological well-being
+ Minimize cardiovascular disease development.

Additional benefits of training for clients with neurological problems may include a reduction in spasticity, and a reduction of pain from musculoskeletal origin.[8]

The role of exercise in neuromuscular disease, however, is a topic of debate. Some earlier literature advised against exercising neurologically weakened muscles, based on case reports of the development of overuse weakness following vigorous activity in patients with progressive neuromuscular conditions.[9,10] Thus, strenuous physical activity was not advised in this client group as little was known about its effect on the motor neurons. It has been hypothesized that the physiological by-products of exercise may contribute to the degeneration of the vulnerable motor neurons through increased exposure to neurotoxins.[11]

This view has been challenged by many authors who have conducted studies on exercise in patients with ALS and other neuromuscular disorders. In 1996, Wright *et al.*[12] looked at a 12-week aerobic walking programme in patients with slowly progressive neuromuscular diseases (this study did not include clients with ALS). They wanted to see how diseased skeletal muscle responded to exercise, and looked at maximal and submaximal cardiovascular, respiratory and work capacity variables. They found a positive training effect in five out of eight subjects, with no subjective indication of overwork weakness.[12]

Two studies investigated whether moderate or high resistance exercise is more beneficial in clients with slowly progressive neuromuscular disease.[9,10] The results found the moderate resistance programme of greater benefit than high-resistance training, with significant gains in strength after 12 weeks of concentric muscle training. One negative finding was possible overuse fatigue of the elbow flexors with eccentric high-resistance work.[9]

New research is looking at the effects of exercise in the transgenic mouse population, where mice have a *SOD-1* gene mutation form of ALS. The authors found that transgenic mice undergoing therapy with insulin-like growth factor-1 had a longer lifespan if they exercised regularly whilst receiving gene therapy, suggesting that physical activity may actually enhance the therapeutic effect of this treatment.[13]

Liebetanz et al.[14] also found survival times to be longer in an exercising population of transgenic mice than that of the sedentary group, with no detrimental effect from vigorous exercise.

Therefore, exercise of the right kind, and at the correct time during the course of the disease might be beneficial in ALS. Evidence exists to support this in mice experiments[14] but further research is required in the human population. Individual programmes will need to be designed for the patient according to their ability and fatigue levels, but a few basic principles should be adhered to.

Points to consider when prescribing exercise to patients with ALS

- ◆ Moderate rather than maximal strength training[9,10]
- ◆ Care with eccentric strengthening of muscles[9]
- ◆ Cardiovascular (CV) training three times a week – moderate CV work[12]
- ◆ Strength training is not recommended in muscles which are less than 10% of maximum strength[15]
- ◆ May reduce spasticity[8]
- ◆ May not affect pain levels[8]
- ◆ Resistance training is not proven to affect Activities of Daily Living[10]
- ◆ May reduce fatigue.[8]

Tone management

ALS is an unusual neurological condition in which patients may present with both increased and decreased muscle tone due to the progressive loss of both upper and lower motor neurons.[16]

The upper motor neuron (UMN) consists of the neurons which form the descending tracts travelling from the brain through the spinal cord and control the lower motor neurons. Loss of the upper motor neurons can lead to hyperreflexia and spasticity, as well as reducing the central drive onto the motor unit, resulting in weakness. Loss of the lower motor neurons (LMN) causes hyporeflexia and muscle atrophy and it has been found that this LMN loss has the greatest effect on muscle weakness.[16] Most individuals with ALS will encounter spasticity at some point during the course of the disease, whereas all will have progressive LMN symptoms.[17]

Spasticity

Literature on the management of spasticity in ALS is scarce, with only one randomized controlled trial available.[17] Thus most of the following information has been extrapolated from literature on the management of spasticity in other neurological conditions and opinions from experts in the field of ALS regarding medication.

The medical management of spasticity, in general terms, consists of the use of centrally acting anti-spasmodic agents such as benzodiazepines, baclofen, tizanidine, and dantrolene,[18] given either in oral or intrathecal form. Such systemic agents, although efficacious in other patient groups, have a known side-effect of causing muscle weakness. Thus in patients with ALS, where muscle weakness is often the primary symptom, they need to be administered with care. There was a favourable case report in 1999 on the use of an intrathecal baclofen pump to treat a patient with ALS, who had intractable spasticity, with claims that after pump insertion the client was able to walk unaided and climb stairs, compared with only mobilizing a few steps before intervention.[19] Another case report on the use of gabapentin to treat spasticity in two patients with ALS found that in uncontrolled observations, both patients had positive functional gains from using gabapentin compared with conventional anti-spasticity agents.[18]

To avoid systemic side-effects from anti-spasticity medications, focal spasticity has been successfully treated in recent years with botulinum toxin, which is now licensed for use in specific pathologies. It may be useful for treating isolated spastic muscles which may otherwise shorten and lead to joint contractures.[20]

The physiotherapeutic management of spasticity consists of positioning and posture management, splinting, orthotic use and maintenance of muscle length and ROM.

Repetitive ROM exercises have been shown to have a positive effect on the reduction of spasticity.[21] Drory *et al.*[8] also found that active ROM exercises significantly reduced spasticity as measured by the Ashworth scale after three months.

Lower motor neuron signs

Features of lower motor neuron dysfunction are evident in patients with ALS, as it is a disease that affects the anterior horn cells and thereby causes LMN impairment. The features of LMN dysfunction include: muscle atrophy, muscle weakness, fasciculations, hypotonia and cramps. The extremities are usually the first areas to be affected by this LMN loss, and thus the feet and hands may require early therapeutic management to maintain their functional use as long as possible.

Orthotics, splinting and collars

In the upper limb, weakness may cause joint hypermobility and secondary subluxation, particularly at the wrist and shoulder girdle.[11] Shoulder slings, collar and cuff, strapping techniques and other supports are available for attempts to support the shoulder and prevent traction injuries.[22] The effectiveness of each needs to be assessed individually, based on its fit and the stability it will provide. It is possible to splint the hand to support the medial and longitudinal arches in order to assist grip strength and function by improving thumb opposition.[1] Splints can be fabricated with Soft Cast™ by

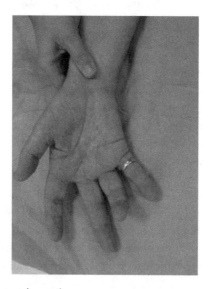

Fig. 7a.1 Hand with muscle wasting.

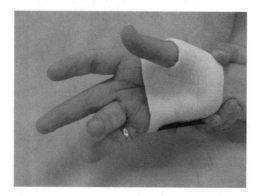

Fig. 7a.2 Soft-cast splint.

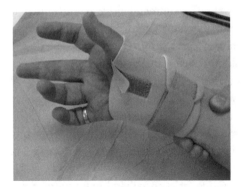

Fig. 7a.3 Neoprene splint.

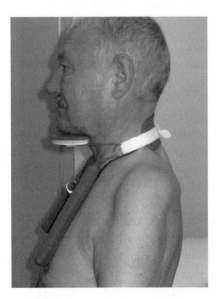

Fig. 7a.4 Example of a collar.

an experienced therapist. Off-the-shelf neoprene wrist splints can also be useful to assist with thumb opposition.

Orthotics may assist in maintaining mobility for clients suffering from foot drop in the early to mid stages of the disease. An ankle foot orthosis (AFO) is commonly prescribed to help correct this problem by holding the weakened ankle in dorsiflexion when mobilizing and preventing the client from tripping and falling during gait.[1,23] Due to the progressive nature of ALS orthotic departments often prioritize these referrals. Other off-the-shelf or fabricated orthoses are available if recommended by an orthotist, but there is limited literature on the use of orthotics in the ALS population.

Progressive weakness can also affect the neck muscles: this becomes most evident after prolonged periods of being upright, resulting in an inability to hold the head up against gravity. Different collars can be useful to maintain head position and prevent muscle fatigue. A simple soft collar can be sufficient but pressure on anterior structures can increase the shortness of breath that is caused by inspiratory muscle weakness. The two most frequently used collars are the Headmaster™ and SALT™ collars (see Figure 7a.4). The Motor Neurone Disease Association also provides information on their web site (www.mndas-sosciation.org) on a wide variety of collars but for more complex lateral instabil-ities custom made collars may be more appropriate. Collars can be used for the largest part of the waking day or for shorter periods, for example in the car.[11,24]

Mobility

The maintenance of mobility is an important factor for all patients with ALS. The independence achieved through mobility is an indicator of quality of life and perceived well-being.[11,25] As mobility becomes more difficult and the risk of falls increase, sticks, crutches, frames and rollators can aid the individual and maintain safety when walking.[1] There is no definitive time frame in the progres-sion of the disease as to when mobility may be affected, so it is up to the individual clinician to determine at what stage intervention is required. Early consideration and discussion of walking aids will help with acceptance of these when pro-vision becomes necessary.[2] Environmental adaptations might be needed to enable independence at home, for example rails, ramps or a stair lift, and referral to an occupational therapist is essential for the most appropriate advice.

With further deterioration of mobility or increased upper limb weakness, transfers between surfaces will become more difficult. It is therefore essential that the carer is educated with regards to manual handling policies when assisting with these. Transfers can be aided by the use of sliding boards and if more assistance is needed, a hoist may be indicated.[11] There are a variety of hoists available and an occupational therapist will be able to advise on the most appropriate type.

Early referral to wheelchair services is vital because wheelchair prescription is required for almost all patients with ALS and users report increased ability to interact in the community.[26] Wheelchair provision can be perceived as a negative milestone, thus sensitivity needs to be exercised when broaching the subject. Wheelchair use can also play an important role in energy conserva-tion.[1,24] Wheelchairs can be used intermittently for community access or as the main seating and positioning option during the day. A wide variety of wheelchairs are available and the needs of the individual will determine the specific wheelchair prescribed. Because of the sometimes rapid progression of ALS, frequent reassessments will aid the provision of the most appropriate seating option.[1] The chair can vary from a lightweight self-propelling chair to, in the later stages of the disease, an attendant-propelled, reclining chair with a head rest, pressure-relieving cushion, lateral trunk supports and arm rests. Good posture in the chair can help to minimize respiratory distress and achieve optimal pressure relief.[11] Electric wheelchairs with various environmental controls are also available and provide users with greater independence and an improved sense of well-being.[26]

Respiratory management

All people with ALS will experience respiratory muscle weakness at some stage during disease progression.[6] To compensate for the muscle weakness, accessory muscles are used to maintain sufficient oxygenation levels and the breathing pattern is altered.[23] A reduction of physical activity will lead to decreased airflow through the lung fields and progressive inspiratory and expiratory muscle weakness will lead to reduced chest expansion. During the night, when the respiratory drive is lower, the changed breathing patterns are more evident and will result in morning headaches; this is an early sign of respiratory failure.[1] Non-invasive positive pressure ventilation (NIPPV), is an adjunct used to assist ventilation that relieves shortness of breath, improves the quality of life and may also extend the lives of patients with this disease[27,28] (see Chapter 4a). Respiratory failure is a major cause of morbidity and mortality in this client group because it can result in airway obstruction, aspiration, pneumonia and repeated hospital admissions.[29-32]

In individuals with ALS the swallowing mechanism can be impaired. This increases the risk of aspiration and thereby the necessity to cough to maintain the airway.[30] The risk of aspiration can be minimized by close collaboration with the speech and language therapist to establish the difficulties experienced and provide advice on safe swallowing, as well as information on what consistency food should be in order to prevent aspiration.[11]

Weak respiratory muscles and poor function of the glottis will result in a reduced ability to create sufficient pressure prior to and sufficient force during a cough, to effectively clear the secretions.[30] The weak cough can be optimized and made more effective by using an assisted cough manoeuvre.[6,33] Contra-indications to this manoeuvre are a paralytic ileus, internal abdominal damage, a bleeding gastric ulcer and rib fractures.[34]

Self-assisted cough

The patient uses his upper limbs to assist or replace the weak abdominal muscles. One forearm is placed flat against the stomach, below the ribs, and the other hand is crossed over it. As the individual initiates the cough he presses with the forearm in and up to push the diaphragm up and create the necessary pressures for an effective cough. If the upper limbs are not strong enough for this manoeuvre a carer-assisted cough is required.

Carer-assisted cough while sitting

This follows the same principles as above and the carer positions one forearm on the stomach, just underneath the ribs and the other behind to create counter pressure. It can be helpful to lock the fingers on the opposite side. The flat aspect of the forearm is used and as the cough is initiated the carer pushes in and up to assist the cough. Timing between the initiating of the cough by the patient and the pressure of the carer is crucial to achieve an effective cough (see Figure 7a.5).

Carer-assisted cough while supine

The same principles apply as described above. The carer now uses their forearm to mimic the action of the abdominal muscles in one of two ways, as demonstrated below using both forearms to push up and in or by placing both hands under the ribs and pushing up and in when the cough is initiated (see Figure 7a.6).

Physiotherapy intervention in the case of respiratory failure due to an opportunist infection should be aimed at maximizing ventilation and aiding

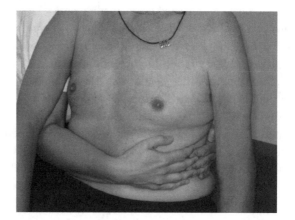

Fig. 7a.5 Carer-assisted cough while sitting.

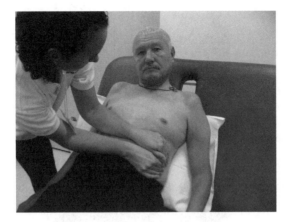

Fig. 7a.6 Carer-assisted cough in while supine.

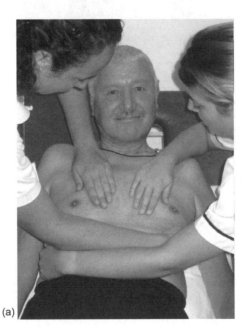

(a)

Fig. 7a.7 (a) Assisted cough with two therapists.

the removal of secretions. Various approaches can be used to optimize ventilation and promote airway clearance, for example active cycle of breathing and forced expiratory techniques. If, however, muscle weakness has advanced and an effective cough or huff is not achievable, an assisted cough will be more appropriate to aid the removal of secretions.[24] Intermittent positive

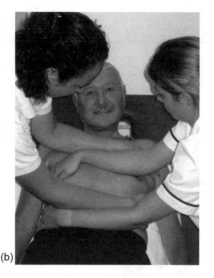

(b)

Fig. 7a.7 (b) Assisted cough with two therapists.

pressure breathing (IPPB) can be used to help prevent atelectasis and achieve a maximal inspiration when the primary problem is inspiratory muscle weakness. An assisted cough can also be used in conjunction with IPPB. For clearance of secretions modified postural drainage can be used,[11] but toleration of the positions can be difficult[24] and the intervention often proves to be too tiring for patients.[35] Suction to clear secretions is invasive and distressing and can increase shortness of breath, but is sometimes required in the acute setting.

Positioning can be important to optimize ventilation–perfusion matching during a chest infection and reclined or tilted positioning in a wheelchair can improve the alignment of the trunk and reduce shortness of breath by changing the effect gravity has on the diaphragm and abdominal mass.[11]

If the manually assisted cough is not effective, the Cough Assist Machine or mechanical insufflator/exsufflator (CoughAssist™, Emerson, Cambridge, MA) is a machine that can aid the clearance of secretions from the central airway and improve perceived quality of life.[36,37,38] Positive pressure is used to achieve maximal lung inflation followed by a sudden negative pressure to the upper airways. This procedure mimics a cough by producing more effective peak cough flows and assisting with the clearance of secretions.[35,36] To achieve adequate pressure build-up in the production of a cough some bulbar function needs to be preserved.[33,36] These machines are not currently widely available in the UK.

In case of difficulties with saliva management due to an impaired swallow mechanism the combined use of medication, e.g. Hyoscine, and home suction can be useful.[39]

Pain management

Pain is a frequent complication in ALS.[40] The pathological process of ALS does not usually cause pain, however in the later stages of the disease, progressive muscle wasting and reduced mobility can cause pain due to adverse stresses on the musculoskeletal system by poor alignment of joints and the inability to regularly change position.[2,40] Muscle cramps and spasms might also be a cause for discomfort.

Pain management is complex and may require the intervention of a doctor, physiotherapist, psychiatrist and the pain team.[40] Physiotherapy management is aimed at prevention of malalignment and contracture formation and this can be achieved by providing stretching exercises for the patient and educating the carer to perform regular passive movements. Advice on adequate support for all joints in sitting and lying is important and provision of the correct wheelchair, mobile arm supports and hospital beds may help to prevent complications. Carers need to be advised to change the position frequently to prevent pain and need education on the best manual handling techniques to prevent undue stresses on the joints during handling.[1,11]

Conclusion

Physiotherapy intervention encompasses a variety of aspects and is aimed at prevention of complications as well as symptomatic relief.[1] The treatment plan needs to be flexible to allow activities of daily life to take precedence over exercises provided by the therapist when fatigue levels need to be considered. Increasingly emphasis is placed on ensuring management should be person-centred and the client is involved and actively participates in all decision-making processes.[2,5]

As ALS is such a multifaceted disease, the involvement of the multidisciplinary team is vital to provide the most efficient care.[1,6] Research into care of the patient with ALS has increased over recent years, but further research is needed to consolidate our knowledge about the intervention we can offer.

Acknowledgements

We wish to thank Philippa Smith, Emma Willey, Professor Nigel Leigh, Jackie Anderson, Sam Prisley and Bryan Vickery for their critical revision of the manuscript.

References

1. Francis K., Bach J. R., DeLisa J. A. (1999) Evaluation and rehabilitation of patients with adult motor neuron disease. *Arch Phys Med Rehabil* **80**: 951–63.

2. Borasio G. D., Voltz R. (1997) Palliative care in amyotrophic lateral sclerosis. *J Neurol* **244** (Suppl. 4): 11–17.

3. Miller R. G., Rosenberg J. A., Gelinas D. F. *et al.* (1999) Practice parameter: The care of the patient with amyotrophic lateral sclerosis (an evidence-based review). *Neurology* **52**: 1311–23.

4. Dal Bello-Haas V., Kloos A. D., Mitsumoto H. (1998) Physical therapy for a patient through six stages of amyotrophic lateral sclerosis. *Physical Therapy* **78** (12): 1312–23.

5. NSF, Department of Health. *National Service Framework for Long-term Conditions*. Available online at http://www.dh.gov.uk/PolicyAndGuidance/HealthAndSocialCareTopics/LongTermConditions/fs/en.

6. Leigh P. N., Abrahams S., Al-Chalabi A. *et al.* (2003) The management of motor neuron disease. *J Neurol Neurosurg Psychiatry* **74** (Suppl IV): 32–47.

7. Carr J. H., Shepherd R. B. (2003) Strength training and physical conditioning. In Carr J. H., Sherpher R. B. (eds) *Stroke Rehabilitation*, pp. 233–58. Edinburgh. Butterworth-Heinemann.

8. Drory V. E., Goltsman E., Goldman Reznik J., Mosek A., Korczyn A. D. (2001) The value of muscle exercise in patients with amyotrophic lateral sclerosis. *J Neurol Sci* **191** (1&2): 133–7.

9. Kilmer D. D., McCrory W. A., Wright N. C., Aitkens S. G., Bernauer E. M. (1994) The effect of a high resistance exercise program in slowly progressive neuromuscular disease. *Arch Phys Med Rehabil* **75**: 560–63.

10. Aitkens S. G., McCroroy M. A., Kilmer D. D., Bernauer E. M. (1993) Moderate resistance exercise program: Its effect in slowly progressive neuromuscular disease. *Arch Phys Med Rehabil* **74**: 711–15.

11. Peruzzi A. C. and Potts A. (1996) Physical therapy intervention for persons with amyotrophic lateral sclerosis. *Physiotherapy Canada* **48** (2): 119–26.

12. Wright N. C., Kilmer D. D., McCrory M. A., Aitkens S. G., Holcomb B. J., Bernauer E. M. (1996). Aerobic walking in slowly progressive neuromuscular disease: Effect of a 12-week program. *Arch Phys Med Rehabil* **77**: 64–9.

13. Kaspar B. K., Frost L. M., Christian L., Umapathi P., Gage F. H. (2005) Synergy of insulin-like growth factor-1 and exercise in amyotrophic lateral sclerosis. *Ann Neurol* **57**: 649–55.

14. Liebetanz D., Hagemann K., von Lewinski F., Kahler E., Paulus W. (2004) Extensive exercise is not harmful in amyotrophic lateral sclerosis. *Eur J Neurosci* **20**: 3115–20.

15. Forrest G., Qian X. (1999) Exercise in neuromuscular disease. *Neurorehab* **13**: 135–9.

16. Kent-Braun J. A., Walker C. H., Weiner M. W., Miller R. G. (1998) Functional significance of upper and lower motor neuron impairment in amyotrophic lateral sclerosis. *Muscle Nerve* **21**: 762–8.

17. Ashworth N. L., Satkunam L. E., Deforge D. (2005) Treatment for spasticity in amyotrophic lateral sclerosis/motor neuron disease (review). *The Cochran Collaboration*

18. De Carvalho M. (2001) Gabapentin for the treatment of spasticity in patients with amyotrophic lateral sclerosis. *Amyotroph Lateral Scler Other Motor Neuron Disord* **2**: 47–8.

19. **Marquardt G., Lorenz R.** (1999) Intrathecal baclofen for intractable spasticity in amyotrophic lateral sclerosis. *J Neurol* **246**: 619–20.

20. **Sheean G. L.** (1998) The treatment of spasticity with botulinum toxin. In Sheean G. L. (ed.) *Spasticity Rehabilitation*, pp. 109–26. London Churchill Communications, Europe.

21. **Katz R. T.** (1988) Management of spasticity. *Am j Phys Med Rehabil* **67**: 108–16.

22. **Edwards S., Charlton P.** (2002) Splinting and the use of orthoses in the management of patients with neurological disorders. In Edwards S. (ed.) *Neurological Physiotherapy a Problem-solving Approach*, 2nd edn, pp. 219–53. Edinburgh: Churchill Livingstone.

23. **O'Gorman B.** (2000) Physiotherapy. In Oliver D., Borasio G. D., Walsh D. (eds) *Palliative Care in Amyotrophic Lateral Sclerosis*, pp. 105–11. Oxford: Oxford University Press.

24. **O'Gorman B., Oliver D., Nottle C., Prisley S.** (2004) Disorders of nerve 1: Motor neuron disease. In Stokes M. (ed.) *Physical Management in Neurological Rehabilitation*, pp. 233–51. London: Elsevier Mosby.

25. **MNDA** (2002) *Movement and Mobility. Your Personal Guide to Motor Neuron Disease.* Patient information leaflet available at http://www.mndassociation.org/full-site/publications/listing.htm.

26. **Trail M., Nelson N., Van J. N., Appel S. H., Lai E. C.** (2001) Wheelchair use by patients with amyotrophic lateral sclerosis: a survey of user characteristics and selection preferences. *Arch Phys Med Rehabil* **82** (1): 98–102.

27. **Benditt J. O.** (2002) Respiratory complications of amyotrophic lateral sclerosis. *Semin Respir Crit Care Med* **23** (3): 239–47.

28. **Gruis K., Chernew M. E., Brown D. L.** (2005) The cost-effectiveness of early non-invasive ventilation for ALS patients. *BMC Health Services Research* **5** (58), online.

29. **Lyall R. A., Donaldson N., Fleming T., Wood C.** *et al.* (2001) A prospective study of quality of life in ALS patients treated with noninvasive ventilation. *Neurology* **57**: 153–6.

30. **Hadjikoutis S., Wiles C. M., Eccles R.** (1999) Cough in motor neuron disease: a review of the mechanisms. *Q J Med* **92**: 487–94.

31. **Bach R.** (1993) Amyotrophic lateral sclerosis. Communication status and survival with ventilatory support. *Am J Phys Med Rehabil* **72** (6): 343–9.

32. **Lechtzin N., Wiener C. M., Clawson L., Chaudhry V., Diette G. B.** (2001) Hospitalization in amyotrophic lateral sclerosis: causes, costs, and outcomes. *Neurology* **56**: 753–7.

33. **Sancho J., Servera E., Díaz J., Marín J.** (2004) Efficacy of mechanical insufflation-exsufflation in medically stable patients with amyotrophic lateral sclerosis. *Chest* **125**: 1400–5.

34. **Bromley I.** (1998) *Tetraplegia and Paraplegia – A Guide for Physiotherapists*, 5th edn. Edinburgh: Churchill Livingstone.

35. **Chatwin M., Ross E., Hart N., Nickol A. H., Polkey M. I., Simonds A. K.** (2003) Cough augmentation with mechanical insufflation/exsufflation in patients with neuromuscular weakness. *Eur Respir J* **21** (3) : 502–8.

36. **Bach J. R.** (2002) Amyotrophic lateral sclerosis: prolongation of life by non-invasive respiratory aids. *Chest* **122**: 92–8.

37. **Lahrmann H., Wild M., Zdrahal F., Grisold W.** (2003) Expiratory muscle weakness and assisted cough in ALS. *ALS Other Motor Neuron Disord* **4**: 49–51.

38. **Winck J. C., Gonçalves M. R., Lourenço C., Viana P., Almeida P. V. J., Bach J. R.** (2004) Effects of mechanical insufflation-exsufflation on respiratory parameters for patients with chronic airway secretion encumbrance. *Chest* **126**: 774–80.

39. **Simmons Z.** (2005) Management strategies for patients with amyotrophic lateral sclerosis from diagnosis through death. *Neurologist* **11** (5): 257–70.

40. **Newrick P. G., Langton-Hewer R.** (1985) Pain in motor neuron disease. *J Neurol Neurosurg Psychiatry* **48** (8): 838–40.

Chapter 7b

Multidisciplinary care:

occupational therapy

Chris Kingsnorth

The occupational therapy (OT) assessment of a person with ALS involves consideration of the domains of occupational performance as described by Rennie and Thornton.[1] Occupational performance is 'an individual's ability to perform activities of daily living, influenced by their environments, within a satisfactory time frame and at an age appropriate level, to fulfill life roles'. Activities of daily living are 'the range of everyday tasks an individual needs to perform to fulfill their occupational roles in self-care, work and leisure'. In the occupational therapy model, the performance components comprise the skills necessary for personal activities.

In the management of ALS, aspects of the domain of concern impact the sufferer's ability to fulfil desired roles. It is important the OT recognizes the uniqueness of each disease experience and incorporates this into assessment of their abilities and needs;[2] however there are some common strategies. Some equipment which enables the individual to achieve a desired occupational role is expensive. It can be argued, however, that due to the short duration of the condition, rapid changes and the small number of patients, a selected equipment collection will be recycled economically. An equipment system such as that of the Irish Motor Neurone Disease Association[3] is effective.

Domain of concern

Age

Age at onset affects the extent of life roles influenced by impairments. For example male patients under 45 years referred to OT may have issues such as paid employment, parenting and outdoor activities. They are more likely to have a partner able to assist them in their roles and self-care. These younger patients may not accept impairments and seek to 'keep ahead' of the disease by strategies, techniques and equipment to compensate for the changes. This provides a challenging and satisfying partnership with the OT. It can also be frustrating when the required equipment is unavailable, expensive, or not yet invented! Younger patients also may have a greater tolerance of assistive technology. Older patients are often more accepting of their fate and because of this or a reluctance to place demands, require encouragement to accept assistance. The older person is more likely to have an aged carer who may themselves have a disability and their needs are greater. These patients, however, do not usually have the same scope of life roles.

Environment

OT intervention will be influenced by both the social and the physical environment. Where the patient is socially isolated, there is greater need for access to community services, immediate response to equipment needs and the possibility of being unable to remain at home in the terminal stages. The cultural/social milieu may be one in which the 'sick' role requires that the sufferer be assisted in all aspects of daily living even though independence could be maintained. In this situation, intervention will be aimed towards assisting the carer to carry out their role, for example training the carer in practical skills, such as manual handling and use of assistive equipment.[4]

The physical environment requires regular evaluation as abilities and needs change. It is difficult to plan ahead while being sensitive to the patient and carer's need to be positive and hopeful. It is also important to assess the patient and family's ability to cope with these changes and challenges,[5] as introduction of equipment before the patient is prepared may lead to rejection because it is 'symbolic of disability and reminds him of his deteriorating condition'.[2] Deterioration in ambulatory ability suggests future need for a wheelchair; it may be necessary to suggest measuring for ramps when the patient is still walking. The ability to remain independently mobile at home, where lower limb weakness is the major symptom, is affected by access (steps/stairs), width of doorways and circulation space. Where they live alone there are the added issues of ability to open doors and use a key.

The problem of a suitable bed may be as simple as providing blocks to raise the existing bed to a height easier to rise from, or be level with the wheelchair, or a board between mattress and base for a firmer base. The more complex needs of adjustable height and postural control can be met with a hospital bed (not readily available) or purchasing their own electrically controlled bed. It is important that this has height and both head and leg adjustment. In one case where the patient's mother was the primary carer she was exhausted through having to adjust his posture throughout the night. The expense of an electric bed meant he could adjust his posture independently and his mother was then better able to cope with the demands of the day. Community nurses and carers were also more able to adhere to occupational health and safety guidelines in providing ongoing assistance.

Time

Progression of ALS means that needs change rapidly. Complex systems of funding and purchasing equipment mean that equipment or service is often not provided in a timely fashion. It is often necessary to develop an equipment resource, such as electric wheelchairs, which can fill a need until other sources are available. Voluntary support groups, such as the Motor Neurone Disease Association, can help.

Performance components

Those most commonly related to OT intervention are motor and social. Complete loss of motor ability is linked with all aspects of daily living. Sophisticated environmental controls allow a patient to continue social interaction and make changes in their environment with the subtlest input.

Motor

Muscle strength and active range of movement (ROM)

There are associated wasting and dysfunctional joint positions. Custom-made thermoplastic resting splints for the wrist and hands maintain optimum muscle length and functional joint positions. These would be worn at night or when watching TV, for example. ALS patients have a low tolerance for static splints with poor compliance for wearing them. A compromise is to have them wear them on alternate hands on alternate nights.

Shoulder supports alleviate joint stress during ambulation where there is loss of strength in antigravity muscles (see the list of suppliers in Appendix 1). They have also been useful in relieving pain.

Compensatory devices which allow optimum use of residual muscle power may be needed. This may be to provide distal support in the upper limb, i.e. wrist and fingers, thus allowing effort to be channelled into controlling the shoulder, for example when eating or using a keyboard. Alternatively, the shoulder and elbow may be assisted with a gravity-eliminating device allowing use of residual wrist and finger function. These perform a dual role of enhancing independence while maintaining joint ROM. Another simple example is providing raised seating for the toilet and sitting room to allow larger proximal muscles to be utilized for standing up.

Loss of endurance

It may be necessary for the patient to make choices about which activities they continue to expend energy on, and which they will accept help with. It has been noted that 'there is no correlation between independence in Activities of Daily Living (ADL) and quality of life'.[6] Patients may be counselled to accept self-care help, allowing more time and energy for quality time with family and leisure or work, in this way 'lowering their expectations regarding their physical disabilities and by focusing on life areas that are independent of physical capabilities'.[7] Work simplification principles can be applied in early disease, for example sitting for tasks such as showering and washing dishes, thus conserving energy.

Hand function

Specific examples will be given in the section on Activities for daily living, but there are some general principles. In the early stages where grip strength and precision is affected by loss of intrinsic function, large handles and lighter tools may be useful. Devices to hold items allowing more gross grip or movement may be useful, such as a palmar cuff to hold cutlery or a pen holder for writing.

Mobility

Consideration needs to be given to both patient and carer when deciding on a wheelchair. Initially a manual wheelchair may suffice, but a six-week waiting period for an electric wheelchair means forward planning is required. Change in status from walking to wheelchair is devastating to some, and preparing them for this requires sensitive handling by all. Where patients are able to walk short distances at home, a successful interim solution is a scooter. They are more acceptable as less 'disabled-looking' than a wheelchair and soften the blow of not being able to continue driving a car.

Manual wheelchairs need to be lightweight, with easily removed wheels so it is easier for a less able carer to lift. Removable and adjustable height armrests reduce the weight while allowing for transition from standing transfer to side for slideboard transfers. Friction grip on the push-rims allows longer-term independent wheeling as grip strength deteriorates. Pressure points must be addressed with cushioning, together with considerations such as cushion covers. For example, shiny Lycra cushion covers facilitate slideboard transfers and removal of pants for toileting.

If an electric wheelchair is inappropriate or unavailable, a pushchair is useful. Where trunk and head control deteriorate, these provide the option of 'tilt in space'. This is preferable to recline from a postural viewpoint as it allows a change in seating pressure while supporting the trunk and head and maintaining stable pelvis position. Subtle changes of tilt in space can negate the need for external head fixation such as forehead straps or neck collars. Consultation with the speech pathologist regarding head position is vital where swallowing is compromised. When the patient is unable to self-propel, a pushchair is easier for carers.

Most patients with lower limb involvement require an electric wheelchair. There are many options. Choice will be governed by availability, cost, portability, postural requirements and additional attachments, for example a lightweight folding demountable chair, or a fixed chair with customized seating, electric tilt and recline and additional head support. The type of controller will depend on motor ability and range from a standard hand control, hand control with arm support, to head control, knee or foot control, with different switching options. The optimum chair allows them to have some control over their life, independent mobility, ability to change position and to access other areas, such as communication and environmental control equipment.

Posture

Maintenance of posture has implications for control of pain, access to equipment and pressure care. Pelvic stability is central to functional sitting posture. As muscle strength deteriorates it is vital cushioning supports the pelvis in a stable position. Lateral trunk support may be required through customized cushioning or choice of wheelchair. In the later stages the position of the trunk most conducive to breathing or to allow head control, is with the body tipped back as with tilt in space. This makes it difficult to see a communication device or computer screen, modifications are required to position these items and posture needs to be changed for eating. A simple, adjustable neck brace has been used as a short-term measure to support the head forward for eating or while traveling in wheelchair transport. A wheelchair with electrically controlled postural adjustment increases the ability to independently adjust posture and reduces anxiety associated with breathing difficulties.

Bed mobility

In the early stages, difficulty moving in bed may be assisted by a firm base by use of a bed board, a simple bed rail which slides under the mattress or wearing satin nightwear. As abilities decrease, a suitable pressure mattress may preclude the necessity to move at night, when there is assistance to manually posture during the day. Other options include an electric bed (see Environment): some find it more comfortable to sleep in a recliner lounge chair.

Transfers

The critical factor in facilitating independent transferring is the height of surfaces. When there is lower limb weakness, seating needs to be raised (see Performance component 1). When a wheelchair is in use, positioning of items to allow safe transfers is important. For example, the bed may be moved to allow the chair to be positioned appropriately. Chairs and beds which have been raised to assist standing transfers may need to be lowered to the height of the wheelchair, if side or slide-board transfers are introduced. Slide-mats and transfer belts are useful for assisted slide-board transfers. Standing and side transfers to the car may be assisted by a wedge cushion on the car seat to level it out, with a Lycra cover to assist slide and swivel. Where dependent standing transfers are used a swivel board or turntable may assist the carer. As complete dependence in transfers occurs, a hoist, either electric or hydraulic, may mean the difference between staying at home or being cared for in an institution. There are many hoists and slings therefore careful choice must reflect the patient, carer, and environment. When the patient can weight bear with assisted support, standing hoists have been used. They allow easy access for all hygiene activities and the patient maintains an upright posture. As the disease progresses a more dependent hoisting is required. This transition may not be accepted by the patient or the carer; but continuing to use the standing hoist puts both at risk.

Driving

The patient must be advised with regard to driving ability and an assessment necessary. Where the disease process has been slowly affecting lower limbs only, hand controls may allow continued driving; aids such as hand grips for the steering wheel, for example a spinner knob, may help.

Social

This includes skills to maintain communication and social contacts.

Writing

see Hand function above.

Typing

Mobile arm supports and suspension arm slings assist access to keyboards for typing or augmentative communication (see the list of suppliers in Appendix 1). Most success has been gained by customizing them with thermoplastic functional wrist splints. Typing splints to the fingers may be required (Figure 7b.1.) Arm supports can facilitate reading the newspaper or magazines and software

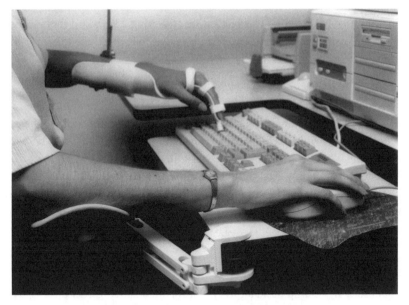

Fig. 7b.1 Left hand showing a modified overhead sling support and typing splint. The right hand is using the computer mouse with the Ergorest.

can minimize the physical activity required to access the patient's PC, for example the use of word prediction and single switch access.

Telephone use

Modifications can be made to hold the phone, and modified telephones are available, for example with large pressure-sensitive keys. There are hands-free telephones which allow communication to continue by telephone. An answer-phone attachment is helpful as speech deteriorates, as it allows a message to be taken without embarrassment or confusion for the caller or the patient. The telephone may also be linked to the computer.

Activities of daily living

Self-care

There has been a great deal written on solutions for self-care deficits. This section will be limited to ideas in response to individual problems. The deficits vary according to the type and onset of ALS. Those with bulbar involvement remain ambulatory for longer; initial motor problems are usually in the upper limbs. This may result in difficulty with eating, toileting, dressing and using a keyboard or communication device. Those with involvement of the lower limbs have problems with transfers and mobility. By the time their upper limbs are involved enough to affect eating and using a keyboard they require assistance in all areas of self-care. The ideas that follow include those for the upper limb primary involvement first.

Personal hygiene: toileting

Where grip strength is diminished, moist towelettes instead of toilet paper can help. Simplified clothing without fastenings, and loops on the waist or the use of braces, assist with clothing. More expensive options include a bidet with sensor which both washes and dries after toileting.

The most commonly used equipment includes an over-toilet frame (to raise the seat), hand rails and later a wheeled shower/commode chair. The latter can be wheeled by patients or carer over the toilet and then into the shower, limiting the transfers required. It can be used with standing, slide-board (side) transfers, or hoist transfers.

Bathing

Liquid soap in a pump pack, a thermostat for water, a tap-turner or lever taps and a soap mitt may be useful. There are shower and bath seats, fixed or adjustable to allow the patient to be raised and lowered, which contribute to safety and energy-conservation. The wheeled commode/shower chair is invaluable where the shower is accessible or there is drainage in the bathroom floor. A tilt and recline shower commode, with a hoist, allows a patient who is dependent in posture and head control to shower while being safely supported.

Dressing

Simplified clothing, and easy fittings with minimal fastenings are advisable. Loops on trousers and socks, hook and loop fastening or slip-on shoes aid dressing. Some women find wearing a skirt proves easier for toileting.

Feeding

Mobile arm supports can be adjusted for independent eating. More success has been found with the suspension arm positioners and customized wrist support. The most successful and flexible combination for one patient used mobile arm supports for the keyboard and reading the paper, and a counter balance sling attached to his chair for eating and teeth cleaning. Weights could be added as motor ability declined. The Neater Eater has been used success-fully by some. It is clamped to the table. There are individual models and adjustments which allow the user to bring food to the mouth with little physical input. Some are reluctant to try it because of the 'robotic' appearance, perhaps reinforcing their loss of function; while others are pleased to maintain their ability to share mealtimes with the family.

Work

The duration that work can be maintained is determined by the nature of the work, the standing of the employee, and employer willingness to adapt to the patient's changing ability. Where the work requires keyboard skills and is sedentary, adaptations are easier (see Typing, above). For example, one patient worked as a merchant banker for many months with an electric wheelchair for independent mobility. He was delivered to the building goods entrance by wheelchair taxi so that he could access his office through a door using a modified key, as the main doors were too heavy. Circulation-space, desk orientation and height were altered for easier access. Initially he transferred to a suitable office chair and later worked from his wheelchair. Provision was made for an Ergorest (see the list of suppliers in Appendix 1) to assist with typing, and typing splints were made.

The suspension arm sling was used for one-handed typing and this enabled another young man to stay working with an understanding employer until his general strength deteriorated. He continued to use this at home for his computer and later, one was fitted to his wheelchair to be used with his communicator (Lightwriter).

Occupational therapy intervention requires partnership with the patient to problem-solve, identify and adapt to, the rapid changes and the individual needs of the sufferers. Optimal service is dependent on recognition by funding bodies of their unique needs for services and equipment in a flexible and timely manner.

Acknowledgement

Thanks to my colleague Carmelle Lipman for assistance in locating reference material.

References

1. **Rennie H., Thornton C.** (1988) Activites of daily living, an area of occupational expertise. *Australian Occupational Therapy Journal* 35: 44–58.
2. **Doman C.,** (2002) Motor neurone disease. In Turner A, Foster M, Johnson S. (eds) *Occupational Therapy and Physical Dysfunction: Principles and Practice*, 5th edn, pp. 489–505. Edinburgh: Churchill Livingstone.
3. **Corr B.,** *et al.* (1998) Service Provision for patients with ALS/MND: a cost-effective multidisciplinary approach. *Journal of the Neurological Sciences* 160 (Suppl.1): S141–S145.
4. **Naughton V.** (2002) Prepare to care, Education and Training Package. Western Australia. Independent Living Centre of WA - unpublished personnal communication.
5. **Copperman L., Farrell S., Huges L.** (2002) Neurodegenerative Diseases In Trombly M., Randanski M. (eds). *Occupational Therapy for Physical Dysfunction*, 5th edn. pp. 898–902. Baltimore: Lippincott Williams and Williams.

6. **Cardol M., Elvers J. W. H., Oostendorp R. A. B., Brandsma J. W., de Groot I. J. M.** (1996) Quality of life in patients with amyotrophic lateral sclerosis. *Journal of Rehabilitation Sciences* 9: 99–103.

7. **Foley G.** (1994) Quality of life for people with motor neurone disease: a consideration for Occupational Therapists. *British Journal of Occupational Therapy* 67 (12).

Chapter 7c

Multidisciplinary care:

speech and language therapy

Amanda Scott and Maryanne McPhee

Summary

The speech and language therapist has an important role in the multidisciplinary assessment of the person with ALS. This includes the assessment of both speech and swallowing and advice and support to cope with these issues. There is a specific role in the provision and support of augmentative and alternative communication systems, as well as in the support of swallowing and secretion care, in collaboration with other members of the multidisciplinary team.

Introduction

The ability to communicate is a fundamental human activity, enabling us to share our thoughts covering the full range of life experiences. In ALS, speech may become unintelligible and sometimes language and cognitive functions become impaired. These problems can lead to difficulties interacting with family and loved ones, carers and health professionals. Those caring for people with ALS have a responsibility to provide the most effective means of communication possible.

This chapter outlines the speech and language therapist's role in ALS, and focuses on aspects of speech impairment and communication as the disease progresses. In early bulbar impairment, focus on speech production for short periods may help but alternative means of communication are more important later in the disease. Because communication always includes other people, optimizing communication should include family, friends, health professionals and carers.

The ability to communicate declines gradually, which allows time for adjustment to loss and the impact these have on relationships. Early recognition of declining speech intelligibility and communication makes it easier for the person to convey decisions regarding the disease and the changes it imposes. It also provides the opportunity for timely strategies to facilitate communication.

Description of speech impairment in ALS

Bulbar impairment is one of the most important clinical problems because it impacts swallowing and communication. In about 20–25 per cent symptoms begin in the bulbar musculature.[1] Over 90 per cent will develop bulbar symptoms.[2]

Bulbar dysfunction and related communication, secretion and respiratory complications are major issues and impact on quality of life.[3] The impairment may range from mild dysarthria, presenting as a slight slurring of speech, to anarthria, or no speech. According to Aronson[4] mixed dysarthria is most common, because of involvement of both upper and lower motor neurons.

Normal speech depends on adequate functioning of the respiratory system, vocal cords, tongue, pharynx and soft palate and lips. In ALS, these become impaired due to reduced rate, range, strength and accuracy of muscle movement. This may result from loss of upper motor neurons, leading to spastic muscles, or of lower motor neurons, causing flaccid muscles, or, more commonly, a combination of both. The specific effects are as discussed next.

Respiratory function

Weakness of the muscles of respiration can be due to either upper or lower spinal motor neuron loss. The impairments described above frequently co-occur with bulbar symptoms. Impaired respiratory support for speech decreases volume and the prosodic features of communication, such as stress, rhythm, intonation and rate. It may also reduce phrasing – in the number of words per breath, making speech more effortful with a strained–strangled quality. Decreased volume of speech causes difficulties communicating against background noise. This restricts the ability to socialize in groups and interrupt others. The reduction in the prosodic features limits the expressive communication, such as irony or excitement.

Laryngeal function

The larynx, which houses the vocal cords, is at the top of the trachea. During respiration, the vocal cords are open. To produce voice, or phonate, the vocal cords come together in the midline and vibrate as the airstream passes through. This closure is necessary for a strong, clear voice. Changes in pitch depend on the flexibility of the vocal cords, which lengthen, as the larynx raises and tilts forwards, to produce higher pitch sounds, and shorten, when the larynx is lowered to produce lower pitch sounds.

Lower motor neuron impairment results in a soft, weak voice with a breathy quality. The voice may sound low pitched and monotonous.[5] Upper motor neuron impairment causes the voice to be harsh and strained. People with phonatory impairment also experience problems communicating against background noise. Vocal fatigue, which further restricts conversation, is common.

Soft palate and pharyngeal function

Most speech sounds are produced with airflow directed through the oral cavity. Closure of the nasopharyngeal opening is achieved through elevation of the soft palate and contraction of the pharynx. During production of 'n', 'm' and 'ng' (as at the end of song) the soft palate is lowered against the elevated back of the tongue to allow air flow through the nose. This results in the nasal quality of these sounds. Impaired soft palate/pharyngeal closure results in nasalization of all speech sounds and loss of clarity and intelligibility. Nasal emission reduces oral airflow, and inefficient use of air leads to fading at the end of words and phrases, shorter phrases and fewer words per breath. Velopharyngeal incompetence with resulting hypernasality and nasal emission is common.[3]

The tongue

The tongue is the principle articulator of speech. A range of subtle movements produce speech. During the production of the 'k', 'g' and 'ng' the back of the tongue elevates. The sounds 's', 'z', 't', 'd', 'l', 'r' and 'n' require elevation of the tip. The sides elevate during the production of 'sh', and to produce 'th' the tip projects forward between the teeth. The generalized tongue weakness is the major cause of reduced speech intelligibility. Mild tongue impairment is associated with slurring. As tongue function deteriorates, fewer sounds can be accurately produced and eventually speech becomes unintelligible. They become more dependent on augmentative and alternative communication with reduction in the quality of many aspects of communication.

Lip function

Lip closure is required for the production of 'm', 'p' and 'b', while rounding is required to produce 'w'. During the production of 'f' and 'v' the lower lip approximates the upper teeth. Spastic lips have a retracted appearance with the teeth visible, and difficulty with lip closure. Flaccid lips result in weak sound production and drooping at rest. Poor oral closure is associated with drooling, which can cause embarrassment and reluctance to speak.

The cheek muscles are usually affected when lip impairment is present. When the muscles are spastic, the inside of the cheeks press against the teeth and problems associated with biting the cheeks occur. This can become exacerbated if the person has a bite reflex. Swelling, pain and ulceration result.

Other problems which affect communication

Positioning and general comfort

The effectiveness of communication may depend on physical comfort. Appropriate positioning decreases abnormal tone, reduces effort required to maintain a sitting position, minimizes reflexive responses and clonus, facilitates access to communication devices and optimizes respiratory function. Liaison with physiotherapists and occupational therapists about seating, head, neck and trunk support and upper limb function is essential.

General comfort also relies on basic needs being met often by others, e.g. drinking, toileting, blowing their nose etc. A quick and efficient method of communicating attention to these tasks must be established.

Pathological laughing and crying

Pathological laughing and crying is recognized occasionally but poorly understood.[6] It is not known why some cry while others laugh or experience a mixture of the two. It has been considered a disturbance of motor affective behaviour, but is probably related to frontal lobe dysfunction. Poeck[7] highlighted three primary features: loss of voluntary emotional control, in response to non-specific stimuli, and lack of association with prevailing mood.

Pathological laughing and crying, also referred to as emotional lability, is associated with spastic bulbar impairment. This presents as unconstrained triggering of an emotional response, appropriate in type but excessive in magnitude. Once initiated, the response is difficult to stop. Clinical experience suggests discussing emotive issues is more likely to trigger pathological crying, and in severe cases, pathological laughter or crying even with mildly emotional topics. Pathological laughing or crying can impede verbal communication and social activity. McCullagh and Feinstein[6] described three cases of pathological laughing and crying, where the affect changed from a predominance of crying to laughter. Pathological laughing and crying can be conceptualized as perseveration of the motor responses for emotion. Changing the motor response by changing the pattern of breathing may enable them to regain control. This may be achieved by concentrating on inspiration during uncontrolled laughter and expiration during uncontrolled crying. In mild cases, simple strategies include a reassuring but not excessive response and a change of topic to help break the pattern. Participants in Murphy's study[5] described how thinking positively assisted them in breaking the pattern. For some, antidepressants can be of assistance. Smith and Brooks[8] reported patients with ALS and pseudobulbar affect responded to treatment with Neurodex (dextromethorphan and quinidine sulphate) and all reported improved quality of life.

Cognitive and language impairment

Although once considered uncommon, cognitive impairment is common – see Chapter 4c. The impairments reported range from florid personality changes with severe impairment of frontal lobe executive functions to mild cognitive deficits. Frontal and temporal lobe involvement have been identified post mortem[9–11] and through neuropsychological testing.[11,12,13] The problems detected using neuropsychological testing included deficits of verbal fluency, spelling, the ability to generate concepts or shift mind sets and problem-solving.

Specific deficits of language function have been identified with a small number of patients with aphasia in association frontotemporal dementia.[11] Problems with comprehension and production of verbs, with progressive non-fluent aphasia, have been identified. In some language impairment has advanced to complete mutism. This occurs with and without other features of frontotemporal dementia.[14]

Cognition and language impairments are thought to be under-reported because they may be masked by dysarthria or behavioural abnormalities. However, they have implications for both verbal communication and use of augmentative and alternative communication. For these reasons communication partners may not recognize the extent of these deficits Therefore cognitive impairment needs to be considered in breakdowns in communication. These may include:

- A deterioration in spelling
- Inappropriate responses to questions
- Introduction of seemingly unrelated topics in conversation
- Poor eye contact, attention directed to peripheral aspects, e.g. fidgeting in handbag during conversation
- Difficulty switching topic in conversations

- ◆ Loss of organization skills, e.g. losing things, difficulty managing finances, missing appointment times
- ◆ Will continue to write a message even though the content has been accurately predicted
- ◆ Over-formalized pedantic communication style.

As cognitive and linguistic functions deteriorate the communication partner must assume more responsibility. Inaccurate responses, inability to write concise messages or to write key words of a verbal message to improve the efficiency of communication hinder the flow of an interaction. Where these problems occur the communication partner may interpret incomplete messages or take responsibility for maintaining the topic.

Cognitive and linguistic functions need to be considered when selecting the appropriate communication device.

Problems of oro-pharyngeal secretions

In normal function, 600 ml of saliva is produced and swallowed per day.[15] This is a largely subconscious activity. In MND, problems with oro-pharyngeal secretions often co-occur with speech difficulties and usually with impairment of swallowing.

Typically, individuals with oro-pharyngeal secretion problems begin the day with a dry mouth and the retention of thick, tenacious secretions in the pharynx. When these are a problem; the individual may find moistening the mucosa by humidifying the atmosphere helpful. This can be achieved using a vaporizer, inhaler, or the steam from the shower. Sipping fruit juices, which contain mucolytic enzymes, such as dark grape juice, pineapple juice and papaya juice may help. Papaya enzyme tablets are available from health food shops and clinically useful. A light oil, such as grapeseed oil, can be beneficial for lubricating the oro-pharyngeal structures and facilitating oral movements during speech.

As the day progresses, they often have increased difficulty swallowing secretions, leading to pooling and/or drooling of saliva. This is frequently worse following meals (including enteral feeds), and towards the end of the day, when the postprandial increase in digestive secretions and fatigue may contribute to poor saliva control. At this time, individuals may be reluctant to engage in communication for fear of spitting or dribbling.

In mild cases increased saliva can be managed by regular, volitional swallowing. Sipping a drink during interactions to swallow pooled saliva, or deliberately swallowing before speaking can help. As swallowing problems progress drooling may become so troublesome that medication is necessary to reduce saliva. Usually anticholinergic medications such as atropine and probanthine are prescribed. Care must be taken because their effectiveness may reduce over time.[16] Their most effective use is often situational for short periods, e.g. before a social event.

Other management approaches for managing saliva include injection of botulinum toxin into the salivary glands[17] or radiation.[18] Both methods reduce the production of saliva, however, further multicentre studies are required. When managing saliva control consideration needs to be given to the importance of moist mucous membranes of the structures involved in speech. The use of artificial saliva, frequent sips of fluid or small amounts of oil is recommended.

Intervention

Environmental considerations

Environmental factors include any external influences on functioning and on the disability. The environment can provide both positive and negative influences.[19] Persons may require assistive technology for several life functions, including wheelchairs or scooters for mobility, adaptive equipment for eating, a hoist for transfers, specialized vehicles for transport, ramps and home modifications for mobility/accommodation of equipment and the option of life-extending treatments (such as non-invasive ventilation or mechanical ventilation). Both the person and their family/carers must then be open to each new environmental adaptation, and this can be challenging, especially with rapid deterioration. Timely introduction of equipment that the patient and family require is vital.

With regard to patients with dysarthria, background noise or a group setting can pose difficulties. It may result in reduced intelligibility or the person straining. Simple listener strategies such as turning off the television and radio, shutting doors or moving to a quieter location make speaking and listening easier. When conversing, seating arrangements should facilitate communication by ensuring people are face to face and that lighting is adequate. Having the light source e.g. a lamp or window, behind the person with dysarthric speech should be avoided, as this makes it difficult for the listener to see facial expressions to supplement intelligibility.

The role of direct speech therapy in ALS

Speech is much more than the encoded linguistic message. Speech, as part of communication, conveys personality, such as sense of humour and feelings towards the subject of the conversation. With progressive loss of speech, there is a corresponding loss of the ability to converse. This encompasses loss of control of the environment, loss of identity, change in self-image and self-esteem and a loss of purpose. This impacts on relationships within the family and broader community. Open discussion regarding these changes to the person's speech and the impact on relationships and everyday life can help. This can lead into a discussion of the expectations of alternative and augmentative communication.

Degenerative conditions require special consideration when choosing therapeutic interventions. Four out of five people with MND will require intervention regarding their communication.[20]

Many of the aspects of speech impairment discussed respond to traditional speech therapy, such as prolonging speech to reduce respiratory effort, and assist with initiation problems,[21] or modified 'yawn/sigh' exercises to reduce vocal tension.[22] Rate reduction strategies and vocal rest are also important.[19] However, careful consideration of the rate of disease progression in relation to the timing of therapy and the duration of intervention is important. The desire to ameliorate speech problems by setting up programmes which include repetitive speech and muscle exercises, has the negative effect of providing a means by which the person can monitor their own deterioration. Research from Watts and Vanryckeghem[23] found that resistance exercises, oral motility and strengthening activities, isometric exercises and loudness activities may cause decreased voice quality and rapid rate of decline in speech intelligibility. However, all the participants in Murphy's study[5] expressed a strong desire to use their own speech for as long as possible, so functional speech strategies need to be encouraged.

Facilitating techniques

Facilitating techniques such as vibration, brushing and ice to the muscles involved in speech can modify abnormal muscle tone and improve intelligibility for short periods.[24] There has been little investigation into their efficacy, but they are helpful. The effects are thought to be transient so they should be used ahead of a situation where communication is envisaged, such as before the arrival of visitors.

Augmentative and alternative communication (AAC)

Speech does not disappear suddenly. As it deteriorates, people make adjustments. Changes may include reducing phrase length to accommodate a reduction in respiratory support for speech, or slowing speech and using deliberate articulatory movements as the speech muscles become weaker.

Eventually speech may be augmented using pen and paper, an alphabet board, a word and phrase board or an electronic communication device. When speech becomes unintelligible, they become totally reliant on an alternative method of communication.

Determining when to intervene with AAC options has been based on the individual's intelligibility and, more recently, on reduction in speaking rate.[19] Speakers maintain 100 per cent intelligibility until their rate is reduced from 200–250 words per minute to approximately 100–120 words per minute. There is then an abrupt drop in sentence intelligibility. Data collected by Beukelman and Ball[25] indicated a rapid decline in speech intelligibility associated with a decline in speaking rate: this occurs in all types of ALS. Persons with bulbar onset reach rapid decline 14 months post-diagnosis, those with mixed onset 22 months post-diagnosis and those with spinal onset at 34 months post-diagnosis.

The authors recommend therapists are involved from diagnosis to ensure an ongoing relationship which will facilitate the measurement of changes in speaking rate and anticipate communication needs.

Communication, whether via gesture, verbal, written or using a communication device, conveys information at various levels of complexity. Table 7c.1 provides a summary of activities within a framework for conceptualizing the range of communication requirements using AAC.

Table 7c.1 Communication activities

Face to face conversation. Rapid, informal, exchange of thoughts and feelings. Small talk between two or more partners.
Social closeness. To establish, maintain and/or develop personal relationships.
Social etiquette. To conform to social conventions of politeness, e.g. please, thank you.
Quick basic needs/wants. Rapid communication of needs/wants, e.g. change position, change the channel, wipe the mouth.
Detailed needs/wants. Conveying at least a few sentences about a need/want to be sure that the partner understands, e.g. indicate what you want to do on an outing.
Detailed information. Conveying considerable information, e.g. tell someone how you feel about him/her; give your opinion on an issue or topic.
Personal stories/anecdotes. Telling a personal story or anecdote during a communication interaction for purposes of illustrating a point, exchanging experiences, telling a joke, etc.
Referring to the past. Telling stories of past events. Adults over 65 years of age refer to the past almost as often as they refer to the present.
Telephone. Using a voice output device or an interpreter to communicate over the phone.
Written communication. Producing 'hard copy' for correspondence, work, creative writing.

Mathy,[26]

The introduction of AAC

The appropriateness and timing of AAC devices plays a significant role in acceptance and enables the person to have time to learn how to use the device before it becomes a necessity: this may not, however, be appropriate for psychological and emotional well-being. Individual coping styles need to be respected. Some like to plan and find early introduction reassuring, others prefer a 'wait and see' approach. For these people, early introduction can be confronting and conflicts with their coping strategies. It may also cause anxiety and stress by indicating they will lose their speech.[5] However, the AAC system must be available when the person is ready.

As well as ensuring AAC devices are provided in a timely manner, it is essential they are reliable, portable, have good quality voice output and are available for an appropriate loan period. Murphy[5] highlights the importance of spending time discussing vocabulary and the types of messages people want. This requires regular monitoring and review as needs and circumstances change. Appropriate modifications or new strategies may need to be found. Occasionally, a person may not perceive their loss of speech to be significant and will therefore be less likely to embrace AAC.

Inclusion of communication partners

Communication does not occur in isolation, and any intervention should include the communication partners. Adjustment to dysarthric speech or AAC impacts on everyone with whom the person interacts. For this reason, family, friends, carers and health professionals should be included in therapeutic interventions.

Many people find communicating with someone who is difficult to understand or using a communication device stressful, and may avoid interactions. Training listeners in strategies that assist in the process is essential. Training can include skills in asking questions to define a topic, framing yes/no questions in a systematic way, and understanding the differences between communication to meet basic needs versus free conversations and exposition of issues. Dependency on others to facilitate communication leads to a loss of control and sufficient time allowed for in-depth discussions.

When an AAC device is used, effective communication is dependent upon the active participation of all. Their job can include ensuring the device is maintained; the device is appropriately set up and positioned and batteries are charged. This is not always easy, since many people are unfamiliar with electronic equipment. Introduction of additional equipment can be overwhelming in the daily workload of carers. For these reasons, patients and their families and carers should be supported when AAC is used.

During normal speech around 150–250 words are communicated per minute (Goldman-Eisler, 1998).[27] An efficient electronic communication device user communicates 15–20 words per minute.[28] Whilst there have been considerable improvements in electronic communication devices, with features such as word prediction and phrase and sentence storage, no device can match normal verbal communication. The time required should be adjusted to allow for different communication activities.

Types of AAC

Various AAC devices are available. Physical disability, linguistic functioning, cognitive status and the rate of disease progression need to be considered when determining the device to be recommended. Consideration of the portability, durability and maintenance of communication systems is necessary when deciding on which is most appropriate and functional for an individual.

Simple methods such as voice amplifiers, pen and paper and magnetic writing boards are quick, convenient and portable and require little training. Many find these low-tech AAC methods suitable. For more advanced physical deterioration and when fatigue, and/or cognitive impairment become an issue, pre-recorded message boards, alphabet boards and picture boards help.

GEWA Laser pointers™ fixed to a pair of glasses, a headband or a hat and utilized with individually designed alphabet/phrase boards can be effective for some in advanced disease.

Etran boards™, which only require eye movements to indicate target letters, are useful. Since these depend on appropriate training and practice for both the person and their communication partners, intensive training for all concerned is important to facilitate effective communication.

More technologically advanced systems include text to speech software computer packages and electronic communication devices such as the Lightwriter™. These have the advantage of voice output, which enables telephone communication, with young children and in groups. Prediction functions can assist people with poor keyboard skills or impaired dexterity. Scanner options can make these more appropriate as they can be added at a later stage if upper limb function deteriorates. It is important to liaise with the occupational therapist when setting up scanning systems to find the best switch access.

An Eye gaze computer system, such as that by LC technologies, is operated entirely with the eyes. Eye movements are calibrated and by looking at control keys on a screen, a person can synthesize speech, control environment (lights, call bells, etc.), type, run computer software, operate a computer mouse and access the Internet and email. These systems are costly but effective.

High-tech AAC options may never be suitable for some while for others they can enhance communication significantly. Artificial, high-tech communication systems cannot give words intonation, spontaneity, humour and wit. An investigation of why people chose not to use an electronic device found a variety of reasons.[5] Some felt that by not using speech they were admitting defeat, others would rather say it than write. The shared understanding of daily events in close and long-term relationships was considered to reduce the need for things to be said. It was reported that as the disease progresses communication becomes restricted to familiar people and communicating with unfamiliar people is too tiring. Because a significant amount of communication is non-verbal, some felt the AAC device would remove closeness. The slowness of the speech output and the voice quality of electronic devices were deterrents. Others complained the learning requirements were too complex and time-consuming.

Communication during the later stages of the disease

The speech and language therapist, with the multidisciplinary team, must facilitate and support the person and their family to ensure quality communication throughout the disease. Communication options need to reflect the wishes and needs of the person, their family/carers, and the rate and progression of the disease.

It is imperative to focus on the persons' needs and allow them to cease use of high tech devices and consider other options without feeling they are letting someone down. Some will persist with options that are no longer suitable because they are causing frustration or fatigue. The speech and language therapist should gently introduce more appropriate AAC.

Efficient methods of communicating the needs of day-to-day living should be well established early in the disease and modified as required. These should be clearly documented to ensure that others are aware, particularly if the person moves from their home to facility-based care. This ensures communication boards and electronic devices can be updated and relevant yes/no questions asked. This avoids anxiety and frustration when the person has to repeat directions to meet changing needs.

Other strategies found helpful during this stage are:

+ Lists of daily needs, likes/dislikes.
+ Digital photos of comfortable positions (the person can then indicate with Yes/No if they want to vary. The photo is used as the starting position). This is useful for people who have difficulty finding a comfortable position.

- Photos of various sleeping positions. (helpful if the person is waking at night and needs to adjust their position).

- List of possible reasons the person may wake at night. Yes/No responses can be used to confirm the current issue. This increases the speed of communication for cares/nurses at night.

In care settings, such as a hospital, a nursing home or a hospice, the provision of staff that are familiar with the patient can become a point of contention. When communication is difficult, either because speech is difficult, or communication via an alternative means requires cooperation from the communication partner, individuals often express a preference for specific staff, usually those who are best able to communicate with that person. This illustrates the importance of the speech pathologist's role regarding training in AAC for all those who care for people with ALS.

Conclusion

The role of the speech pathologist in the final stages of the disease should encompass patient support and advocacy. As a member of the multidisciplinary team we have the expertise and knowledge to solve communication issues and ensure the patient's wishes and needs are respected.

References

1. **Haverkamp L., Appel V., Appel S.** (1995) Natural history of amyotrophic lateral sclerosis in a database population. Validation of a scoring system and a model for survival prediction. *Brain* 118: 707–19.

2. **Shaw C.** (2000) Amyotrophic lateral sclerosis/motor neuron disease: clinical neurology and neurobiology. In Oliver D., Borasio G., Walsh D. (eds) *Palliative Care in Amyotrophic Lateral Sclerosis,* pp. 1–19 Oxford: Oxford University Press.

3. **Yorkston K., Beukelman D., Strand E., Bell K.** (1999) *Management of Motor Speech Disorders in Children and Adults,* 2nd edn. Austin, TX: Pro-Ed.

4. **Aronson A.** (1980) Definition and scope of communication disorders. In Mulder D. (ed.) *The Diagnosis and Treatment of Amyotrophic Lateral Sclerosis,* pp. 217–223 Boston, MA: Houghton Mifflin.

5. **Murphy J.** (2004) 'I prefer contact this close': perceptions of AAC by people with motor neuron disease and their communication partners. *Augmentative and Alternative Communication* 20 (4): 259–71.

6. **McCullagh S., Feinstein A.** (2000) Treatment of pathological affect: variability of response for laughter and crying. *The Journal of Neuropsychiatry and Clinical Neurosciences* 12: 100–2.

7. **Poeck K.** (1969) Pathophysiology of emotional disorders associated with brain damage. In Vinken P., Bruyn G. (eds) *Handbook of Clinical Neurology,* vol 3, pp. 343–367 Amsterdam, North Holland.

8. Smith R., Brooks B. (2005) Treatment of pseudobulbar affect in ALS. *Lancet* **4**: 270.

9. Hudson A. (1981) Amyotrophic lateral sclerosis and it's association with dementia, Parkinsonism and other neurological disorders: a review. *Brain* **104**: 217–47.

10. Wilson C., Grace G., Munoz D., He B., Strong M. (2001) Cognitive impairment in sporadic ALS: a pathological continuum underlying a multi-system disorder. *Neurology* **57**: 651–7.

11. Strong M., Lomen-Hoerth C., Caselli R., Bigio E., Yang W. (2003) Cognitive impairment, frontotemporal dementia, and the motor neuron diseases. *Annals of Neurology* **54** (Suppl. 5): S20–S22.

12. Massman, Sims, Cooke, Haverkamp, Appel & Appel (1995)

13. Moretti R., Torre P., Antonello R., Carraro N., Cazzato G., Bava A. (2002) Complex cognitive disruption in motor neuron disease. *Dementia and Geriatric Cognitive Disorders* **14**: 141–50.

14. Bak T., O'Donovan D., Xuereb J., Boniface S., Hodges J. (2001) Selective impairment of verb processing associated with pathological changes in Brodmann areas 44 and 45 in the motor neuron disease – dementia–aphasia syndrome. *Brain* **124**: 103–20.

15. Watanabe S., Dawes C. (1988) The effects of different foods and concentrations of citric acids on the flow rate of whole saliva in man. *Archives of Oral Biology* **33**: 1–5.

16. Mathers S., Reddihough D., Scott A. (2004) Medical management of saliva. In Scott A., Johnson H. (eds) *A Practical Approach to the Management of Saliva*, 2nd edn, pp. 115–22. Austin TX: Pro-ed.

17. Porta M., Gamba M., Bertacchi G., Vaj P. (2001) Treatment of sialorrhea with ultrasound guided botulinum toxin A injection in patients with neurological disorders. *Journal of Neurology, Neurosurgery and Psychiatry* **30**: 534–40.

18. Harriman M., Morrison M., Hay J., Ravonta M., Eisen A., Lentle B. (2001) Use of radiotherapy for control of sialorrhea in patients with amyotrophic lateral sclerosis. *Journal of Otolaryngology* **30**: 242–4.

19. Ball L., Beukelman D., Pattee G. (2003) Communication effectiveness of individuals with amyotrophic lateral sclerosis. *Journal of Communication Disorders* **37**: 197–215.

20. Saunders C., Walsh T., Smith M. (1981) Hospice care in the motor neuron diseases. In Saunders C., Summers D., Teller N. (eds) *Hospice: the living idea*, pp. 127–147. London: Edward Arnold Publishers.

21. Ingham R.J. (1984) *Stuttering and Behaviour Therapy: Current Status and Experimental Foundations*. San Diego, CA: College – Hill Press.

22. Boone D., McFarlane S. (1994) *The Voice and Voice Therapy*, 5th edn. Prentice Hall.

23. Watts C., Vanryckeghem M. (2001) Laryngeal dysfunction In Amyotrophic Lateral Sclerosis: A review and case report. *BMC Ear, Nose, Throat Disorders* **1** (1): access as www.biomedcentral.com/1472-6851/1/1.

24. Scott A., Staios G. (2004) Sensory-motor approaches to oro- facial facilitation. In Scott A., Johnson H. (eds) *A Practical Approach to the Management of Saliva*, 2nd edn, pp. 65–73. Austin, TX: Pro-ed.

25. Beukelman D., Ball L. (2002) Improving AAC use for persons with acquired neurogenic disorders: understanding human and engineering factors. *Assistive Technology* **14**: 33–44.

26. Mathy P., Yorkston K., Gutmann M. (2000) AAC for Individuals with Amyotrophic Lateral Sclerosis. In Beukelman D., Yorkston K., Reichle J. (eds) *Augmentative and*

Alternative Communication for Adults with Acquired Neurologic Disorders, pp. 233–270. Baltimore: Paul Brookes Publishing Company.

27. **Goldman-Eisler F.** (1986) *Cycle Linguistics: Experiments in Spontaneous Speech.* New York: Academic Press.

28. **Foulds R.** (1987) Guest editorial, Augmentative and alternative communication, 3: p. 169.

Chapter 7d

Multidisciplinary care:

psychology

Jos Kerkvliet

Summary

The clinical psychologist can play different roles within the team caring for someone with ALS: diagnostician, researcher, external consultant, psychosocial therapist and team facilitator. All team members will provide psychosocial support for patients and their families and may need support in this role. The clinical psychologist may be well placed to provide this support and to help in the coordination of care and the support of team members in the more complicated interactions.

Good psychosocial care of the patient with ALS and their family is essential in the success of the ALS team. Every member must have a good understanding of the process of adjustment for the patient and family from the onset of symptoms. Psychosocial care is not the exclusive territory of social science; on the contrary, they should only be called upon in specific circumstances.

There are limited numbers of clinical psychologists, and their skills need to be used carefully and to best effect. It is rare to find a clinical psychologist who works exclusively with ALS. Most likely to offer services to people with ALS are those who work in health psychology specialties, elderly services or delivering services to people with chronic illnesses. Recommended activities for clinical psychologists are assessment of complex cases, supervision, consultation and teaching.[1] The main strength they bring to bear is their training in and knowledge of psychological theories to explain human behaviour, including the brain–behaviour relationship.

The following psychological issues must be considered: the effect of ALS on the patient, patient neuropsychology and reactions to the symptoms (diagnosis, chronicity and facing death), coping strategies of the family and the effects of individual coping strategies of family members on each other. Another is the social support network, reactions of friends and the wider community. The clinical team will also react to the patient and family and their way of coping. Team effectiveness will depend on the members' ability to express their reactions constructively. The clinical psychologist may have a role in the management of the cognitive changes of ALS, the psychological impact on the person with ALS, and in the role of facilitator within clinical ALS teams.

Cognitive changes in ALS

There is increasing awareness of cognitive changes in ALS. Chari *et al.*[2] suggested there may be ALS with subclinical cognitive impairment, only detected in research through neuropsychological screening. Twenty-five per cent of 50 patients with ALS had non-verbal visual attention difficulties, suggesting frontal neurological damage, although they had not been diagnosed with dementia. Abrahams *et al.*[3] confirmed these findings with neuropsychological tests of word fluency. Patients and carers were unaware of these difficulties. Other studies[4] have suggested cognitive impairment may approach 50 per cent of all people with ALS. Most commonly impairments are subtle in presentation, primarily in frontal and temporal functions. It is likely that there is a continuum from subtle to full-blown frontotemporal dementia. The latter only affects about 5 per cent, with 10 per cent of those with frontotemporal dementia developing ALS.[5] The subtle cognitive changes are thought to develop relatively slowly. Mild cognitive impairment may be a precursor of dementia and may even indicate the stage of the disease. It is also possible that those with mild cognitive impairment have a different category of disease. Language and communication may be impaired and forms the particular concern of speech and language therapists – see Chapter 7c.

In larger ALS centres, cognitive impairment may be more likely to be detected. In local services, which deal with small numbers of ALS patients, and have less access to neuropsychology services, such changes may be missed. There are significant implications for patient management if there is cognitive impairment and dementia.

Worthington[6] stresses that some dementia patients will have neurological problems that should be neither neglected, nor exaggerated. He points out that most patients who have both ALS and dementia presented with a personality disintegration or psychological dysfunction before recognizable physical symptoms. They already had full-blown dementia before ALS symptoms developed. It is therefore likely that some ALS patients go undetected in health facilities for people with dementias.

Whether to inform the patient and the family about the possibility of cognitive involvement needs to be evaluated in the light of the devastating effect this information may have. Silverstein *et al.*[7] found that patients with ALS who might suffer from memory impairment, were more likely to choose not to be resuscitated in a hypothetical scenario, than those with ALS alone. To lose cognitive functions or to anticipate this loss is distressing. Remember that most patients do not have to face any cognitive involvement in their disease.

What was previously considered good practice – giving assurances that ALS does not affect the mind – is misplaced. There is an ongoing interesting debate on this issue taking please in care for the elderly.[8] Recent research[5] has shown that carers report less cognitive dysfunction compared with controls. Among the reasons for this low level of reporting on the effects of cognitive deterioration on everyday life it is postulated that this may be due reduced demands from physical disability and defensive responses to investigations into cognitive status. This raises the question of whether patients with ALS and their relatives want to know about the possibility of cognitive deterioration.

This may be further illustrated by the relative frequency of dementia in ALS by Catherine Lomen-Hoerth.[9] A cohort of 100 diagnosed ALS patients were tested with word generation tests and 31 tested abnormally. Just over half (17) agreed to have a full neuropsychological and neuropsychiatric work-up. Of the 69 who had normal tests on the word generation tests, 27 agreed to have the full work-up. The paper does not report the degree to which patients were offered further tests even though word tests were normal. In other words, of the initial 100 subjects 56 did not want to know more about cognitive changes and 44 did. These figures indicate the ambivalence people have about wanting to know the effects of ALS and protecting themselves and their relatives from difficult organically induced changes in mind and identity.

The particular ways in which cognitive impairments manifest themselves, must be known to the multidisciplinary team:[10]

- Changes in personality (rigidity or aggressiveness).

- Slow psychological processes like decision making, answering questions, memory.

- Emotionality (uncontrollable crying, laughter or anger).

- Difficulties with new information, due to distractions and language comprehension difficulties.

- Difficulties with problem-solving, and generating new ideas and strategies when old ones prove unsuccessful.

- Difficulties in divided attention (unable to do two things at once, like walking and talking).

If team members suspect some of these, these should be shared in the team to establish if other members have the same view. A discussion with the patient and/or the relatives needs to be considered remembering that frontal lobe impairment causes lack of insight into their own difficulties, and they may not recognize symptoms easily. Their relatives may also be reluctant to consider the possibility.

When patients or relatives ask questions about behaviour changes or psychological status, an educational approach is appropriate. A clinical psychologist could combine this with advice on how to manage the environment, and strategies to enable optimum performance.

The task of assessing cognitive and behavioural changes will be most appropriately carried out by a clinical psychologist to establish neuropsychological status and consider whether the behavioural change could be a coping style or premorbid psychopathology.

The psychological impact on the person with ALS

Early research into the psychological impact has been of doubtful quality, but findings have been widely quoted. It is possible this has led to service providers underestimating the need for psychosocial interventions. Based on observation of only 10 patients Brown and Mueller[11] concluded that ALS patients displayed a stoic personality, independence, internal focus of control and ability to exclude dysphoric affect from awareness. The fashion was to look for personality traits as contributory factors in specific illnesses. Gould *et al.*[12] tried to replicate this study, but found no link between personality and ALS. In fact they reported that 22 per cent of the 40 subjects they studied had depressive symptoms.

Other research focused on the possibility that neurological disease could cause depression. Shiffer and Babigian[13] reviewed psychiatric records in ALS and MS. They found 19 per cent of 365 patients with multiple sclerosis had depression, against 5 per cent of 124 with ALS. Although the sample sizes were large, the method had serious bias and the conclusions doubtful.

There was one early report of the impact of ALS on the patient and the family which still stands. Bregman[14] reported on her experiences of living with six families with ALS. She highlights the impact of the disease progression on social roles, loss of status and friends, and personal experiences of embarrassment and feeling a burden. Quantitative research does not capture these well nor describe the disease experience over time.

The first substantive piece of quantitative research was by Montgomery and Erikson.[15] They studied 38 patients and found 50 per cent had elevated anxiety and depression scores. They found no association between elevated depression and anxiety scores and disease severity.

The relationship between disease severity and psychological status is complex. The general population (including health care professionals) assumes that people who are disabled must be emotionally disturbed. The focus of research is often on those who have evidence of psychological distress, but not on those who do not. It would be as enlightening to explore which factors contribute to psychological well-being, as it is to know more about which increase psychological distress – for example, the role hope can play in the disease process.[16] The Montgomery and Erikson[15] study leads to the conclusion that functional impairment is related to psychological distress. However, severe depression is not related to disease severity.

In contrast Bocker et al.[17] concluded there is a significant link between disability of daily living function and severity of mood disturbance. This was based on 21 patients, all in advanced disease, and therefore must be limited to end stage disease.

A methodologically sound study was carried out on a cohort of 181 ALS patients,[18] using the National Register of Patients. They found substantial psychological distress in 75 per cent and estimated 16 per cent to have severe psychological problems. They did not find a strong relationship between functional disability or dependence and psychological distress. However, they used two measures, the General Health Questionnaire (GHQ) and the Barthel Index, both of which can be criticized. The GHQ is sensitive to recent changes in health status, but not to chronicity of a condition; the Barthel Index is insensitive to pain or speech problems. They found no connection between psychological status and type of ALS.

The complexity of the relationship between psychological distress and severity of disease is further complicated by the sampling methods of the studies. Hogg et al.[19] studied 59 ALS patients. They had a low incidence of speech problems (12 per cent). Most (52 per cent) had been diagnosed between 1 and 2 years; 17 per cent more than 4 years. This found a connection between physical impairment and psychological distress: with increased physical impairment there was more depression and for patients with severe speech problems, an increase in anxiety. They also reported a relationship between depression and use of denial as a coping strategy. This may be clinically important, necessitating a study of the effectiveness of strategies aimed at reducing denial.

The other complicating factor in the relationship between ALS and depression is the variety of measures used to assess depression. Jau-Shin Lau et al.[20] reported depression in 44 per cent consistent with the ALS Patient Care

Database. Both use the Center for Epidemiologic Study-Depression (CES-D) as their measurement. Lou et al.[20] concluded that disease severity did not correlate with Quality of Life measures.

Unfortunately the study by Rabkin et al.[21] does not compare the two measures used: the Beck Depression Inventory and a Structured Clinical Interview for DSM-IV. This would have allowed a comparison of a self-rated measure with a clinician measure of depression They report low levels of psychiatric impairment and of psychological distress. There is no relationship between distress and severity of disability or length of illness. They conclude: 'Clinical depression or significant depressive symptomatology is not an inevitable or common outcome of life-threatening disease, even in the presence of major disability' Rabkin et al.[21]

Recent research in psychological adaptation to chronic illness focuses on how patients understand their diagnosis in terms of causality, severity and progression, and the way these influence how they cope. Their coping style may in turn influence their disease representations. Earl et al.[22] point out that health professionals should be warned about assuming they can anticipate the patient's view or that their perspective on the disease is the medical one. Patients individual representations of their disease vary and do not relate to objective severity. The level of distress and willingness to adhere to treatments are related to disease representation and this is, in part, why the new research is important. No relationship has been found between coping style and emotional outcome. Another way in which illness representation research may prove useful is the effect the psychological profile may have on survival. McDonald and Carpenter[23] showed that patients with a poor psychological status had shorter survival. They interviewed 144 patients and followed them for 2–3 years. The psychological profile was constructed using seven scales. The scales measured hopelessness, depression, perceived stress, anger, depression, purpose in life, health focus of control and satisfaction with life. They controlled for duration of disease, severity of the disease, and age. The sample used by McDonald and Carpenter may have been biased by over-representation of patients who survive longer.

A study by Johnston et al.[24] controlled for this bias, by studying a cohort of 38 patients, prior to admission for diagnosis, at six weeks and six months. They conclude that their study supports McDonald and Carpenter's earlier findings. Johnston et al. state that patients with a more positive mood survive longer than those with a more negative mood. This study demonstrates increased survival is unrelated to the individual's experience of the disease per se (patients were all recruited at diagnosis, and the symptoms and level of disability at diagnosis was unrelated to survival). Johnston *et al.* propose three possible mechanisms for shorter survival of low mood patients: different health behaviours (diet, physical activity, symptom monitoring); they induce health professionals to behave differently (not offer additional procedures, not offer support to accept additional procedures) or a physiological mechanism relevant to disease progression (e.g. neuroendocrine immune function). All need further investigation.

Clinically there is not enough evidence to justify protocols to systematically attend to and influence coping styles and disease representations, although research is moving in that direction. There is enough evidence of the effectiveness of treatment of depression in other neurological conditions, to warrant routine assessment of and treatment for depression.[25] A newer concept of hopelessness in relation to ALS[26] is important particularly because it might mediate between depression and suicidal intent and predict intensity of suicidal ideation and intent better than depression itself. Severity of illness, length of illness and socio-economic, demographic variables are not significant predictors of hopelessness. External locus of control and low sense of purpose in life are. Assisting patients to find meaning and acquiring a sense of control over their health are valuable.

Teamwork in ALS: the role of the clinical psychologist

The role of a clinical psychologist in a team may encompass that of assessor (for cognitive changes and adjustment styles of individuals), researcher (to assess the effectiveness of psychosocial approaches) and psychosocial therapist working with family systems (see Chapter 7d) and team facilitator (working with the impact the disease and family have on the team). This section will address the role of team facilitator.

Research on stress in the health professions is vast.[27] Personal perceptions of stress may be influenced by workload, physical strain, responsibility, relationships at work, work and home demands, role ambiguity and role conflict. Role ambiguity may particularly apply to psychosocial care, as all members of the team provide it, and family members may choose to express distress to team members less equipped to deal with it, than the identified psychosocial worker (social worker, counsellor or clinical psychologist).

Working with dying patients is stressful.[28,29] Working in the caring professions is stressful. Menzies[30] described a teaching hospital using social defence systems against the inherent stress undermine the staff's abilities to cope, rise to the challenge and face their anxieties. In recognition of work stress numerous approaches have proliferated. Stress management interventions[31] – or "therapeutic" organizational approaches[32–34] may be useful in a multidisciplinary team. In that role the clinical psychologist may review recurrent difficulties in the team. Unconscious defences can be explored and discussed, leading to a change in organizational structure and processes. This is the role of an organizational consultant, which the psychologist would take up to promote change in team structure or processes. This role is not compatible with that of assessor, researcher or psychosocial therapist.

As a participant in the multidisciplinary team it is important for the psychologist to be aware of the social forces in the organization and encourage open discussion of frustrations and anxieties, to strengthen the team's confidence and mutual support. (See later the case example, Mrs Johns.) The cultural changes in industrialized nations affect our tendency to construct our role as a responsibility to give shape to the end life. For instance Pasetti and Zanini[35] discuss the unique aspects of ALS requiring staff to address ethical dilemmas around informed consent, communication of diagnosis and prognosis and the decision making process in advanced disease. They point out the use of jargon and evasive language as a defence against the emotions from the message of death the disease invokes. Decision-making anxiety may lead to extreme or opposite solutions such as euthanasia or over-treatment. They limit their discussions to the physician, but in multidisciplinary services, these dilemmas fall to all involved. Another example is provided by Ganzini et al.[36] They explored the health care experiences and palliative care needs of ALS patients in their final months. They looked at preferences for end of life care, completion of advance directives, preparation for death, which life sustaining treatments were administered and which withheld or withdrawn.

Rabkin et al.[21] explore patients' interest in hastening death and assistance in dying. They found depressive symptoms were associated only with refusal of the least invasive interventions, like non-invasive ventilation. Depressive symptoms were unrelated to more invasive interventions like tracheostomy with mechanical ventilation. The willingness to consider asking for a lethal prescription in the future was not associated with depression or distress. Such findings force teams to consider the reality of the patient's experience, irrespective of the legal context of the service or the moral values of the staff.

In terms of the stress experienced and perceived by staff working with ALS, the study by Carter et al.[37] is interesting. They compared the responses of 195 health care professionals working with both MS and ALS. Health care professionals were more negative about ALS than MS patients in terms of their perception of how much they could offer the patient, their confidence and their ability to convey hope. They report that their ability to convey hope depended on the patient's ability to cope. Rapid progression of the disorder made it difficult to convey hope as did the inevitable overall progression. MS patients were seen as more stressful due to changes in cognition, mood and personality, the unpredictable course of the disease and a (perceived) tendency to be difficult or demanding.

The possibility of a reciprocal relationship between the team and patient's ability to cope with ALS is important in the light of the studies by McDonald and Carpenter[23] and Johnston *et al.*,[24] which indicate that patients with a more positive mood survive longer. The health care team may inadvertently exacerbate the loss of hope. It may be that health professionals tend to associate hope with the absence of disease or lack or progression. Carter *et al.*[37] suggest "it is important that health professionals be given opportunities within their work environments to reflect on their practice, so they remain open to new ideas and concepts".

Another interesting conclusion from the same study[37] is that what health care professionals find most useful for themselves in coping is supportive, well coordinated teamwork. One of the frustrations was the inability to track members of the team. Regular meetings provide opportunities to coordinate care, reflect on the way families cope and on how the team responds. The clinical psychologist can play an important role in team meetings, enabling them to reflect on their own process, particularly with families who display complicated reactions. Systems theory is helpful in this context, e.g. Altschuler.[38] The strength of the feelings experienced by families and team members is illustrated in the case history of Mrs Johns.

Case history

Mrs Johns

Mrs Johns was diagnosed with ALS when she was 47 years old. She had a husband and two teenage children taking exams before going to university. Her husband was a nurse and wanted to look after his wife by carrying out the professional duties of a nurse. Initially the family did not want much involvement from the team. Mrs Johns' physical deterioration did not really warrant more involvement as she was relatively well. The couple were hopeful of a cure. They were religious and belonged to a church, which inspired hope of a cure through prayer. When the cure did not come and the disease progressed, contact with the family was complicated because Mr Johns refused to speak to staff and when he did it was often to criticize nursing staff for particular aspects of care.

(A) Mrs Johns learnt to use a Lightwriter and would come to day care. She would get professional staff to read and listen to her prepared text. Mrs Johns got depressed at times. The text would often be expressing suicidal ideas and wishes to die. Whilst the text would play, Mrs Johns would smile at the professional, leaving an incongruent communication.

(B) Towards the end of Mrs John's protracted illness, it transpired the couple had not been able to process emotional difficulties before the diagnosis of ALS. Couple conflict seemed to be ended by Mrs Johns harming herself (e.g. cutting herself by breaking a window). Conflict resolution continued to be problematic for them.

Mrs Johns expressed distress about a particular way her husband cared for her and invited the professionals to convey this for her. At the same time she was unwilling for any team member to address these complaints with them together.

(C) As the disease progressed and Mrs Johns became more dependent, the relationship between the two seemed to improve. Mrs Johns however expressed her despair in the Day Hospice. On a few occasions she howled loudly for an hour whilst in the bath.

(D) In the end Mrs Johns died peacefully at home. Mr Johns did not avail himself of the bereavement service. The family participated in some fundraising events.

In the work with Mrs Johns, the team was frustrated because members could not get supportive roles because the family held different beliefs (a cure would emerge), or were criticized – Point A. It was important for team members to discuss their feelings of frustration, anger and powerlessness. They came to the conclusion that their frustrations and powerlessness mirrored those in the family, and the anger was a displacement from that towards the disease (or God) to the team. Later (Point B), many team members talked about their feelings of awkwardness and fear when Mrs Johns played her suicidal ideas to them on her Lightwriter. They felt powerless because she did not want them to do anything, say more herself, nor want staff to get antidepressant medication. Euthanasia was not an option for Mrs Johns herself, because of her religious beliefs (there was a glimpse of a spiritual crisis, when she put on the Lightwriter "God, where is he now"?) and because euthanasia is illegal in this health care system. The team concluded we were supposed to feel the despair and awkwardness she felt about the cruelty of her disease and her abandonment, combined with guilt for being unable to do anything to alleviate the pain.

It was a relief for the team to find out that conflict resolution had always been a problem in the couple's relationship. This was recognized as a release from some guilt about being isolated from the family. Team members had spoken previously about feeling de-skilled and guilty about being unable to help. Isolation was also the way the couple protected their children from the disease. The children could not approach the team for their own needs, again leading to guilt in the staff. When (Point C) individual team members were invited to get involved in the marital conflict, it was as messenger. Mr Johns would get angry with the messenger and ignore the message. Team discussion led to the strategy to encourage Mrs Johns to communicate directly with her husband or get her husband's agreement to talk with a social worker. After this was explained to Mrs Johns the complaints ceased and Mr Johns began to contact members of the team to request specific help with the care of his wife.

Towards the end of Mrs Johns' life she had episodes of howling with despair in the bath – (Point D). This was hard for the Day Hospice staff and other visitors. When we talked this through we concluded that the only place Mrs Johns felt safe enough to let her feelings flood her, was in the bath on her own in the Hospice. This made it possible to see the expression of despair in a more positive light, as trust in the Day Hospice allowed her to express herself.

Conclusion

Depending on the team, the role of the clinical psychologist may be as diagnostician-researcher, external consultant, psychosocial therapist and team facilitator, and ALS teams must decide what is most important within the resources available. For all teams it is important that all team members provide psychosocial support and the team meets regularly for the coordination of care and the support of each other in their complicated interactions with patients, families and other professionals.

References

1. MAS (Management Advisory Service) (1989) *Review of Clinical Psychology Services.* London: Department of Health.
2. Chari G., Shaw P., Sahgal A. (1996) Non-verbal attention, but not recognition memory or learning processes are impaired in motor neurone disease. *Neuropsychologia* 34 (5): 377–85.
3. Abrahams S., Goldstein L. H., Al-Chalabi A., Pickering A., Morris R. G., Passingham R. E., Brooke P. J., Leigh P. N. (1997) Relation between cognitive dysfunction and pseudobulbor palsy in amyotrophic lateral sclerosis. *Journal of Neurology, Neurosurgery and Psychiatry* 62 (5): 464–72.
4. Strong M. J., Lomen-Hoerth C., Caselli R. J., Bigio E. H., Yang W. (2003) Cognitive impairment, frontotemporal dementia, and motor neuron disease. *Annals of Neurology* 54 (Suppl. 5): S20–S23.
5. Abrahams S., Leigh P. N., Goldstein L. H. (2005) Cognitive change in ALS. *Neurology* 64: 1222–6.
6. Worthington A. (1996) Psychological aspects of motor neurone disease: a review. *Clinical Rehabilitation* 10: 185–94.
7. Silverstein M. D., Stocking C. B., Antel J. P. (1991) Amyotrophic lateral sclerosis and life-sustaining therapy; patient's desire for information, participation in decision making and life-sustaining therapy. *Mayo Clinic Proceedings* 66: 906–13.
8. Drickamer M. A., Lachs M. S. (1992) Should patients with Alzheimer's be told their diagnosis? *New England Journal of Medicine* 326 (14): 947–51.

9. **Lomen-Hoerth C.** (2004) Characterization of amyotrophic lateral sclerosis and frontotemporal dementia. *Dementia and Geriatric Cognitive Disorders* 17: 337–41.

10. **Grossman A., Bradley W.** (2003) Psychosocial factors and cognition in amyotrophic lateral sclerosis. *ALS and Other Motor Neuron Disorders* 4: 225–31.

11. **Brown W. A., Mueller P. S.** (1970) Psychological function in individuals with amyotrophic lateral sclerosis (ALS). *Psychosomatic Medicine* 32: 141–52.

12. **Gould B. S., Houpt J. L., Morris F. H.** (1977) Psychological characteristics of patients with amyotrophic lateral sclerosis (ALS). *Psychosomatic Medicine* 39: 299–303.

13. **Schiffer R. B., Babigian H. M.** (1984) Behavioural disorders in multiple sclerosis, temporal lobe epilepsy and amyotrophic lateral sclerosis: an epidemiological study. *Archives of Neurology* 41: 1067–9.

14. **Bregman A. M.** (1983) Living with ALS: major concerns of patients and families. In Charash L. I., Wolf S. G., Kutscher A. H., Lovelace R. E., Hale M. S. (eds) *Psychosocial Aspects of Muscular Dystrophy and Allied Diseases, Commitment to Life, Health and Function*, pp. 137–47. Springfield, Illinois-Chas Thomas.

15. **Montgomery G. K., Erikson L. M.** (1987) Neuropsychological perspectives in myotrophic lateral sclerosis. In Brookes B. R. (ed.) *Neurologic Clinics*, 5, pp. 61–81. Philadelphia, PA: W. B. Saunders.

16. **Centers L. A.** (2001) Beyond denial and despair: ALS and our heroic potential for hope. *Journal for Palliative Care* 17 (4): 259–64.

17. **Bocker F. M., Seibold I., Neundorfer B.** (1990) Disability in everyday tasks and subjective status of patients with advanced amyotrophic lateral sclerosis. *Fortschriffe der Neurologie – Psychiatrie* 58: 224–36.

18. **Hunter M. D., Robinson I. C., Neilson S.** (1993) The functional and psychological status of patients with amyotrophic lateral sclerosis: some implications for rehabilitation. *Disability and Rehabilitation* 15: 119–26.

19. **Hogg K. E., Goldstein L. H., Leigh P. H.** (1994) The psychological impact of motor neurone disease. *Psychological Medicine* 24: 625–32.

20. **Lau J., Reeves A., Benice T., Sexton G.,** (2003) Fatigue and depression are associated with poor quality of life in ALS. *Neurology* 60: 122–3.

21. Rabkin J. G., Wagner G. J., Del Bene M. (2000) Resilience and distress among myotrophic lateral sclerosis patients and cargivers. *Psychosomatic Medicine* 62: 271–9.

22. **Earl L., Johnston M., Mitchell E.** (1993) Coping with motor neurone disease – an analysis using self-regulation theory. *Palliative Medicine* 7: 21–30.

23. **McDonald E. R., Carpenter C. L.** (1994) Survival in amyotrophic lateral sclerosis. *Archives of Neurology* 51: 17–23.

24. **Johnston M., Earl L., Giles M., McClenahan R., Stevens D.** (1999) Mood as a predictor of disability and survival in patients diagnosed with ALS/MND. *British Journal of Health Psychology* 4 (2): 127–36.

25. **Mohr D. C., Goodkin D.** (1999) Treatment of depression in multiple sclerosis: review and meta-analysis. *Clinical Psychology Science and Practice* 6 (1): 1–9.

26. **Plahuta *et al.*** (2002) Amyotrophic lateral sclerosis and hopelessness. *Soc Sci Med* 55: 2131–40.

27. **Hardy S., Carson J., Thomas B.** (ed.) (1998) *Occupational Stress, Personal and Professional Approaches*. Cheltenham: Stanley Thornes Ltd.

28. Tyler P. A., Cushway D. (1992) Stress coping and mental well-being in hospital nurses. *Stress Medicine* 8: 91–8.

29. Vachon M. L., Lyall W., Freeman S. (1978) Measurement and management of stress in health professionals working with patients with advanced cancer. *Death Education* 1: 365–74.

30. Menzies I. E. P. (1959) The functioning of social systems as a defence against anxiety: a report on a study of the nursing service of a general hospital. *Human Relations* 13: 95–121.

31. Carson J., Knupers E. (1998) Stress management interventions. In Hardy S., Carson J., Thomas B. (eds) *Occupational Stress, Personal and Professional Approaches*, pp. 157–74. Cheltenham: Stanley Thornes Ltd.

32. Stapley L., Cleavely E., Dartington T. *et al.* (1995) *Organisational Stress in the National Health Service.* London: Health Education Authority.

33. Stapley L., Cardona F., Cleavely E. *et al.* (1996) *Organisational Stress: Planning and Implementing a Programme to Address Organisational Stress in the NHS.* London: Health Education Authority.

34. Huffington C., Brunning H. (1994) *Internal Consultancy in the Public Sector. Case Studies.* London: Karnack Books.

35. Pasetti C., Zanini G. (2000) The physician-patient relationship in amyotrophic lateral scerosis. *Neurological Science* 21: 318–23.

36. Ganzini L., Johnston W. S., Silveira M. J. (2002) The final months of life in patients with MND. *Neurology* 59: 428–31.

37. Carter H., McKenna C., McLeod R., Green R. (1998) Health professionals' responses to multiple sclerosis and motor neurone disease. *Palliative Medicine* 2 (5): 383–94.

38. Altschuler J. (1997) *Working with Chronic Illness.* London: Macmillan Press.

Multidisciplinary care:

nursing care

Dallas Forshew

Summary

The nurse is a generalist who needs the ability to be all things to all people at an ALS centre and must have the qualities of flexibility, creativity, warmth, empathy and more, acting as a specialist practitioner, manager, counselor, coordinator, educator, supporter, researcher, mentor and innovator. The nurse has an essential role in the support of the person with ALS, their family and the other members of the multidisciplinary team.

Introduction

The role of the nurse in ALS is as varied and complex as the needs of the patients and their families. The nurse cares for and gives guidance from the time of the initial diagnosis through to the terminal stage of the illness. This includes a large spectrum of needs including emotional and psychological, education regarding the disease process, referrals to community agencies, sorting through insurance and governmental regulations, the rationale for and practical aspects of interventions such as feeding tubes and non-invasive ventilation and symptom management.

In addition, the nurse in a multidisciplinary team is often responsible for the general coordination and management of the team members and clinic organization.

At the time of diagnosis

The period of investigation, while the diagnosis is unclear, may well be the most emotionally difficult time for all concerned.[1] While the diagnostic work-up is in process, there is a sense of 'hanging in the air'. Lives may be put on hold while the reason for the patient's symptoms are sorted out. Most patients know that there is something seriously wrong: when the diagnosis is given, the reaction may be tinged with some relief because "At least now we know what we are dealing with."[1,2]

However, the overwhelming feelings of the patient and family revolve around the knowledge that their lives are changed forever. Their hopes and expectations for the future are shattered. It is our responsibility, as a team, to help them find ways to readjust their expectations to meet their new reality. In fact, this readjustment must happen over and over again throughout the disease process as every loss of function is grieved.[3] ALS is not a static disorder – it is dynamic and it seems that every time an adjustment is made to a new loss, another loss comes forward and adjustment is needed again and again.

There are two main goals of the nurse at the time of diagnosis. First, the patient needs to leave the clinic with knowledge of the disease: second, the patient needs to feel supported and secure in the belief that he will be cared for well.[4]

The physician gives the diagnosis and initial teaching but, no matter how sensitive and skilled the physician is, the patient may not hear much after the diagnosis is initially discussed. If available, the patient will immediately benefit from a session with the nurse. The nurse can augment the physician's discussion by quietly listening to the patient's interpretation of what was said and then talking in plain language about what ALS is and what it is not. The role of dispelling myths about the disease is just as important as giving new information. Written information should be given and the patient told that they may telephone with questions or concerns. Many clinics have a packet of materials that is given to every new patient. Referral to the local support agencies, including the ALS and MND associations, is critical.

Attention to the family

ALS affects the patient but also the family and close friends: many patients will admit that they believe the disease is harder on their family than on them. It will give patients a great deal of comfort to know that their family will be given attention. This can be accomplished in many ways. It is important to consider the family members and simply ask how they are doing, such as enquiring if they are getting enough sleep, as the nurse can make suggestions to ease many sleep issues. Do they have someone to talk to? Do they need counselling? Are they attending to their own medical care? Many caregivers let their own health decline because they are so focused on caring for their loved one. Do they get out of the home and the caregiving role frequently enough? They must remain rejuvenated in order to provide the best care. Are they keeping close ties with their friends? They will need these friends throughout the disease but even more after their loved one is deceased.

Who attends clinic appointments with the patient is, of course, at the patient's discretion. Encouraging family and even friends to attend clinic appointments will contribute to better follow-through on recommendations because the others will reinforce the recommendations at home. Everyone will have a better understanding of the rationale for the recommendations if several people have heard the discussion.[5]

Of course, the patient is always addressed directly during the interview, even if they have difficulty with their speech. A professional would never direct questions to the family if the questions should be directed to the patient. However, family will often contribute to the clinic interview by supplementing what the patient says and it may be appropriate to direct some questions to family. This can bring important information to light.[6]

Patients and family members will often admit that they protect each other from certain information or feelings. They will both feel better supported if each are given private time during the interview. This can be extraordinarily empowering to each individual.

Coordination with support agencies

The role of support agencies is integral to the well-being of the patient and family. These agencies attempt to reach every community. They include such organizations as the ALS and MND Associations throughout the world. Internet access has the ability to reach out to those areas that are too remote for a local group – see Appendix 2, which contains a list of web sites.

The strength and range of services of the support agency will vary in each community. The basic services usually include education materials, support groups and lending of equipment. Those agencies that are better funded may offer special programmes for children, transportation and funding for lodging to attend clinic appointments, help in the home for bathing and dressing of the patient, a nurse or other professional to visit the home, or a visiting programme to provide a companion while the caregiver goes out.

It is the responsibility of the nurse to know which services are available in the community and to coordinate with the agencies. The nurse can seek out information from the agency about their interactions with the patient and family that would be useful in their clinical care. Likewise, the nurse can coordinate with the agency after the patient's clinic visit or telephone contact. The nurse can request a home visit or recommend a piece of equipment and may ask the agency to reinforce a clinic recommendation.

Referral to and coordination with home care and palliative care/hospice

Home care services may be available to support someone at home – depending on local facilities and funding. It is most often the nurse who will carry out the referral and then keep in close communication with the agency. The services are provided to the patient in their home and may include a home nurse, physiotherapist, occupational therapist, social worker, or home health aid. The clinic nurse should clearly state the needs of the patient and then keep in contact with the agency to make sure the needs are being met. Likewise, the agency may identify additional needs and seek approval from the clinic nurse to provide extra services. The nurse coordinates with the physician and team members to keep them informed and to seek their input. The patient is best served if the nurse and agency keep in close contact and coordinate care.[7]

Like home care services, the initiation of palliative care and hospice services requires further discussion and involvement of the wider multidisciplinary team. It is often the nurse who will make the referral and give details to the hospice of the patient and family needs. In turn, the hospice will discover additional needs and keep in close contact with the nurse. The nurse will then communicate this information to the other team members, enabling the palliative care team and hospice and the clinic to collaborate and inform each other of the care they are providing.

Palliative care will provide a wide variety of services, including assessment and recommendations from professionals such as the hospice nurse, physiotherapy, occupational therapists, dietitian, speech and language therapist, social worker, pastoral care and hospice physician.

Most ALS centres in the US will maintain their close relationship with the patient for all disease-related issues such as nutrition, breathing and symptom management. Hospice agencies have particular expertise in such areas as pain management, constipation, urinary tract infections, prevention of decubitus ulcers and the social issues that surround this final and very natural stage of life.

Patient education

Education of the patient and family is fundamental to the role of the nurse in every disease state. ALS is no exception. Armed with accurate information, the patient and family are better equipped to cope with every stage of the disease. Education starts on the day of diagnosis and occurs with every interaction. Patients are more likely to accept recommendations if they understand the reasoning behind the recommendation and it is explained in language the patient understands.[8]

The nurse needs to make sure that the patient and family have a good understanding of the disease and its progression, the rationale for all interventions and all aspects of medication use.

Compliance with interventions is enhanced if the subject is brought up early within a broad framework and then, as the time comes closer for needing that intervention, more direct information is given. For example, high compliance with feeding tubes can be had through a step-wise approach. Near the time of diagnosis, the patient can be empowered with the knowledge that nutrition is an important part of care for ALS, that they have control over this area, and the clinic will give them the information they need along the way. As the patient progresses, they are given information about how to enhance their diet to prevent weight loss. When it is difficult for the patient to keep up with their caloric needs and it is deemed that they will eventually need a feeding tube, mention of an alternative to oral intake can be made well before a feeding tube is needed. Small pieces of information given over time will help the patient become aware that the eventual need for a feeding tube is natural and thus acceptance is more likely to be easy.

A basic part of the nurse's own education revolves around techniques used to teach the adult learner. Attention must be paid to the patient's readiness to learn. The day of diagnosis may not be a good time to teach more than the basics of the disease and then teach further at another visit in a few weeks. Some ALS centres in the US offer an orientation class for patients with a new diagnosis. This might be given monthly by the nurse or through the local support agency.

The levels of education and understanding are important consideration in the discussion with patients and families. Not all will be literate and even a person with several university degrees may have trouble with concepts that are far from their field. The nurse must use language, free of all jargon, that the patient can understand. Educational materials should be written at a reasonable level, using simple words and short sentences but without 'dumbing down' the material.

Awareness of cultural differences needs to inform the communication approach that the health care team members use with the patient. In some cultures, difficult medical information is given to the family and not the patient. In others, it is not polite to look the patient straight in the face while talking. Although some of these examples are very difficult to carry out in today's age of openness and full information, cultural differences must be respected. There are ways to get the information to the patient that are still respectful of their heritage.

Written material is needed to reinforce what is taught in clinic. Patients will often forget the details of what was said because they are overwhelmed. It is recommended that information be given verbally with time to ask questions and then reinforced with written literature. The nurse may write multiple information handouts that cover topics such as medication rationale, potential side-effects and dose escalation schedules, rational for interventions such as non-invasive positive pressure ventilation, instructions for use of the feeding tube, summary of recommended Internet sites, books, and agencies, summary of the ongoing research that encourages the patient to take part and many more. The nurse may also mentor team members in writing handouts pertinent to their specialty.

It is incumbent upon the nurse and all team members to remember that the patient and family will need further reinforcement of all teaching. It is the nature of any serious disease that the patient can only remember so much at any given time.

Outreach education to community agencies

ALS remains a rare disease but with the advent of specialty clinics, there are now centres of excellence for patient care. This is not true for home care or hospice agencies, where a patient with ALS is infrequent. It is in the best interest of our patients that we reach out to community agencies and provide specialized education about the disease and the varied needs of its patients. This can be accomplished by talking to one's counterpart at the agency whether it is nurse-to-nurse or therapist-to-therapist. The nurse has an excellent opportunity to do this when the referral is initially telephoned into the agency and the nurse sets up expectations for further communication. Such opportunities continue as a cooperative relationship develops between the clinic and the agency.

The nurse can also offer to provide educational activities for the agency staff whenever a patient is referred, especially if it is an agency that has not been used in the past. This is an excellent way to build relationships and educate at the same time.

Coordination and management of the ALS centre

The multidisciplinary team approach has become the standard of care for people with ALS.[9] The organization, coordination and management of such a team are often the responsibility of the centre's nurse.[4,5]

Attention is given to the entire patient experience from the first phone call through to the last clinic visit. Every aspect of the centre should be welcoming. Patients do not look forward to coming to the centre, because they know that they will be confronted with more news of weakness and loss. We must do everything possible to make patients want to come again. Building strong personal relationships and always finding something positive to say to the patient will help in this regard.

An ideal centre will give a high priority to having the telephone answered by a person rather than a machine. The reception area should be quiet and the receptionist warm. The clinic area should afford privacy within a professional atmosphere. It is often the role of the nurse to set these as required expectations for the staff.

Staff education is important for the patient's sake but also for the professional satisfaction of each team member. Team members are more likely to be invested in the centre if they feel that the centre is invested in them. It is recommended that there are regular opportunities for a team meeting that involves a particular clinic issue. Articles can be distributed every week or so. There can be a journal club for the staff. The nurse can organize these activities and act as an advocate for the staff. The director can make time available for such activities and provide funds for attendance at conferences. The director can show their interest in the staff by participating in these efforts. The director can also support the nurse as the nurse supports the staff. The nurse should attend ALS conferences on a regular basis and have the opportunity to develop collegial relationships with nurses in similar roles.

A yearly retreat provides time for team building, education, staff support and addressing administrative issues. It is advisable to hold the retreat away from the ALS centre. Sections might be devoted to discussion of difficult clinical issues, ethical problems, communication and coordination amongst staff, research, stress reduction, or others. Staff will feel more invested in the process if they are asked to contribute to forming the agenda.

Burnout among staff can be devastating for the patients, team and the individual team member. The nurse manager can take measures to prevent this. Providing staff education, as above, is important. Everyone in medicine is stretched and works very hard. The nurse can be watchful and make sure that the work is distributed in a reasonable fashion. A regular or occasional support group for the staff indicates the high value that the centre places on their well-being. The support group might be led by the nurse, social worker, psychologist, or someone from outside the centre. In general, the nurse needs to be available to the staff for any concern that they might have.

The flow of the patients and the staff through the clinic should be organized such that the patients are taken into their rooms quickly and have little waiting time between seeing team members. Team members will appreciate a simple but well organized system by which they know where they go next so that their time is used efficiently. Every clinic handles these issues differently but the nurse can assure that they are managed well.

In terms of management of the centre, it is the nurse's responsibly to coordinate with the director and carry out the director's wishes. It is the director's responsibly to use the nurse as a partner in the management of the clinic, for the nurse will have the ear of the team members and an overall sense of the centre's coordination.

Research

Many ALS centres in the US are in academic institutions. These centres will be actively involved in drug studies or clinical research aimed at improving care. Patients appreciate obtaining care at a centre that is involved in research: it gives them a sense that they are being cared for by professionals who are very knowledgeable and who are doing important work. This is important work and should be acknowledged as such by every team member.

The benefit of drug studies is obvious: the benefit of sound clinical research is just as important and can carry even more benefit. When a question is asked about clinical management of ALS, it has the potential to radically change the patient's outcome. This is changing management practices and leading to increased quality of life and greater longevity in ALS patients.

The nurse and medical director of the centre can inspire staff interest in clinical research. Staff can be taught how to critically read a research article. Staff can also be integrated into clinical research at the centre. The nurse is often already involved in this research and can be a strong resource. The nurse might help the team member think of a clinical question and assist, along with the medical director, with the design of the project. With nurturing, clinical research projects can become a routine aspect of the centre's activities.

Patient care during and between clinic visits

It is advisable that the nurse telephones each patient a week or two before the scheduled clinic visit. This will provide invaluable information that will enhance the patient's care.

The nurse can perform a variety of duties during the clinic. The nurse might be the organizer and only see patients who have specific issues that are not addressed by the other team members. More often, the nurse has individual time with the patient and family and may perform a general assessment of the patient at the beginning of the visit and determine which team members the patient will see at that visit. The nurse may focus on patient and family education regarding new or ongoing issues. This might prepare the patient for a more thorough discussion with an individual team member. An example might be noting the patient's weight loss and stressing the importance of nutrition to the patient in a general way. This may help the patient to be more receptive to the specific recommendations of the dietitian later in the visit.

Nurses will often review medications with the patient and obtain the patient's perception of their efficacy and side-effects.

Each team member will make recommendations throughout the patient's visit. The nurse needs to make sure that the patient is given written recommendations and discusses these recommendations with the patient at the end of the visit. This gives the patient an opportunity to ask questions and the nurse an opportunity to be sure that the patient leaves with all the necessary paperwork and understands all of the instructions. The nurse can develop forms for this and a variety of other purposes.

If a team member is absent from clinic, the nurse should have enough knowledge of that team member's specialty to be able to fill in. In most centres, the entire team is only available on a particular day every week or two but the nurse is in the centre full time. The nurse must be able to assess and give recommendations in every area. This often includes performing bedside pulmonary functions tests, demonstrating the use of equipment such as a walker, and assessing the patient's nutrition status.

It is good clinical care for the entire team to meet after clinic to discuss each patient. The nurse might be designated to organize this meeting. The physician usually leads such meetings with ample time allotted for each team member to contribute. The purpose of the meeting is to coordinate patient care and to be clear on what needs to be done by who to follow-up on the patient's needs. It is often the nurse who is responsible for seeing that every team member completes their task. An offshoot of the meeting is that staff education can be a prominent part of the discussion. The rationale for a recommendation might be explained or the difference between one kind of motor neurone disease and another such as ALS and primary lateral sclerosis (PLS).

The nurse may telephone the patient about two weeks after their clinic visit, allowing review of the recommendations and assessment of follow-through. This is a suitable time for problem-solving and further education.

The nurse has many responsibilities between the patient's clinic visits and is often the person who handles most of the patient phone calls and gives guidance or arranges referrals. Again, education is a mainstay of the nurse's role. The nurse can refill prescriptions under the direction of the physician and complete many of the forms sent by equipment companies or agencies. Patients and families take great comfort in the knowledge that the nurse is available for support and counseling.

Impact of frontotemporal dementia

It is now recognized that frontotemporal dementia (FTD) and related cognitive disorders are prevalent in ALS[10] – see Chapter 4c, page 111. It is imperative that all professionals working with ALS patients are aware of this issue and are given tools to better work with these patients and support their families. Patients with FTD will learn in an entirely different way than patients with only ALS and may be unable to make sound decisions regarding acceptance of interventions.[11] However, techniques used to work with people with traumatic brain injury of the frontal lobe can bring about remarkable results. An invaluable resource for professionals and families dealing with this is the book *What if it's Not Alzheimer's: A Caregiver's Guide to Dementia* edited by Lisa Radin.[12] It defines clear strategies that are successful when dealing with this issue.

It is important that the centre nurse and physician to make sure that all team members are aware of this overlap syndrome and the techniques needed to work effectively with these patients. Extra support and insight are needed for the family. The family is able to cope with the behaviour and/or judgement changes much better if they understand the nature of the problem. The Family Caregiver Alliance web site, www.caregiver.org, provides downloadable education materials on FTD and behavioural changes. However, information should be given to the family only if they are ready to accept this additional problem. Some families will chose to ignore or deny the problem. These family members should not be confronted with information that they are not prepared to handle.

Bereavement rituals for families and staff

Nearly all patients with ALS will be referred for hospice care. Every hospice has a bereavement program for families after the patient's death and the nurse can reinforce the utility of this programme to family members.[13] Family members may feel better faster if they take advantage of the bereavement programme and this is important for all family members, not just the spouse.

Members of the multidisciplinary team also need time and space to grieve. The work with the patient is intense and the staff will become attached and have feelings for the patient. Every time a patient dies, the staff feels a loss.

Many clinics have rituals that are helpful to both the families and to the team members. One simple ritual is to send a condolence card to the family on which each team member has written a small personal note. This tells the patient's family how much the staff cares and it helps to bring closure for the staff. Some centres hold a yearly memorial for families of patients who have died under their care. This can be quite meaningful for the families and perhaps even more meaningful for the staff.

Taking care of the nurse

Just as burnout can be a problem for other team members, so it can be for the nurse as well. It may be that while the nurse is taking care of everyone else, she may neglect caring for herself. By nature, many nurses will do their best to work until all of the staff and patients' needs are met. This is an impossible task because the work is never finished and never will be. The nurse must heed the advice that she gives to the staff; prioritize, pace yourself, take your holiday time, seek rejuvenation though outside activities and use the medical director or other appropriate person for support.

Conclusion

The nurse has a crucial role in the activities of the ALS centre and the coordination of the patients care and support. The nurse will hold the centre together and move it forward while partnering with the physician director. To a great extent, it is the nurse who is responsible for implementing the principles of excellence in the conduct of ALS centres.

References

1. Borasio G. D., Sloan R., Pongratz D. E. (1998) Breaking the news in amyotrophic lateral sclerosis. *J Neurol Sci* **160** (Suppl. 1): S127–33.
2. Miller R. G., Rosenberg J. A., Gelinas D. F., Mitsumoto H., Newman D., Sufit R., Borasio G. D., Bradley W. G., Bromberg M. B., Brooks B. R., Kasarskis E. J., Munsat T. L., Oppenheimer E. A. (1999) Practice parameter: the care of the patient with amyotrophic lateral sclerosis (an evidence-based review): report of the Quality Standards Subcommittee of the American Academy of Neurology: ALS Practice Parameters Task Force. *Neurology* **52** (7): 1311–23.
3. Andersen P. M., Borasio G. D., Dengler R., Hardiman O., Kollewe K., Leigh P. N., Pradat P. F., Silani V., Tomik B., EFNS Task Force on Diagnosis and Management of Amyotrophic Lateral Sclerosis (2005) EFNS task force on management of amyotrophic lateral sclerosis: guidelines for diagnosing and clinical care of patients and relatives. *Eur J Neurol* (12): 21–38.
4. Van den Berg J. P., Kalmijn S., Lindeman E., Veldink J. H., de Visser M., Van der Graaff M. M., Wokke J. H., Van den Berg L. H. (2005) Multidisciplinary ALS care improves quality of life in patients with ALS. *Neurology* **65** (8): 1264–7.

5. **Traynor B. J., Alexander M., Corr B., Frost E., Hardiman O.** (2003) Effect of a multidisciplinary amyotrophic lateral sclerosis (ALS) clinic on ALS survival: a population-based study, 1996–2000. *J Neurol Neurosurg Psychiatry* 74 (9): 1258–61.

6. **Oliver D.** (2004) The development of an interdisciplinary outpatient clinic in specialist palliative care. *Int J Palliat Nurs* 10 (9): 446–8.

7. **Houde S. C., Mangolds V.** (1999) Amyotrophic lateral sclerosis: a team approach to primary care. *Clin Excell Nurse Pract* 3 (6): 337–45.

8. **Simmons Z.** (2005) Management strategies for patients with amyotrophic lateral sclerosis from diagnosis through death. *Neurologist* 11 (5): 257–70.

9. **Borasio G. D., Voltz R., Miller R. G.** (2001) Palliative care in amyotrophic lateral sclerosis. *Neurol Clin* 1: 829–47.

10. **Lomen-Hoerth C., Anderson T., Miller B.** (2002) The overlap of amyotrophic lateral sclerosis and frontotemporal dementia. *Neurology* 59 (7): 1077–9.

11. **Olney R. K., Murphy J., Forshew D., Garwood E., Miller B. L., Langmore S., Kohn M. A., Lomen-Hoerth C.** (2005) The effects of executive and behavioral dysfunction on the course of ALS. *Neurology* 65 (11): 1774–7.

12. **Radin L.** (ed.) (2003) *What If It's Not Alzheimer's: A Caregiver's Guide to Dementia.* Amherst, New York: Prometheus Books.

13. **Hebert R. S., Lacomis D., Easter C., Frick V., Shear M. K.** (2005) Grief support for informal caregivers of patients with ALS: a national survey. *Neurology* 64 (1): 137–8.

Chapter 8

International aspects of care

David Oliver

The care of people with ALS may vary across the world according to the resources available, the health care systems and the cultural and societal attitudes to chronic illness and ALS in particular. The following organizations were contacted for their opinions on the care provided for people with ALS in their own country:

Motor Neurone Disease Association of Australia

There are seven state-based Associations and there is a coordinating organization which deals with literature, advocacy and awareness.

Motor Neurone Disease Association – England

Established in 1979 and has 85 local branches, with a membership of 6000.

Japan ALS Association (JALSA) – Japan

Established in 1986 and has 6,500 members, including people with ALS, families and professionals.

Vereniging Spierziekten Nederland (VSN) – Dutch Association of Neuromuscular Disorders – Netherlands

ALS is included with other neuromuscular disorders and there is a total membership of 10,000.

Yugoslav ALS/MND Association – Serbia

Has 200 patients as members and a very small budget, allowing advice and information on ALS and limited contact. Liaises with neurological services from the Institute of Neurology in Belgrade.

Motor Neurone Disease Association of South Africa

Established in 1990 and has two nursing advisors and nine volunteers. Works closely with palliative care providers throughout the country.

ALS Association (USA)

The ALS Association is the only national not-for-profit voluntary health organization dedicated solely to improving the lives of people with ALS and finding a cure.

The organizations were asked to respond to several questions about the care of people with ALS in their country and the role of the Association:

- Brief description of the organization
- Examples of good practice and care
- Difficult aspects of care
- End of life issues and care.

Examples of good practice

Australia

The Association provides a 'navigator' role, helping people with ALS understand the system, identify their needs and then determine services that can meet these needs.

- The help provided varies across Australia but relationships have developed with service providers allowing:

  (i) People to be cared at home for longer

  (ii) Community-based and palliative care-focused teams offering care

  (iii) Clinics

  (iv) Links with palliative care providers

  (v) ALS care advisors

  (vi) Equipment provision

  (vii) Empowerment of people with ALS

- Support for carers – the 'Living Well' project
- Health professional interest groups to enhance professional knowledge and skills
- Weekends away for carers and families of people with ALS
- Use of volunteers to provide respite and activities for people with ALS.

England and UK

The Association has established itself as a significant service provider, influencer and partner with statutory services:

- Information for people with ALS, their carers and professionals
- Equipment loan and campaigning for improved availability
- Financial support people with ALS
- Education and training opportunities
- Development of care centres to improve care
- Development of Standards of Care to achieve quality of life for people with ALS – from diagnosis to death
- Regional Care Advisors providing support and advice.

Japan

- Local support systems have developed – to coordinate the care provided by the professionals, carers and volunteers
- Experience has developed in the care and support of people requiring respiratory support – up to 30 per cent of all people with ALS
- Care programmes for ALS patients aim to continue throughout the progression of the disease, and may include invasive ventilation when respiratory failure occurs. The care provided may include the provision of communication devices and other interventions to maintain their quality of life
- Development of social security systems to support care in the community.

The Netherlands

- Specialist multidisciplinary ALS teams have developed based within rehabilitation services
- Patient information has been important resource for people with ALS and their carers
- Support groups for people with ALS and their carers – often in collaboration with the ALS rehabilitation team.

Serbia

- The Association is able to provide information and guide people with ALS to the most appropriate neurological service and professional carers
- Telephone contact with people with ALS and their families can be helpful in supporting them, particularly in rural areas.

South Africa

- The Association liaises with specialist palliative care providers, who are able to visit people with ALS more easily and in their own community, allowing care to be provided for people with ALS across large distances and within very limited resources

- Information is provided for people with ALS and their carers, both informal and professional
- Education of professionals allows greater awareness of the problems faced by people with ALS and facilitates referral for support – this has included the support from other countries.

USA

The ALS Association provides comprehensive services for people with ALS, their families and caregivers through a network of Chapters, ALSA Certified Centers, which are located at many of the most renowned health care institutions in the US, and a nationally directed programme of research, advocacy and public education.

The ALSA Delivers Program includes:

- Public education and awareness
- Family support groups – caregiver support and respite care
- Equipment loan
- Coordination of care at clinics and at home
- End of life care
- Information and education
- Advocacy on behalf of people with ALS politically
- Development of ALSA Certified Centers of Excellence allows high quality care to be provided
- The ALSA Centers work closely with the ALSA Chapters based on the National Standards of Care and provided through a multidisciplinary clinical care model
- The ALSA Certified Centers are distinguished nationally recognized institutions, known as 'the best in the field'
- The ALSA Center Medical Directors participate in clinical research studies
- A cohesive relationship among the ALSA Certified Centers is promoted, facilitating the sharing of best practices and clinical outcomes.

Common themes

The care of the person with ALS that develops in each country is dependent on the existing medical and social care system. However, all areas stress the need for the provision of information for people with ALS, their families and their professional carers. In many areas there are problems encountered by people with ALS within the existing systems and there is a need for a coherent care pathway, provided by experienced and knowledgeable health and social care professionals. The team approach is helpful – the team coming from within neurological services, rehabilitation, palliative care or specialist services.

Difficulties experienced in providing care for people with ALS

Australia

- ◆ Access to funded services is often difficult – in particular personal care at home and respite care
- ◆ Funding of services is complex and confusing
- ◆ Palliative care may be difficult to access earlier in the disease progression and in some areas is restricted to end of life care
- ◆ Nursing homes are often unable to provide the appropriate care, in the best way
- ◆ The long distances restricts access to care services.

England/UK

- ◆ Services find it difficult to respond to the speed of progression of ALS and the changing needs of people with ALS
- ◆ Coordination of services is limited – especially as the number of people with ALS within any one area is small.

Japan

- ◆ There are limited resources for psychological care for people living with ALS
- ◆ The ability to provide information for people with ALS may be restricted as there is often a reluctance to speak the truth about the diagnosis and ALS.

The Netherlands

- ◆ Palliative care is limited at home and services are not always able to support people with ALS and their families, resulting in exhaustion of carers
- ◆ The services do not always respond to the progression of the disease and the changing needs of the person, including all the aspects of care.

Serbia

+ Admission to hospital may occur, but the person with ALS may be required to pay for specialized procedures and few receive specialist help

+ There is limited palliative care and the only care may be from local nursing services

+ There is little funding to support the work of the Association, restricting the care that can be provided.

South Africa

+ The health care system – state care provided at a basic level for 70 per cent of the population and private care providing specialized and complex care, as long as the medical insurance is sufficient, for 30 per cent

+ The vastness of South Africa makes personal contact with the majority of people with ALS very difficult. The infrastructure is often limited and the diversity of languages, education and the increased risk of crime and violence restrict the care provided

+ A wide array of cultural and religious beliefs alters the perceptions regarding the disease, the ways of treatment and the attitudes to deterioration and death

+ Funding of the Association is very limited and there are few people involved across the country

+ Palliative care is not always available across the country

USA

+ Access to obtain the resources people with ALS and their carers need can be difficult

+ The time taken for a diagnosis to be made is often lengthy and difficult for patients. There are often numerous tests and procedures to rule out other diseases

+ There is a need for new approaches to provide services to a great number of patients through alternative care delivery models

+ There is a need to ensure general neurologists facilitate referral to specialist ALS neurology services.

Common themes

All areas describe the problems encountered by people with ALS as the disease progression is faster than for the majority of other neurological conditions. This is accentuated by the variability of the coordination of services and the lack of resources – both in health and social care and palliative care.

End of life issues

Australia

- Most people would like home based palliative care and in a survey in one State 70 per cent of people were at home at one month before death and 53 per cent one week before death
- The Associations provide follow-up to families and refer for counselling if required
- One area provides group sessions for bereaved carers, addressing issues of loss, death and planning for the future.

England/UK

- Many people with ALS are unable to access palliative care – in 2005 a survey showed that only 39 per cent of people with ALS had access to palliative care
- There are pronounced geographical variations in palliative care provision.

Japan

- Palliative care within hospital is not widely available for people with ALS, as the services provide care primarily for cancer patients in the last six months of life
- Care at home for ALS patients is provided by primary care physicians and nurses
- Physicians and other health care professionals are often reluctant to discuss end of life issues, such as the withholding and withdrawal of medical treatment, or palliative care in the terminal stages
- Many of the patients with ventilatory support die from pneumonia
- Most patients with ALS die in hospital.

The Netherlands

- The aim of care at the end of life is on quality of life
- Medication is often given to reduce symptoms
- Euthanasia is provided for many people with ALS, and their life is ended at their request.

Serbia

- Seventy per cent of people with ALS die at home, and are cared for by their families, local doctor and neurologist.

South Africa

- Most people die at home and are cared for by their local doctor – who may have limited experience in the care of ALS
- A few people have non-invasive ventilation – only if they can afford to pay for this themselves.

USA

- People with ALS and their families need support in the decision-making as the disease progresses
- Further education would be helpful for people with ALS and their families in the completion of Advance Directives
- There is a need for increased education of health care professionals involved in ALS care. There is often a reluctance to discuss end of life issues and there may be limited knowledge of palliative care and symptom management for ALS patients – including the use of opioids, withdrawal of treatment and need for psychosocial and spiritual support
- There is frequently an absence of coordination between carers and they often become exhausted with the burden of care.

Common themes

The care at the end of life varies greatly and would appear to depend on cultural and societal mores as well as resources. The acceptance of the inevitability of death is an issue within many societies. There are extreme variations from people receiving assisted death and euthanasia to long-term ventilation. There is no 'right' or 'wrong' answer to these issues but it is essential to consider these deeper cultural issues in caring for a person with ALS. As communication opens up across the world, especially with the use of the Internet, these differences may be highlighted and further dialogue will need to be encouraged.

Conclusion

Many areas – regardless of the health service provision and resources – have developed appropriate services for people with ALS. It is helpful for any service to link and liaise with the general care services in primary and secondary care to improve the care for these people. Moreover the development of standards of care is able to support all carers involved in the day to day care – so that people with ALS are provided with the most appropriate care.

Acknowledgements

The information for this chapter was provided by the following Associations:
Motor Neurone Disease Association of Australia – Rod Harris
Motor Neurone Disease Association of the UK – Tricia Holmes, Director of Care Development, Sarah Fitzgerald, Head of Public Relations and Media
Japanese ALS Association – Kimiaki Kanazwa, Secretary General
Dutch Association of Neuromuscular Diseases – Anja Horemans
Yugoslav MND/ALS Association – Dr Zorica Stevic
MND Association of South Africa – Vivien O'Cuinneagain
ALS Association – Jennifer Brand
The editors also wish to acknowledge the contributions to the first edition of this book on these international issues:
Andrea Versenyi, USA
Hideaki Hayashi, Japan
Zbigniew Zylicz, The Netherlands
Diane Heron, South Africa

Chapter 9a

End of life care:

ethical issues

Leo McCluskey and Lauren Elman

Summary

Many ethical issues are faced when caring for patients with ALS and their families – in the making of decisions, especially regarding nutrition and respiratory support, and at the end of life. Increasingly, in certain parts of the world, there is increasing discussion and practice of assisting dying – by assisted suicide or euthanasia. All of these areas need to be considered carefully while caring for someone with ALS, and all involved in the care of patients and families need to be aware of the ethical issues involved.

Case history

Mr M is a 59-year-old man sent to you for evaluation of progressive dysarthria. He is highly educated and has worked for years as an engineer. He was recently fired because bizarre behaviour and dysarthria caused his company to suspect alcoholism. He is in the process of divorce from his wife of 38 years, with whom he has four grown sons. His wife claims he has become aggressive and 'changed' over the last three years. Mr M's biggest complaint is that he is unable to focus on words while reading. Evaluation reveals bulbar onset ALS with frontotemporal dementia (FTD) as the presenting feature.

Initially he has no life-threatening complications, but lacks insight into his condition. He has not designated a durable power of attorney and is unwilling to do so. His wife has told their children that he is 'faking' a disease to avoid a large divorce settlement and they are currently estranged from the patient. After long conversations he gives you permission to speak to his sons about his condition. After they are educated about the disease and the dementia they become more involved.

Over the ensuing months, Mr M develops dysphagia with weight loss. He decides to proceed with gastrostomy tube placement but insists on continuing to live independently. He progresses to anarthria and communicates by writing. His language significantly deteriorates and you become concerned about his ability to make end of life decisions. You request that his oldest son attend the next clinic visit so advance directive decisions and durable power of attorney can be established while he is still capable of communicating his wishes.

Shortly thereafter, progressive dementia requires admission to a nursing home with subsequent hospice care. His sons were responsible for all decisions during the end stages of his disease.

Introduction

Morality refers to a shared set of beliefs about norms of right and wrong that prevail in a particular culture or subculture. Various cultures exhibit great differences in their customary morality. The term ethics, used by philosophers, refers to a method of examining and understanding morality. No single ethical vision prevails in Western pluralistic societies. The two extremes of imposing the morality of the group on those who differ, and non-interference in the moral lives of others, may coexist. Clinical ethics is usually framed as system by which one examines morality, conduct and social practices. The aim is to arrive at an answer to the questions 'Why should I (or we) do X or Y?' and 'What reasons would justify such action and why?' rather than to 'What ought I (or we) to do in this and similar situations?' Four broad principles form the basis of ethical obligations:

1. *Beneficence* refers to the duty to benefit and further the welfare of patients.
2. *Non-malificence* refers to the obligation to prevent harm and minimize risks.
3. *Autonomy,* also referred to as *respect for persons,* refers to the duty to protect and defend informed choices of patients with decision-making capacity.
4. *Justice* refers to an obligation to protect health care access.

In addition to these principles the established clinician patient relationship includes implicit moral obligations of respect for privacy and confidentiality, honest communication about diagnosis, treatment and prognosis, determining patient capacity to participate in shared decision-making, and providing ethical valid informed consent. Paternalism, imposition of the physician's personal view of the patient's best interests, undermines autonomy and should be avoided. A moral dilemma may arise when an ethical obligation exists on both sides of a choice to perform or not perform an action and ethical analysis provides a reason to support both alternatives. Clinical ethics offers a framework to justify, interpret, analyse and hopefully resolve moral dilemmas that arise within the context of patient care. A complete discussion of clinical ethical analysis is beyond the scope of this chapter. We favour the method of clinical pragmatism, a case method of problem-solving.[1-3]

Ensuring a good death is an essential aspect of ALS care but presents a multitude of ethical issues. Depending upon disease trajectory, life-threatening features of bulbar and or respiratory muscle dysfunction may occur early or follow months or years of progressive weakness.[4–7] Delay in diagnosis, common in ALS, may confound recognition of their life-threatening potential until bulbar and/or respiratory dysfunction are fully manifest.[8,9] Once ALS is confirmed, the patient is faced with the inevitability of death, though the time frame may range from weeks to years. This reality forces the patient to choose between life extension via gastrostomy tube insertion and/or mechanical ventilation and terminal comfort care.[4,10,11] Ability to make this choice may be compromised by frontotemporal cognitive dysfunction.[12–14] Optimally, clinicians caring for these patients should recognize life-threatening symptoms, monitor decision-making capacity, manage potential end of life scenarios, and provide comfort and hope while aggressively managing terminal symptoms.

Decision-making

Autonomy

In societies that emphasize autonomy, an informed, adult patient who possesses capacity usually makes all medical decisions. A patient with decision-making capacity understands their condition and potential treatment options and effects, demonstrates reasoning consistent with the medical facts and their own values and communicates their choice and its potential ramifications. Individuals with capacity are free to refuse any medical intervention before (withholding) and after (withdrawing) it is initiated even, for example a gastrostomy tube or tracheostomy, if this leads to death.[1,2,15,16]

Delegated decision-making

In societies where individual autonomy is paramount an ALS patient may appoint a surrogate decision-maker in the event that they become incapable of making or communicating medical decisions. This may be informal, but is most effective if legally binding by appointment of a durable medical power of attorney. The delegated surrogate's decisions are usually honoured as if the incapacitated patient themselves had made them. Optimally the surrogate exercises substituted judgment by making decisions using the known and expressed values or expressed choices of the patient. This should apply even if this decision conflicts with the choice the surrogate would make for themselves in the same situation. If patient values or choices are unknown the surrogate can choose based upon their own opinion of the patient's best interests.[1,2,17]

In some societies and ethnic groups an ALS patient may delegate medical decisions to a spouse, adult child, adult children, a family elder, a family group, a friend or other trusted individual even if the patient has decision-making capacity. The ALS patient may refuse to be informed of the diagnosis and prognosis. While this may be considered an abdication of individual autonomy, it can also be viewed as an autonomous choice to delegate decision-making based upon established social or ethnic practices. Whether breaking the news of the diagnosis or informing the patient of progression of disease, the clinician should anticipate the possibility of ethnic or cultural differences in handling medical information and respect the patient's wishes. This may require the clinician to communicate with the person or persons designated by the patient to make decisions for the patient.

Impaired capacity

Frontotemporal lobar dementia (FTD) is now recognized as part of the clinical and neuropathological spectrum of ALS – see Chapter 4c. This may present as a progressive change in personality with changes in social and personal conduct often with dysinhibition causing impulsive, inappropriate and compulsive behaviours for which the patient has little insight or less commonly as a language disorder characterized by word-finding difficulty and poor category naming that may progress to muteness. Subtle cognitive impairment may be evident only with formal testing for mental flexibility, verbal fluency, abstract reasoning, verbal memory and visual .memory. Early detection is best accomplished by asking caregivers.[12–14,18–24,25]

FTD may be present at diagnosis or it may develop during the disease course. Once present it will progress in severity, but it is difficult to predict to what extent FTD it will compromise capacity. As demonstrated in Alzheimer's disease, ALS patients with FTD may lose decision-making capacity as behavioural and language deficits progress.[26,27] It cannot be assumed that an ALS patient will be capable of a discussion of advance directives when life-threatening complications of dysphagia and respiratory muscle weakness develop. For this reason clinicians should discuss advance directives with willing ALS patients with capacity before the development of life-threatening complications and before FTD develops or progresses. Optimally recognition of FTD should prompt ALS clinicians to encourage patients to legally appoint one or more willing and knowledgeable medical surrogates and discuss treatment preferences with them in advance of cognitive decline.

An ALS patient with decision-making capacity can communicate a choice and discuss the potential ramifications. This may be significantly compromised in individuals who are unable to speak because of bulbar dysfunction and limited in their ability to use their hands for writing or typing on a computer keyboard. Some individuals can utilize alternative and adaptive communication (AAC) devices to overcome these obstacles. For patients willing and able to utilize these devices, personal and community resources may limit their access. Meanwhile, progressive motor dysfunction will limit the usable time frame of AAC devices. Early impairment of communication should prompt clinicians to discuss advance decision-making with willing patients before effective communication is lost. Clinicians should also encourage the appointment of surrogate decision-makers from within the family, if appropriate.

End of life

Discussion triggers

Many aspects of ALS are inconvenient, demoralizing and even painful, without being life-threatening. Whereas some may present with life-threatening bulbar or respiratory dysfunction, others have a more chronic, progressive course. The timing of discussion of end of life issues varies by patient. It depends on the symptoms and signs present, but is also dictated by the patient's desire for and willingness and ability to participate. As noted above FTLD should be considered in the timing of discussion. The first discussion of end of life care may be at diagnosis. This occurs either at the request of the patient or because life-threatening symptoms necessitate it. More commonly, though, the diagnosis includes a brief discussion about the progressive nature of the disease without the details of decisions regarding end of life care. Unless necessary or requested by the patient, excessive focus on terminal disease at diagnosis is considered by many clinicians to be ill advised as this does not foster hope.[10]

Is it near?

Comprehensive care of ALS includes routine symptom screening of bulbar and respiratory dysfunction.[10] Symptoms of respiratory dysfunction include shortness of breath, orthopnea, poor sleep, daytime sleepiness, daytime fatigue and unexplained anxiety. Tachypnoea, low vocal volume, lack of breath support, use of accessory muscles of respiration and paradoxical abdominal motion during inspiration may be evident. In addition, the AAN ALS practice parameter recommends longitudinal measurement of objective respiratory function, such as the forced vital capacity (FVC), but other options exist.[10] The absolute values of the erect and supine FVC and the slope of the change in FVC are indicators of disease progression.[10,11,28] Non-invasive positive pressure ventilation (NIPPV) is usually instituted when FVC falls below

50 per cent of predicted. Discussion of NIPPV should prompt a discussion of progressive respiratory failure and advance decision-making, including both tracheostomy (for long term mechanical ventilation) and palliative care usually via hospice.[10,11]

Life-threatening aspects of bulbar disease include malnutrition and dehydration and inability to handle secretions predisposing to aspiration pneumonia. Weight, swallowing dynamics and handling of secretions inform the physician about progressive bulbar disease. Dysphagia with weight loss of more than 10 per cent of body weight should prompt a discussion of gastrostomy. Hospice and palliative care should be discussed with patients who decline this.[10,11]

Uncertainty

When considering the end of life, clinicians must accommodate to uncertainty regarding the six-month life expectancy of any ALS patient. Uncertainty is commonly present when the FVC is below 50 per cent of predicted in a patient who denies respiratory symptoms and lacks abnormal respiratory signs. Many who have bulbar dysfunction, have difficulty performing spirometry because of poor mouth seal, excessive oral and pharyngeal secretions, and poor laryngeal closure.[29–31] We can supplement spirometry by monitoring respiratory symptoms and signs and employing other tests of respiratory function (nocturnal oximetry, polysomnography and arterial blood gases). There still may be uncertainty about the severity of respiratory muscle weakness and an accurate answer to the question 'Does this patient have six months or less to live?' [32–36] Confidence can be increased by reframing the question as 'Would it be a surprise if this patient were to die within 6 to 12 months?' Truth-telling obliges the clinician to discuss uncertainty while initiating or continuing advance decision-making. It is better to have this discussion too early than too late.

Presenting the options

Informing the willing patient and/or their chosen or legally appointed surrogate(s) about end of life options fulfils ethical responsibilities regarding autonomy, beneficence and truth-telling. Paternalism is avoided by discussing all options in a balanced, unbiased and factual way. An either/or choice paradigm in which the pros and cons of each choice are explored is most practical. When the option of tracheostomy and LTMV is discussed, so is the alternative of palliative and hospice care. The alternative of feeding tube placement is discussed in parallel with the hospice. Regardless of the decision on whether to consider life extension or palliative care options, the patient should not be abandoned and a plan of care put in place – palliative care may be instituted early in the disease progression, alongside other care – see Chapter 2. While these conversations may be difficult for both the clinician and the patient, they should take place in time to allow both patient and family process the information and discuss the issues at home. Follow-up visits should be scheduled quickly to allow for questions and information to be re-presented. The physician must make clear that the patient can change their mind about treatment, and should actively but gently re-solicit the patient's wishes at subsequent visits, as preferences for treatment options change over time.[37–39]

Life extension – pros and cons

Gastrostomy may extend life for those with severe dysphagia at risk for dehydration and malnutrition. The device can be placed with minimal risk and discomfort and is easy to use and maintain. It allows patients to continue to eat by mouth for pleasure and avoid anxiety-provoking and socially compromising coughing and choking. It provides access for medications to manage symptoms of ALS.[40–45] Some patients express concerns about a negative body image and dependency upon medical technology. Non-invasive respiratory aids can extend life and delay tracheostomy.[46] Attitudes regarding this vary between and even within cultures.[47] Tracheostomy for LTMV can extend life after respiratory failure. With good nursing and supportive care patients can be maintained indefinitely.[48–51] Small, portable and rechargeable ventilators can be carried on a motorized wheelchair and afford mobility options to optimize social interactions. Some may continue to work. Unfortunately tracheostomy often renders speech impossible except save for those who can use a Passy-Muir valve.[52–54] Alternative and adaptive communication technologies may allow patients to communicate for a time.[55–57] However, disease progression will eventually culminate in the locked-in state making communication impossible.[58–60] Tracheostomy may compromise swallowing, necessitating a gastrostomy tube and reduction or cessation of oral feedings. If not an issue at the time a tracheostomy is placed, FTD may eventually develop. Because communication may be limited, FTD may be difficult to fully detect. FTD may compromise alternative and adaptive communication technologies. Home long–term mechanical ventilation (LTMV) is possible only for those with willing caregivers or home access to medical professionals. Institutional LTMV is an option for those without these benefits. In societies without universal medical access LTMV has financial ramifications that often limits this to individuals with insurance coverage or significant means.[59,61,62] Despite these limitations, patients on LTMV who can communicate may report a satisfactory quality of life.[63–65] Caregivers are, however, heavily burdened.[64,65]

Case history

A locked-in patient

A new ALS patient, Mrs C is accompanied by her husband who provides all of the history. She is 57 years old and has had ALS for eight years. Because of progressive respiratory muscle weakness she had a tracheostomy for long-term mechanical ventilation four years ago. Currently she is quadriplegic and uses a feeding tube for all liquids and nutrition. She is anarthric.

Her husband states that she communicates by facial and eye movements that only he can decipher. On examination she is sitting in a motorized wheelchair. She has a tracheostomy and is being ventilated with a portable ventilator. She has spastic quadriplegia with facial diparesis. She has slowly roving dysconjugate eye movements and frequent facial grimacing. She does not visually fixate. She does not appear to voluntarily move her eyes or any portion of her face to command. She fails to respond to yes/no questions with ocular or facial movements. Rather her facial and ocular movements appear random.

Other members of the clinic team have examined her and they agree that she manifests no ability to communicate. You gently introduce your concerns to Mr C but he vehemently disagrees stating that only he can decipher his wife's eye and facial movements. You ask whether Mrs C had discussed or considered termination of the ventilator if she became unable to communicate. He does not recall any discussion of this.

On clinic visits over the ensuing six months you and your team become certain of your initial opinion that she is locked-in. On each visit you discuss your concerns with Mr C. He continues to insist his wife is able to communicate with him. On the next visit he reports that while transporting his wife to the clinic he had a motor vehicle accident. She was thrown from the wheel chair onto the floor of the van. Mr C placed his wife back into the chair. He did not notice any injury. During the clinic visit she appears unchanged. However, you notice that there is swelling of the right calf with a step-off deformity over the tibia a few centimetres below the knee. You are concerned about a fracture. An X-ray confirms a displaced tibial fracture. She is treated with casting and analgesics. You indicate to Mr C that the lack of any indication of pain from her fracture further supports your diagnosis of the locked-in state. He insists she is able to communicate. On the next clinic visit Mrs C is neurologically unchanged. Ophthalmologic examination demonstrates severe conjunctival injection and a weeping purulent exudate of the right eye. She does not appear uncomfortable and is not blinking excessively. You suggest antibiotic treatment. You discuss your ongoing concern that Mrs C is locked-in emphasizing that she again manifested no apparent response to a painful disorder. Mr C considers the issue over the next two weeks. After consulting with his daughter he decides that his wife is indeed locked-in and it would be in her best interest to withdraw care. He arranges to admit his wife to a local hospital. Her ventilator is discontinued after administering morphine and lorazepam. She died peacefully.

Hospice and palliative care – pros and cons

Education regarding the benefits of palliative care and hospice involvement should be the focus for patients with life-threatening respiratory muscle weakness electing to forego tracheostomy and life-threatening dysphagia electing to forego gastrostomy tube insertion. There is underutilization of hospice care in some countries and a need to educate patients and families about the effectiveness of hospice care for advanced ALS. The variability of ALS presentation and progression causes an array of end of life problems that are well suited to interdisciplinary, multi-modality comprehensive hospice care.[66] The physician should educate willing patients about the dying process and any potential symptoms they may experience, while emphasizing the potential for treatment. These include dyspnea, air hunger, fear and anxiety, and less frequently pain and choking.[67–71] Physicians should emphasize that they will not abandon the patient, but continue to provide care to minimize suffering during the dying process. If feasible, patients should be encouraged to continue visiting their physician once hospice care is initiated to minimize feelings of abandonment. While surviving caregivers report that despite hospice and palliative care patients suffer significant symptoms at the end, hospice patients are more likely to die outside the hospital, in their preferred place and receive morphine.[68,69] Despite significant symptoms, caregivers report their loved one was at peace, prepared for and accepting of death.[68,69]

Purposeful withdrawal of life-extending measures

In some societies autonomous individuals with decision-making capacity or the selected or legally appointed surrogate may discontinue life-extending measures previously embraced. While withdrawal of treatment may seem and feel different to withholding a medical intervention, most Western societies do not draw an ethical distinction between these choices. Under medical supervision mechanical ventilation can be terminated or weaned over 30 to 60 minutes at home, in a hospice or hospital. The patient and caregivers should be advised that death may occur within minutes, or be delayed for hours or even days, and that medications and supportive care will relieve distress or suffering.[15,72] Patients may also to discontinue food and water by mouth or gastrostomy; this usually leads to death within two weeks.[73–79] In one study nearly all deaths occurred within 15 days of cessation of nutrition and hydration; nurses reported that the median quality of death was 8 on a scale of 0 (very bad death) to 10 (very good death). Nursing and caregiver reports indicate that individuals who choose this usually die a 'good death'.[76]

Case history

Withdrawal of food and water

You have been caring for Ms P, a 77-year-old woman with bulbar onset ALS who is anarthric and unable to eat or drink. She has been using a feeding tube for all nutrition and hydration for the past six months. Recently she developed weakness of her arms and hands, limiting her ability to perform activities of daily living, and leg weakness limiting her ability to walk. Increasing symptoms caused her to move from the independent to the assisted living area of her nursing facility. She is very distressed over her increasing symptoms and waning independence. However, she denies depression. She has no cognitive difficulties.

At a Christmas Sunday holiday gathering you are attending she greets you and scratches you a note that says, 'I am tired of this. I want this to end. Can you help me?' You ask for clarification. She makes it clear she is asking you for assistance in dying. Since her FVC is greater than 70 per cent of predicted, and she is receiving food and water via a gastrostomy tube she is not hospice eligible in the USA. Nonetheless you discuss all aspects of palliative care including a hospice, emphasizing that end of life symptoms can be managed when the time comes. She listens attentively but at the end states that she does not want to wait until she develops even more symptoms. She wishes to end her struggle with ALS quickly. You inform her that physician-assisted suicide and euthanasia are legally precluded and you are morally opposed to these options. You inform her of the option of stopping all food and water emphasizing it is unlikely that she will suffer, that symptoms can be managed with hospice care, and it is likely she will die within two weeks. She thanks you and informs you that she will discuss this with her two sons.

One week later you receive a telephone call from one of her sons. He tells you that his mother has decided to withdraw food and water. You immediately institute hospice care at her nursing facility. You receive daily updates from the hospice nurses that she is receiving routine nursing care and is comfortable without complaint. Ms P dies eight days after stopping food and water. The hospice nurses report death was peaceful. Two weeks afterwards both of her sons call and thank you for honouring their mother's wishes and allowing her to exercise her independence.

Benzodiazepines, opiates and other medications can control suffering that may occur after withdrawal of life-extending measures. Since death is expected, there is no medical, ethical or legal justification for withholding the medications necessary to control distressing symptoms. Side-effects may have the unintended effect of hastening death. This is justifiable and referred to as the ethical principle of double effect.[1–3,80] Administration of medication in excess of doses to control symptoms with the intent of quickening death is euthanasia.[1–3]

Physician-assisted suicide and euthanasia

Physician-assisted suicide (PAS) refers to providing a requested lethal dose of medication that the patients use to end their own lives. In PAS, the physician provides the means for death and the patient administers it. PAS is not euthanasia. Euthanasia refers to a physician both providing and administering a lethal medication dose. Euthanasia can be voluntary, at the request of the patient, or involuntary, without the patient's consent. PAS should be distinguished from terminal sedation, which refers to sedating a terminally ill, suffering patient to unconsciousness, maintaining sedation over the ensuing days, and allowing the patient to die of the underlying disease, starvation or dehydration.[3,74,81–87]

PAS – Oregon

The Oregon Death with Dignity Act (ODWDA) passed as a citizens' initiative in 1994 with 51 per cent in favour. Implementation was delayed by legal proceedings that included a petition denied by the US Supreme Court; the 9th Circuit Court of Appeals lifted the injunction on 27 October 1997. In November 1997, a measure asking voters to repeal the ODWDA was on the general election ballot. The voters rejected this 60 per cent to 40 per cent. PAS has been legal in Oregon since 1997.[88]

The ODWDA stipulates that ending one's life within the rules of the act does not constitute suicide, and physicians providing lethal medication to carry out the act are not guilty of a crime. The act defines PAS as the voluntary self-administration of lethal medications prescribed by a physician for that purpose. It specifically prohibits euthanasia. To be eligible to participate patients must have a terminal disease (less than six months to live), be older than 18 years, be an Oregon resident for greater than six months, and be deemed capable of understanding and making the decision. Patients can receive the lethal medication only after two oral requests to their physician within 15 or more days, followed by a written request signed by two witnesses. If the physician has any concern about decision-making capacity or mental illness that may be influencing the decision, then the patient must be referred for psychiatric evaluation. The physician is obligated to discuss feasible alternatives to PAS, with emphasis upon pain control, hospice and palliative care. The physician can request the patient notify next of kin, but the patient is not obligated to do so.[91]

The number of prescriptions given and patients following through with PAS through ODWDA has more than doubled since 1998 (Table 9a.1). However, the number has remained small compared to the total deaths in Oregon, with about 0.14 per cent dying by PAS. Since 1997, ALS patients have been over-represented. Between 1997 and 2005 8 per cent of all Oregon PAS deaths between 1998 and 2004 were people with ALS. ALS patients who chose PAS constituted 2.7 per cent of all deaths from ALS between these dates. Over the

Table 9a.1 Prescriptions written vs. PAS fulfilled as a result of the ODWDA 1998–2005[92]

Year	Prescriptions	Deaths from PAS	Estimated PAS deaths Per 10,000 total deaths
1998	24	16	5.5
1999	33	27	9.2
2000	39	27	9.1
2001	44	21	7.0
2002	58	38	12.2
2003	67	42	14.0
2004	60	35	12.0
2005	64	38	12.0

eight years, the 246 patients who took lethal medications differed from the 74,967 Oregonians who died from the same underlying diseases. PAS decreased with advancing age, was higher for those divorced or never married, those with more education, and a malignant neoplasm, ALS or HIV/AIDS. The rate of PAS to non-PAS deaths from the same causes was high for ALS (269.5/10,000), HIV/AIDS (218.3/10,000) and malignant neoplasm (39.9/10,000). Chronic lower respiratory disease (emphysema) was associated with the lowest rate (8.7/10,000). ALS patients were 31 times more likely to use PAS than those with emphysema.[91]

The prescribing physicians for PAS indicated that the three most common end of life concerns in patients choosing PAS were loss of autonomy, decreasing ability to participate in enjoyable activities life, and loss of dignity. Of 100 ALS patients surveyed before the ODWDA, 56 per cent indicated they would consider PAS. Those who said they would were more likely to be male, more highly educated, had higher hopelessness scores, were less religious and rated their quality of life as lower.[66] Fifty caregivers of deceased ALS patients from Oregon and Washington indicated that one-third of patients discussed wanting PAS in the last month of life. Those expressing interest in PAS in the last month of life were more likely to have greater hopelessness and expressed interest in PAS earlier in their disease. Compared to patients who did not express interest, those who did had greater distress at being a burden to others, more insomnia, more pain, and more discomfort other than pain.[67]

Euthanasia is illegal in the United States. The US Supreme Court ruled there is no constitutional right to assistance in dying. However, the Court left the decision to legalize PAS to each state. PAS is legal only in Oregon. Many states have had assisted death legislation fail in the legislature. California (1992), Washington (1990), Michigan (1998) and Maine (2000) have had referenda in which PAS was defeated. Thirty-nine states prohibit assisted suicide by specific statute, six through common law. In 2001 the US Justice Department ruled assisting suicide was not a legitimate use of drugs controlled by federal drug laws and that the FDA could stop the prescribing rights, and potentially jail, any physician who authorized drugs for this purpose. The 9th Circuit Court of Appeals upheld Oregon's law in 2004. The U.S. Supreme Court upheld the 9th Circuit decision and rejected the US Justice Department's case, thereby upholding Oregon's law in 2006.

Assisted death – The Netherlands

The Criminal Code of the Netherlands contains provisions prohibiting the intentional taking of human life. However, termination of life upon request and assistance with suicide has been permitted in the Netherlands by a non-prosecution agreement between the Ministry of Justice and the Royal Dutch Medical Association. In 2001, the Parliament passed legislation whereby the long-standing practice of terminating life on request, and assistance with suicide would not be a criminal offense if carried out by a physician fulfilling certain 'criteria of due care'. These stipulate that the physician must:

1. be satisfied that the patient has made a voluntary and well considered request,
2. be satisfied that suffering is unbearable, without prospect of improvement,
3. have informed the patient about his or her situation and prospects,
4. have come to the conclusion, with the patient, that there is no reasonable alternative given the patient's situation
5. consult at least one other physician, who must have seen the patient and given a written opinion on the due care criteria referred to above
6. have terminated the patient's life or provided assistance with suicide with due medical care and attention.

The physician is also required to report the assisted death to the municipal coroner.[90]

Treating physicians in the Netherlands reported that 35/231 (17 per cent) ALS patients chose euthanasia and died by that method, 6 (3 per cent) died from PAS, and 48 (24 per cent) received 'palliative treatment that probably shortened their lives'. Those choosing assisted death were more likely to consider religion as unimportant. There was no association with education, income, level of care or any disease characteristics ALS patients in this study were 10 times more likely to choose assisted death than those in Oregon and preferred euthanasia over PAS.[91]

Assisted death – other nations

Belgium legalized euthanasia limited to adults and emancipated minors in 2002.[92] Although Swiss law does not legalize euthanasia, it does not punish those who aid someone in committing suicide for unselfish reasons. The Council of Europe rejected a draft resolution supporting assistance in dying.[93,94]

In 1995, with the passage of the Rights of the Terminally Ill (ROTI) Act, Australia's Northern Territory became the only jurisdiction in the world with both legalized assisted suicide and euthanasia.[95] The law went into effect in July 1996 but was repealed less than one year later. The Australian Medical Association opposed the Northern Territory legislation while it was in effect and continues to oppose both euthanasia and assisted suicide.

Ethical arguments for and against assisted death

Those in favour of assisted death frequently use the following arguments:

- ◆ Justice: Some terminally ill patients hasten death by refusing or terminating treatment. For others, refusal of treatment will not hasten death. For these the only option for hastening death is suicide, and assisted death should be allowed.

- ◆ Autonomy: Decisions about the timing and the nature of death are personal. Competent, terminally ill patients should be allowed to choose the time and nature of their death.

- ◆ Beneficence: Physicians have a duty to relieve physical or psychological suffering, but this is not always possible. PAS should be allowed in order to relieve terminal unbearable suffering.

- ◆ Liberty: The state's interest in preserving life is reduced when a person has a terminal illness and a desire to end suffering by ending their life. Prohibiting PAS is an excessive restriction on personal liberty.

- ◆ Honesty: Assisted death is occurring, but is now secret. Legalization would permit an open and honest discussion.

Those opposing assisted death frequently make the following arguments:

- ◆ Sanctity of life: There is a long-standing, strong, religious moral and secular prohibition against taking human life.

- ◆ Killing vs. letting die: There is an important distinction between letting patients die of their disease by withholding or terminating care, a passive act, and killing using PAS, an active act.

- Slippery slope: Once legalized, there is no way to contain PAS. People who lack access or means to obtain proper medical care and support would be pushed into PAS. This might be encouraged by overburdened family members, and possibly by physicians. Eventually PAS would become a remedy for the suffering of individuals who do not have a terminal disease.

- Harm to medicine/distrust: The ethical traditions of medicine oppose taking of life. If PAS were legalized, the image of medicine would be harmed and the trust implicit in the physician-patient relationship undermined.

- Doctors are fallible: There is inherent uncertainty in diagnosis and prognosis. Legalizing PAS would lead to the death of patients who are, in fact, not suffering from a terminal disorder.

American Academy of Neurology position on assisted death

The American Academy of Neurology in 1998 published a position statement 'vigorously opposing physician-assisted suicide, euthanasia, and any other actions by neurologists directly intended to cause death. Further, the AAN states that legalization of PAS will not make physician participation 'morally or ethically acceptable ipso facto', and reaffirms its position that 'aggressive and effective palliative care should be provided to all patients who need and desire such care'.

World Medical Association position on assisted death

The World Medical Association, with members representing medical associations (including the American Medical Association) from 82 countries, has adopted strong resolutions condemning both PAS and euthanasia and urging all national medical associations and physicians to refrain from participating in them even if national law allows or decriminalizes the practices.[96]

The request for assisted death

Any request for assisted death should be handled with respect and compassion. The appeal should be explored to understand the motivation and determine if there are any treatable physical or psychological symptoms driving the request. It is essential to determine if there are misunderstandings about the likely course of ALS, and if the patient has particular fears or concerns. It is helpful to review potential end of life scenarios and plans of care, emphasizing that symptoms such as air hunger, anxiety, depression and pain can be treated, and suffering minimized or eliminated. Most patients derive reassurance and some sense of control from these discussions and no longer seek assisted death.[97]

Despite these efforts some will persist in their request for PAS. While the AAN's position makes no exceptions for physician participation in PAS, physicians can consider the issue carefully and decide on their own position. Physicians should be advised there are potential legal and professional consequences to participation in PAS, depending in part on the jurisdiction. Careful reflection ahead of time can prepare you to openly discuss your position with the patient, acknowledging and respecting difference of opinion when it occurs. No physician, however, should feel forced to supply assistance if they are morally opposed to PAS.

Alternatives to PAS

ALS patients should be informed there are legal, and some would argue, more ethically justifiable alternatives to PAS to hasten death. As discussed above, patients can elect to discontinue life-extending measures while medications are used to control suffering and distress. Intractable physical and or emotional suffering close to death can be managed with terminal sedation.[84–90]

Conclusions

There are many ethical issues to be considered in the care of people with ALS. It is essential that these issues are discussed, at the appropriate time and with sensitivity – allowing for the differing cultural values and attitudes in society, with respect for different ethnic and cultural groupings and individual families. The wider multidisciplinary team will also need to consider and discuss these issues and in this way enable patients with ALS, their families and professionals to come to decisions that are acceptable to all.

References

1. Fletcher J., et al. (1997) Introduction to Clinical Ethics, 2nd edn. Hagerstown, MD: University Publishing Group.
2. Beauchamp T. L., Childress J. F. (1994) Principles of Biomedical Ethics, 4th edn. New York: Oxford University Press.
3. Bernat J. L. (2003) Ethical Issues in Neurology, 2nd edn. Boston, MA: Butterworth-Heinemann.
4. Mitsumoto H., Chad D. A., Pioro E. (1998) Amyotrophic Lateral Sclerosis. Contemporary neurology series; 49. Philadelphia: F. A. Davis.
5. Rowland L. (1994) Amyotrophic lateral sclerosis. Curr Opin Neurol 7 (4): 310–15.
6. Rowland L. and the Muscular Dystrophy Association (1991) Amyotrophic Lateral Sclerosis and Other Motor Neuron Diseases, pxxii, 569. Advances in neurology, vol. 56. New York: Raven Press.

7. **Rowland L. P., Shneider n. A.** (2001) Amyotrophic lateral sclerosis. *New England Journal of Medicine* **344** (22): 1688–700.

8. **Eisen A.** (1999) How to improve the diagnostic process. *J Neurol* 246 (Suppl. 3): III6–9.

9. **Swash M.** (1999) An algorithm for ALS diagnosis and management. *Neurology* 53 (8 Suppl. 5): S58–62.

10. **Miller R. G.** *et al.* (1999) Practice parameter: The care of the patient with amyotrophic lateral sclerosis (an evidence-based review). *Muscle Nerve.* 22 (8): 1104–18.

11. **Miller R. G.** *et al.* (1999) Practice parameter: the care of the patient with amyotrophic lateral sclerosis (an evidence-based review): report of the Quality Standards Subcommittee of the American Academy of Neurology: ALS Practice Parameters Task Force. *Neurology* 52 (7): 1311–23.

12. **Lomen-Hoerth C.** (2004) Characterization of amyotrophic lateral sclerosis and frontotemporal dementia. *Dement Geriatr Cogn Disord* 17 (4): 337–41.

13. **Lomen-Hoerth C., Anderson T., Miller B.** (2002) The overlap of amyotrophic lateral sclerosis and frontotemporal dementia. *Neurology* 59 (7): 1077–9.

14. **Lomen-Hoerth C.** *et al.* (2003) Are amyotrophic lateral sclerosis patients cognitively normal? *Neurology* 60 (7): 1094–7.

15. **Borasio G. D., Voltz R.** (1998) Discontinuation of mechanical ventilation in patients with amyotrophic lateral sclerosis. *J Neurol* 245 (11): 717–22.

16. **Schwarz J. K., Del Bene M. L.** (2004) Withdrawing ventilator support for a home-based amyotrophic lateral sclerosis patient: a case study. *J Clin Ethics* 15 (3): 282–90.

17. **Sulmasy D. P.** *et al.* (1998) The accuracy of substituted judgments in patients with terminal diagnoses. *Ann Intern Med* 128 (8): 621–9.

18. **Mitsuyama Y.** (2000) Dementia with motor neuron disease. *Neuropathology* 20 (Suppl.): S79–81.

19. **Nakano I.** (2000) Frontotemporal dementia with motor neuron disease (amyotrophic lateral sclerosis with dementia). *Neuropathology* 20 (1): 68–75.

20. **Neary D., Snowden J. S, Mann D. M.** (2000) Cognitive change in motor neurone isease/amyotrophic lateral sclerosis (MND/ALS). *J Neurol Sci* 180 (1–2): 15–20.

21. **Nestor P., Hodges J.** (2000) Non-Alzheimer dementias. *Semin Neurol* 20 (4): 439–46.

22. **Strong M. J.** (2003) The basic aspects of therapeutics in amyotrophic lateral sclerosis. *Pharmacol Ther* **98** (3): 379–414.

23. **Strong M. J.** *et al.* (2003) Cognitive impairment, frontotemporal dementia, and the motor neuron diseases. *Ann Neurol* 54 (Suppl 5): S20–3.

24. **Vercelletto M.** *et al.* (1999) Frontal type dementia preceding amyotrophic lateral sclerosis: a neuropsychological and SPECT study of five clinical cases. *Eur J Neurol* 6 (3): 295–9.

25. **Wilson C. M.** *et al.* (2001) Cognitive impairment in sporadic ALS: a pathologic continuum underlying a multisystem disorder. *Neurology* 57 (4): 651–7.

26. **Hirschman K. B.** *et al.* (2005) Do Alzheimer's disease patients want to participate in a treatment decision, and would their caregivers let them? *Gerontologist* 45 (3): 381–8.

27. **Hirschman K. B.** *et al.* (2004) How does an Alzheimer's disease patient's role in medical decision making change over time? *Journal of Geriatric Psychiatry & Neurology* 17 (2): 55–60.

28. **Varrato J. et al.** (2001) Postural change of forced vital capacity predicts some respiratory symptoms in ALS. *Neurology* **57** (2): 357–9.

29. **Fallat R. J.** (2002) Vital capacity as an efficacy measure: pro. *Amyotroph Lateral Scler Other Motor Neuron Disord* **3** (Suppl 1): S55–7.

30. **Jackson C. E.** (2002) Vital capacity as an efficacy measure: con. *Amyotroph Lateral Scler Other Motor Neuron Disord* **3** (Suppl 1): S59–60.

31. **Gelinas D. F.** (2002) Vital capacity as an efficacy measure: Summary. *Amyotroph Lateral Scler Other Motor Neuron Disord* **3** (Suppl 1): S61–2.

32. **Morgan R. K. et al.** (2005) Use of sniff nasal-inspiratory force to predict survival in amyotrophic lateral sclerosis. *Am J Respir Crit Care Med* **171** (3): 269–74.

33. **Bach, J. R.,** Amyotrophic lateral sclerosis: prolongation of life by noninvasive respiratory AIDS. *Chest*, 2002. **122**(1): 92–8.

34. **Bach J. R., Bianchi C., Aufiero E.** (2004) Oximetry and indications for tracheotomy for amyotrophic lateral sclerosis. *Chest* **126** (5): 1502–7.

35. **Elman L. B., Siderowf A. D., McCluskey L. F.** (2003) Nocturnal oximetry: utility in the respiratory management of amyotrophic lateral sclerosis. *Am J Phys Med Rehabil* **82** (11): 866–70.

36. **Pinto A. et al.** (2003) Nocturnal pulse oximetry: a new approach to establish the appropriate time for non-invasive ventilation in ALS patients. *Amyotroph Lateral Scler Other Motor Neuron Disord* **4** (1): 31–5.

37. **Albert S. M. et al.** (1999) Prospective study of palliative care in ALS: choice, timing, outcomes. *J Neurol Sci* **169** (1–2): 108–13.

38. **Albert S. M. et al.** (1999) A prospective study of preferences and actual treatment choices in ALS. *Neurology* **53** (2): 278–83.

39. **Silverstein M. D. et al.** (1991) Amyotrophic lateral sclerosis and life-sustaining therapy: patients' desires for information, participation in decision making, and life-sustaining therapy. *Mayo Clin Proc* **66** (9): 906–13.

40. **Silani V., Kasarskis E. J., Yanagisawa N.** (1998) Nutritional management in amyotrophic lateral sclerosis: a worldwide perspective. *J Neurol* **245** (Suppl. 2): S13–9; discussion S29.

41. **Miller R. G.** (2001) Examining the evidence about treatment in ALS/MND. *Amyotroph Lateral Scler Other Motor Neuron Disord.* **2** (1): 3–7.

42. **Mazzini L. et al.** (1995) Percutaneous endoscopic gastrostomy and enteral nutrition in amyotrophic lateral sclerosis. *J Neurol* **242** (10): 695–8.

43. **Howard R. S., Orrell R. W.** (2002) Management of motor neurone disease. *Postgrad Med J* **78** (926): 736–41.

44. **Eisen A., Weber M.** (1999) Treatment of amyotrophic lateral sclerosis. *Drugs Aging* **14** (3): 173–96.

45. **Bradley W. G. et al.** (2004) Changes in the management of ALS since the publication of the AAN ALS practice parameter 1999. *Amyotroph Lateral Scler Other Motor Neuron Disord* **5** (4): 240–4.

46. **Bach J. R.** (1993) Amyotrophic lateral sclerosis. Communication status and survival with ventilatory support. *Am J Phys Med Rehabil* **72** (6): 343–9.

47. **Borasio G. D., Gelinas D. F., Yanagisawa N.** (1998) Mechanical ventilation in amyotrophic lateral sclerosis: a cross-cultural perspective. *J Neurol* **245** (Suppl. 2): S7–12; discussion S29.

48. **Borasio G. D., Miller R. G.** (2001) Clinical characteristics and management of ALS. *Semin Neurol* **21** (2): 155–66.

49. **Cazzolli P. A., Oppenheimer E. A.** (1996) Home mechanical ventilation for amyotrophic lateral sclerosis: nasal compared to tracheostomy-intermittent positive pressure ventilation. *J Neurol Sci* (Suppl.): 123–8.

50. **Escarrabill J.** *et al.* (1998) Long-term mechanical ventilation in amyotrophic lateral sclerosis. *Respir Med* **92** (3): 438–41.

51. **Farrero E.** *et al.* (2005) Survival in amyotrophic lateral sclerosis with home mechanical ventilation: the impact of systematic respiratory assessment and bulbar involvement. *Chest* **127** (6): 2132–8.

52. **Kaut K., Turcott J. C., Lavery M.** (1996) Passy-Muir speaking valve. *Dimensions of Critical Care Nursing* **15**: 298–306.

53. **Manzano J. L.** (1993) Verbal communication of ventilator-dependent patients. *Critical Care Medicine* **21**: 512–17.

54. **Byrick R. J.** (1993) Improved communication with the Passy-Muir valve: the aim of technology and the result of training. *Critical Care Medicine* **21**: 483–4.

55. **Gryfe P.** *et al.* (1996) Freedom through a single switch: coping and communicating with artificial ventilation. *J Neurol Sci* **139** (Suppl.): 132–3.

56. **Beukelman D. R., Ball L. J.** (2002) Improving AAC use for persons with acquired neurogenic disorders: understanding human and engineering factors. *Assist Technol* **14** (1): 33–44.

57. **Yorkston K. M.** (1996) Treatment efficacy: dysarthria. *J Speech Hear Res* **39** (5): S46–57.

58. **Hayashi H., Oppenheimer E. A.** (2003) ALS patients on TPPV: totally locked-in state, neurologic findings and ethical implications. *Neurology* **61** (1): 135–7.

59. **Moss A. H.** *et al.* (1996) Patients with amyotrophic lateral sclerosis receiving long-term mechanical ventilation. Advance care planning and outcomes. *Chest* **110** (1): 249–55.

60. **Ringel S. P.** (2004) Personal history: locked in or locked out? *Neurology* **62** (9): 1650–2.

61. **Hein H., Kirsten D., Magnussen H.** (1996) Possibilities and limits of ventilation in amyotrophic lateral sclerosis. *Med Klin (Munich)* **91** (Suppl.) 2: 48–9.

62. **Narayanaswami P.** *et al.* (2000) Long-term tracheostomy ventilation in neuromuscular diseases: patient acceptance and quality of life. *Neurorehabil Neural Repair* **14** (2): 135–9.

63. **Gelinas D. F., O'Connor P., Miller R. G.** (1998) Quality of life for ventilator-dependent ALS patients and their caregivers. *J Neurol Sci* **160** (Suppl. 1): S134–6.

64. **Kaub-Wittemer D.** *et al.* (2003) Quality of life and psychosocial issues in ventilated patients with amyotrophic lateral sclerosis and their caregivers. *J Pain Symptom Manage* **26** (4): 890–6.

65. **Trail M.** *et al.* (2003) A study comparing patients with amyotrophic lateral sclerosis and their caregivers on measures of quality of life, depression, and their attitudes toward treatment options. *J Neurol Sci* **209** (1–2): 79–85.

66. **Ganzini L., Block S.** (2002) Physician-assisted death – a last resort? *New England Journal of Medicine* **346** (21): 1663–5.

67. **Ganzini L., Johnston W. S., Hoffman W. F.** (1999) Correlates of suffering in amyotrophic lateral sclerosis. *Neurology* **52** (7): 1434–40.

68. **Ganzini L., Johnston W. S., Silveira M. J.** (2002) The final month of life in patients with ALS. *Neurology* **59** (3): 428–31.

69. Mandler R. N. *et al.* (2001) The ALS Patient Care Database: insights into end-of-life care in ALS. *Amyotroph Lateral Scler Other Motor Neuron Disord* 2 (4): 203–8.

70. Oliver D. (1996) The quality of care and symptom control–the effects on the terminal phase of ALS/MND. *J Neurol Sci* 139 (Suppl.): 134–6.

71. Oliver D., Borasio G. D., Walsh D. (2000) *Palliative Care in Amyotrophic Lateral Sclerosis (Motor Neurone Disease)*, pp. xii, 202. Oxford, New York: Oxford University Press.

72. Von Gunten C., Weissman D. E. (2003) Ventilator withdrawal protocol. *Journal of Palliative Medicine* 6 (5): 773–4.

73. Bernat J. L. (1997) The problem of physician-assisted suicide. *Seminars in Neurology* 17 (3): 271–9.

74. Bernat J. L. (2001) Ethical and legal issues in palliative care. *Neurologic Clinics* 19 (4): 969–87.

75. Bernat J. L., B. Gert B., Mogielnicki R. (1993) Patient refusal of hydration and nutrition. An alternative to physician-assisted suicide or voluntary active euthanasia. See comment. *Archives of Internal Medicine* 153 (24): 2723–8.

76. Ganzini L. *et al.* (2003) Nurses' experiences with hospice patients who refuse food and fluids to hasten death. See comment. *New England Journal of Medicine* 349 (4): 359–65.

77. Harvath T. A. *et al.* (2004) Voluntary refusal of food and fluids: attitudes of Oregon hospice nurses and social workers. *International Journal of Palliative Nursing* 10 (5): 236–41; discussion 242–3.

78. Whitney C. (1996) Refusal of food and water by a man with end stage Parkinson's disease. *Journal of Neuroscience Nursing* 28 (4): 267–71.

79. Anonymous (1994) Patient refusal of food and water–a way out of the aid-in-dying debate? *Hospital Ethics* 10 (5): 1–3.

80. Bernat E. (1996) Legal limits of assisted death: exemplified by amyotrophic lateral sclerosis. *Wien Med Wochenschr* 146 (9–10): 195–8.

81. Bernat J. L. (2001) Ethical and legal issues in palliative care. *Neurol Clin* 19: 969–87.

82. Burke A. L. *et al.* (1991) Terminal restlessness–its management and the role of midazolam. *Med J Aust* 155 (7): 485–7.

83. Campbell M. L. (2004) Terminal dyspnea and respiratory distress. *Crit Care Clin* 20 (3): 403–17, viii–ix.

84. Cowan J. D., Palmer T. W. (2002) Practical guide to palliative sedation. *Curr Oncol Rep* 4 (3): 242–9.

85. Cowan J. D., Walsh D. (2001) Terminal sedation in palliative medicine – definition and review of the literature. *Support Care Cancer* 9 (6): 403–7.

86. Krakauer E. L. *et al.* (2000) Sedation for intractable distress of a dying patient: acute palliative care and the principle of double effect. *Oncologist.* 5 (1): 53–62.

87. Morita T., Tsuneto S., Shima Y. (2002) Definition of sedation for symptom relief: a systematic literature review and a proposal of operational criteria. *J Pain Symptom Manage* 24 (4): 447–53.

88. Niemeyer D. (2004) *Seventh Annual Report on Oregon's Death with Dignity Act.* Portland, OR: Department of Human Services.

89. Niemeyer D. (2003) *Eighth Annual Report on Oregon's Death with Dignity Act.* Portland, OR: Department of Human Services.

90. **Anonymous** (2001) Termination of Life on Request and Assisted Suicide Act in The Netherlands.

91. **Veldink J. H.** *et al.* (2002) Euthanasia and physician-assisted suicide among patients with amyotrophic lateral sclerosis in the Netherlands. *New England Journal of Medicine* **346** (21): 1638–44.

92. **Anonymous** (2003) The Belgian Act on Euthanasia of May 28, 2002. *Journal of Health Law* **10**: 329–35.

93. **Mackellar C.** (2003) Laws and practices relating to euthanasia and assisted suicide in 34 countries of the Council of Europe and the USA. *European Journal of Health Law* **10** (1): 63–4.

94. **Sorta-Bilajac I.** *et al.* (2005) Dysthanasia: the (il)legitimacy of artificially posponed death. *Medicinski Archiv* **59** (3): 199–202.

95. **Anonymous** (1995) Rights of the Terminally Ill Act, in Northern Territory Government. Australia.

96. **Anonymous** (2002) The WMA Report on Euthanasia. In World Medical Association Policy: *The World Medical Association Resolution on Euthanasia.* Adopted by the World Medical Association General Assembly, available at http://www.wma.net/e/policy/e13b.htm. Washington, DC: World Medical Association.

97. **Rabow M. W., Markowitz A. J** (2002) Responding to requests for physician-assisted suicide: 'These are uncharted waters for both of us.' *JAMA* **288** (18): 2332.

End of life care

Nigel Sykes

Summary

The care of a person with ALS at the end of life will need particular attention and careful management. This includes not only the need to ensure symptoms are managed as effectively as possible, but also the support of the patient, family and professional carers. Many people with ALS fear a distressing death, but most patients are able to die peacefully with appropriate palliative care and support for all involved.

Case history

Jack was a 75-year-old man with a two-year history of limb onset ALS. By the time he was admitted to a hospice to give his family a period of respite he needed assistance to stand and was beginning to have problems with swallowing. He was, however, disinclined to accept a gastrostomy.

The admission was extended because Jack and his family decided that continued care at home was now too difficult and so a nursing home placement was sought. Over this time his swallowing was deteriorating, although he remained able to take thickened fluids, without evidence of aspiration. On the day before his death he was noted to be generally less well on waking in the morning, complaining of widespread discomfort throughout his body and intermittent breathlessness. It was agreed with him that nursing home transfer, which had been imminent, should be deferred.

Jack accepted administration of medication subcutaneously via a syringe driver, and this was set up at midday with morphine sulphate 7.5 mg/24h combined with glycopyrronium bromide 1.2 mg/24h. His speech became less distinct during the course of the day but he remained able to make himself understood by expressions if not always by words. That evening Jack settled to sleep at his usual time. At 4.30 the next morning he was noted by nursing staff to be peaceful but breathing shallowly. Five minutes later Jack's breathing ceased.

Recognizing the terminal phase

Most people with ALS die as a result of respiratory failure.[1] Consequently, the trajectory of decline in respiratory function is the key to anticipating the final stage of the illness. However, the onset of this stage, when it comes, is often rapid and ALS is a cause of sudden death. In a series of 124 ALS patients cared for until death, 40 per cent deteriorated suddenly and died within 12 hours; a further 18 per cent had died within 24 hours of a change in condition first being noticed.[2] This rapidity has implications for the preparations the caring team must make in order to respond quickly to symptom changes and, particularly, the guidance they must give patients' families in order to prepare them for what may appear to be a catastrophically sudden demise.

Alternatively, the character of end of life ALS care can be altered completely by the use of assisted ventilation in the presence of gastrostomy feeding. It has become clear that non-invasive ventilation (NIV) can extend life significantly,[3] and that tracheostomy ventilation can do so for considerable periods to the extent that functional deterioration continues to the point of a locked-in state. The timing and nature of the terminal event are then the result of physician action in deciding when and how ventilator withdrawal should be achieved.

If death occurs suddenly in ALS it seems most often to happen at night, presumably as a result of an exacerbation of nocturnal hypoventilation. Where there are clinical changes which herald the terminal phase of the illness, these usually take the form of an increase in the feelings of breathlessness, even in the face of NIV and despite adjustments to the ventilator settings, or the onset of a reduced level of consciousness associated with diminished respiratory effort. Medication changes can ease the distress associated with breathlessness, but as respiration fails transition is into loss of awareness and ultimately a state of unrousability. At this point the patient's condition is not significantly different from that seen in the end stage of cancer or other terminal diseases, but in ALS the duration of this period is liable to be shorter than that seen elsewhere.

It seems that although NIV delays the onset of the terminal phase, in most cases it does not greatly alter its character or duration. On the other hand, a minority of patients appear to be sustained in a condition of virtual unrousability over several days. This situation can be a cause of much distress to both family and staff, who perceive it as a pointless dragging out of the dying process and an affront to the dignity of the person concerned. After careful discussion between those involved agreement may be reached that the most appropriate response is to terminate the ventilation, after which death ensues in a very short while.

Supporting the patient

Quality of life may be seen as reflective of the degree of congruence between hopes and expectations and the reality of their achievement.[4] If there is a serious mismatch between activities a person regards as their principal source of satisfaction and their ability actually to pursue those activities, the results are frustration and a sense of meaninglessness. It is the role of carers to work to help the patient to adjust their horizons and focus to achieve enjoyment and a sense of worth out of activities which may be new or may previously have been discounted but which still lie within their capabilities. This type of support is a major contribution of hospice day units and creative living facilities. Naturally the range of such activities becomes increasingly limited over time, but this aspect of care remains important right up to the onset of the terminal phase of the illness. It answers not only to the psychological needs of the individual but probably also the social and certainly the spiritual as well.

'Spiritual' signifies the need to find within present existence a sense of meaning. How this is defined is a matter for each person – see Chapter 6. It may, but often does not, involve a framework of religion and the notion of a God with whom it is possible to have a relationship. If religion is an important feature the participation of the clergy might be appropriate, but carers must also be ready for a person to prefer to talk to them as someone who is not an official representative of religion and is unlikely to have all the answers. It appears that certainty, whether in the existence or the non-existence of God, is associated with the lowest levels of anxiety in dying people.[5] For those in between there may be a need to talk through feelings of anger against the Creator for a condition as dreadful as this, or apprehension about long-suppressed ideas of judgement.

If religion does not provide a context for meaning this must arise from a person's sense of relationship to others, the fulfilment they derive from favoured activities and their perception of personal autonomy and control. All three of these factors can be severely impaired by ALS, and as the disease progresses it is a particular challenge for the carers – professional, family and friends – to demonstrate that the ill person still retains a valued place in a social setting, allow them the maximum degree of personal control practicable, and enable them to adjust their sources of satisfaction. Not everyone has the same ability to make these adjustments and the compromises necessary to coexist with a chronic, debilitating condition. From the lack of such reconciliations, from unresolved personal issues, from the awareness of present losses with more to come both of functions and relationships, comes the suffering which is inevitably a part of any terminal illness.

Only the person himself can achieve a resolution of his suffering. It is not amenable to medical therapeutics or nursing interventions. Nevertheless, the caring environment can be such as to either facilitate or hinder the individual's progress in reaching a resolution of suffering. It is for this reason especially that the framework of care for patient and family must be a multiprofessional team. No one discipline is adequate to meet the whole need, but the mutually complementary skills of professionals who respect and communicate with each other provide the best resource to enable the person with ALS to approach the end of their life with dignity and tranquillity.

ALS imposes huge burdens on those who have it, and on their carers, through the relentless increase in disability it brings about. The extent of non-respiratory disability is not necessarily a reliable guide to prognosis, especially in younger people, but it is claimed that the requirement for physical aids and adaptations marks approximately the half way point of the disease career, with gastrostomy feeding at about 80 per cent and ventilatory support at 80–90 per cent.[6] While the ability of so many with ALS to adapt so remarkably to the ravages of their condition is a source of admiration to those close to them, the sense of physical disintegration, the loss of control and of a great deal of what previously made life worth living mean that death is not necessarily seen as unwelcome by patients in the late stages of the disease.

It can be a consolation to someone greatly disabled by ALS, and whose chest function is deteriorating, to be told that their condition will not go on for much longer. An exact prognosis is impossible to judge, though, and if a time is asked for the answer has to be relatively imprecise. Simply to be told that time appears short is not enough without an assurance of continued support and symptom control, because there is also the issue of continued hope.

Some professionals find it very difficult to be asked by patients for an estimate of prognosis, not only because any attempt at accuracy is likely to be misplaced but also because they fear that the answer will cause the person to give up. Relatives are even more likely to take this view. There is evidence that the grounds for hope change as illness progresses.[7] Because of its inexorable nature this transition is perhaps less pronounced in ALS than in other conditions encountered in palliative care, but there may still be a change from hopes that the disease may be slower in its progression or relatively limited in its scope or that it may be retarded by a therapeutic intervention, to the hope for relief of discomfort and for a peaceful end to life.

For any ill person to achieve a maximum degree of comfort, they must feel esteemed and understood by their carers and confident in the ability of the involved professionals to respond appropriately to their needs for information and physical care. Esteem implies a personal warmth and trustworthiness on the part of caring staff that is more than a professional façade yet not an inappropriate emotional closeness. True understanding of the patient's situation can often be particularly hard to gain in ALS because of the radical degree of disability and, especially, the impairment of communication. The fullest use of communication aids is required, together with all the skills of empathy and patience the carer possesses. Empathy is the imaginative entering into the other person's situation, but not the premature and superficial assurance that "I understand how you feel" which distances and is the enemy of trust. Continuity of professional carers (without a burdensome reliance on a single "favoured" individual) is often important in facilitating communication in advanced ALS, as much depends on knowledge of personality, facial expression and patterns of speech.

Consciousness that death is getting nearer can induce a desire for resolution of outstanding personal conflicts, perhaps of long standing, or for the tidying of personal affairs. Even for someone with intact speech it can be difficult to broach these topics and request help. There needs to be a sensitivity on the part of the caring team to the possibility that such issues might lie behind an appearance of restlessness or anxiety, and a readiness to probe gently for the existence of "unfinished business". Appropriate help can make a radical difference to the closing days or weeks of a patient's life. Conversely, not everyone can identify, share or resolve issues like this, and the resulting anxiety may be relieved only by pharmacological means.

It should be remembered that any persistent discomfort makes any other discomfort worse and is also mentally wearing. Hence attention to detail is important in symptom control, so that by the time end of life care dawns a capacity for competent symptom control should have been demonstrated and maintained. There is much in ALS which cannot be fully alleviated, but patients and families usually accept that there are limits to what medicine can achieve as long as the doctor shows a commitment to stay alongside them and keep trying. Whatever the problems earlier on, it should be possible for the promise to be made that at the end distress can be controlled and that death need be neither painful nor frightening. Provided that the correct drugs are available and are administered in the right doses and combinations this promise can be fulfilled.

Despite this, some people with ALS still receive the information that they will experience increasingly severe pain leading to a death from choking. These are terrifying prospects but the reality is very different – uncontrolled severe pain is exceedingly rare and although choking sensations are indeed common in bulbar ALS, choking is not the cause or the context of death. In O'Brien's series only one person was thought to have died in this way, and even then post mortem examination showed that in fact the airways were clear.[2] A more recent multicentre study of ALS patients at the end of life found no instance of death through choking and 98 per cent of the group were perceived to have had peaceful deaths.[8] Unfortunately in Britain the association between choking and ALS has become established by repeated misinformation in the media, requiring both an active approach to symptom control by doctors, nurses and physiotherapists, and continual reassurance if fears are to be allayed. Accurate information provided at the right time can be a great help in a person's ability to cope with the advance of disease and, particularly, with the prospect of its end.

Supporting the family

By family is meant those who are closest and most significant for the patient, whether they be relatives or friends. It is important, although not always easy, to identify who these are. This is not accomplished simply by obtaining details of the next of kin. A great help is to construct a genogram, or family tree, which allows the professional team to see at a glance who constitutes the family, where they are and what other difficulties the family might be enduring at the moment.[9] Around the edge of the genogram should be included particular friends and "significant others" including – sometimes – pets. Ideally this should have been done well before the terminal phase of the illness.

Being close to someone with ALS is enormously stressful. Family may be at greater risk of depression and social isolation than the patient.[10] The progressive functional deterioration is apparent to all, but family members may not recognize how this links with shortening of the prognosis. In particular they may not realise that death from ALS can be sudden. When the end of life is considered, thoughts may be coloured by unfounded apprehension about symptoms such as suffocation, choking and pain. A family's need for accurate information is at least as great as that of the patient.

The paralysis and loss of speech associated with ALS engender a feeling of impotence in all who care for those with it. This experience, which can be uncomfortable even for knowledgeable professionals, may be disabling and extremely distressing for lay carers. Without guidance as to what to expect as swallowing and respiration deteriorate, and how they can gain urgent help in a crisis, an episode of choking or breathlessness can be terrifying not only to patient but also family. It is notable that in the United States, Japan and Germany a high proportion of those with ALS who receive tracheostomy ventilation do so without prior discussion of the procedure because it was initiated in the midst of a respiratory crisis to which the response had been to take the patient to the hospital emergency room.[11] The same sequence of events occurs occasionally in Britain. This is not the way to begin such an invasive technique with so many grave implications. Prior involvement of a multiprofessional team with 24-hour availability can allow the making of informed choices in anticipation of the event and be a resource for advice and practical help in an emergency. Such access has been stipulated in the UK by the National Institute for Clinical Excellence in their guidance on palliative care[12] and, complementary to this document, the wider availability of specialist palliative care to neurological patients has been recommended in the *National Service Framework for Long-Term Conditions* issued by the UK Department of Health.[13] A properly prepared written advance directive can also do much to ensure that appropriate action is taken in an emergency – see Chapter 3c.

Such a team can also facilitate the continuing care of the patient at home, where most terminally ill people wish to be.[14] As life becomes more difficult the proportion wishing to stay at home diminishes but still remains about 50 per cent.[15] Despite assistance from community nursing services, the brunt of home care is borne by the family. Respite admissions to a hospice, hospital or nursing home can help carers to recuperate and resume their task, or additional respite nursing help may be available for limited periods, but for a significant number of families there comes a point when they feel they can no longer look after the patient at home. In this the patient themself may agree, or there may be divergence.

Even if all are in agreement that admission is needed, family members may still be left with a sense of failure and of guilt that they have let their relative down. This may be especially marked if the person with ALS dies soon after they have been admitted, leading to feelings that "if only we had kept going that little bit longer we could have looked after him to the end". It is important for their response in bereavement that families receive reassurance about the quality of their caring efforts prior to the admission, and the appropriateness of seeking inpatient care now. It is also important that there are the facilities and encouragement to enable them to remain with the patient as death approaches, if that would be helpful to them.

For some families it is important that their relative does not die in their home, because of the memories that would leave for the future. Any service caring for terminally ill patients at home needs to have conversations with patient and family about the preferred place of death if at all possible, so that in case of difference there can be discussion and understanding, if not always agreement, and plans made so that admission does not occur as an acute event in response to the distress of a family who have never been able to reveal their concerns about end of life care of their relative. An instrument such as the Preferred Place of Care document may prompt and assist such conversations.[16] Even when death does take place in a hospice or other inpatient unit, usually at least 80 per cent of the patient's last year of life will have been spent at home, and afterwards the perception of families is that they have indeed cared for the person themselves.[15]

Most bereaved people do not need specific bereavement care: they will work through the feelings of loss which are at some time part of every individual's experience by themselves with the support of their own network of family and friends. For a minority, perhaps up to 25 per cent, their adjustment can be helped by specialist bereavement support. This is increasingly widely available, and in Britain can be accessed through CRUSE, the local hospice or social service department.

Supporting the professionals

Even for professionals committed to palliative care, ALS is perhaps particularly prone to engendering in a pervasive sense of helplessness and failure. The difficulties in communication are a considerable contributory factor, as is the prominence of an irreversible process of functional deterioration which may be in contrast to the patient's continued mental vigour – inwardly they seem "well" but their bodies inexorably weaken in a way the professionals can do little about. This leads to feelings of frustration and de-skilling that can result in avoidance of the patient by carers unless the problem is recognized.

To some extent these tensions are eased in the terminal phase, as the end comes into sight and the situation comes to resemble more closely that of people dying of cancer and other conditions. Afterwards, however, staff memories of the case may be influenced by feelings which persist from earlier stages of care. It is likely that they will have known an ALS patient for longer than the average for palliative care patients as a whole, and so the sense of personal loss might be stronger. These factors risk leaving a residue of distress which might impair professionals' ability to look after people with ALS in the future. The situation is worsened by the relative rarity of ALS, which means that staff can find it difficult to gain and maintain confidence in their expertise in caring for those who have this condition.

Therefore it can be helpful if there is both a programme of staff education covering the management of ALS. Better integration and the extension of joint working between specialists in neurology, palliative care and neurorehabilitation will also facilitate the exchange of expertise and ensure that the right skills are available for the changing needs as they arise. Afterwards it can be useful for staff to meet as a multiprofessional group for a sharing of views on how the care of a particular patient went. This session may well identify ways in which care could be improved in the future, but should in addition be a chance for congratulation on the ways in which things have gone well. It should be a managerial responsibility to identify staff members who have particular problems resulting from the experience of care and, without imparting a sense of inadequacy, enable them to talk through the important issues confidentially either on the ward or with an independent counsellor.

Symptom control

The crucial issue in symptom control at the end of life is preparedness. It is a wholly inadequate response to the onset of a distressing symptom if control has to wait on a doctor's order or the pharmacist's acquisition of the medication required. As respiratory capacity shows evidence of serious decline a stock of key drugs should be made available on the ward or in the home ready for use. If the MNDA Breathing Space Kit is in use it is likely that some of the medication will already be available.[17] The following categories of drug should be to hand:

+ Opioids
+ Sedatives
+ Anticholinergic agents.

If the drugs are to be used at home, it is sometimes possible for family members to administer them in a crisis if the rectal or, particularly, the gastrostomy route is available. Whether or not the family is willing to assume this responsibility following adequate guidance, locally agreed paperwork must be filled out to enable community nurses to give the drugs when needed.

A Care Pathway approach to the management of dying has been developed and is increasingly used in UK hospitals, hospices and nursing homes.[18] Although primarily designed for the care of people with cancer it is also relevant to those dying from ALS. The medication and management actions described below are consistent with this pathway.

Opioids

Morphine is effective in the management of pain, breathlessness and nocturnal discomfort in ALS long before the terminal phase of the illness.[18] Doses are widely variable and not usually high, with a median of 60 mg/day being reported.[19] Even in its use for dyspnoea there is no evidence that morphine shortens life when it is used competently. Oliver's study found a median length of use of 51 days and a maximum of 970 days. Dose stability has been noted over periods of years and it is not inevitable that dose escalation will be required in the terminal phase. However, the morphine dose may have to rise if new symptoms intervene or old symptoms worsen, in particular if breathlessness increases. In this case the dose should be titrated upward in the usual way, making increments of 20–50 per cent of the preceding dose level in order to provide a noticeable therapeutic effect without causing excessive drowsiness. If morphine has not been used before it is appropriate to commence at 5–10 mg four hourly for pain, orally or by gastrostomy, or 2.5 mg four hourly for breathlessness.

If a gastrostomy is in situ the administration of medication can continue as before, but without it many patients will require a change of route from oral to parenteral. This can be accomplished by subcutaneous injections (made less uncomfortable if a plastic cannula is left in place to avoid repeated needle sticks) or more conveniently, if the length of the prognosis appears to justify it, by a subcutaneous infusion delivered by a portable syringe driver.[20] Alternatively, morphine or oxycodone can be given rectally; morphine or phenazocine or can be administered sublingually, and fentanyl and buprenorphine (a partial opioid agonist) are available as transdermal patches.

An important consideration if there is a change of route of an existing opioid is to make an appropriate calculation of the equivalent dose. A change from oral (or per gastrostomy) morphine to subcutaneous morphine involves a halving of the daily dose. All such ratios are subject to individual variation and resulting doses may require upward or downward adjustment according to response. A change to the sublingual or rectal route of the same opioid does not require a change in dose except in the case of oxycodone, whose dose should be doubled in transferring from oral to rectal. Transition from oral morphine to transdermal fentanyl requires division of the morphine dose by 150; unless the opioid requirement is stable, fentanyl, although convenient to give, is a less satisfactory choice of parenteral opioid as dose titration is relatively difficult owing to the wide steps between patch sizes and the long delay (up to 23 hours)[21] in achieving and recovering from steady state blood levels.

A patient who has gained particular analgesic benefit from a non-steroidal anti-inflammatory drug (NSAID) can have it continued by suppository (e.g. in the form of naproxen or ketoprofen) or syringe driver.[20] Ketorolac can be mixed with morphine in an infusion but if, as is usually the case, other drugs are also required it is more reliable to give the NSAID rectally.

Whether in cancer or ALS, pain is not generally a problem at the end of life if it has been adequately controlled previously. In a patient who can no longer

Table 9b.1 Conversion ratios from oral opioids to subcutaneous morphine

Oral opioid	To obtain dose of s.c. morphine divide by
Morphine	2
Tramadol	8
Codeine	16
Oxycodone	1
Hydromorphone	Multiply by 4

indicate their feelings carers interpret non-verbal signs of distress – for instance groaning, grimacing or restlessness. Before increasing medication, it should be checked whether there are remediable causes of discomfort, particularly a full bladder or rectum.

Sedatives

A generalized restlessness, which may be due to pain but also to anxiety, has to be distinguished from focal myoclonic jerks as these may be worsened by opioids, especially in the presence of phenothiazines. Rather than persist with opioid medication for restlessness it is more appropriate to use a benzodiazepine, either instead or in addition, for its anxiolytic and muscle relaxant properties. This may take the form of diazepam suppositories rectally or liquid via a gastrostomy, given as required or two or three times a day, or midazolam subcutaneously. Midazolam combines satisfactorily with morphine or anticholinergic agents in a syringe driver.[20] An initial midazolam dose is 2.5 mg stat or 10 mg/24 h.

In ALS a principal role of benzodiazepines is in the control of breathlessness, where their action is complementary to that of opioids. In an acute deterioration in breathing associated with failing respiratory function it is appropriate to give a combination of morphine (or other opioid) and diazepam/midazolam initially and then to titrate the doses of each. A phenothiazine can be used instead of the benzodiazepine, such as chlorpromazine or the more sedating levomepromazine. Both have an anti-emetic effect, if this is important, and there is limited evidence that chlorpromazine can palliate breathlessness.[22] Watch should be kept for myoclonic jerking, but the lowering of the fit threshold that these drugs induce is not a problem in end of life care in ALS. Levomepromazine can be given by subcutaneous infusion, but chlorpromazine causes too many skin reactions to be given by this route.[20]

Contrary to popular impression, it is rare for good symptom control to shorten life. An exception can be the relief of frightening breathlessness in a patient with severe respiratory compromise, in whom any alleviation of their distressing anxiety may result in an inadequate respiratory effort. To anyone in the presence of such a disabled person the imperative to relieve their anguish is clear, even if this might result (and it is never definite that it will) in a shortening of their already extremely short prognosis. The ethical probity of this stance is endorsed by medical authorities in both Britain and the United States, and by the Roman Catholic church. The doses of drugs used must, of course, be proportionate to the patient's current regime.

Midazolam is also an appropriate choice of drug when it is agreed by patient (if still conscious and capable of making such a decision), family and professionals that life is now being prolonged by assisted ventilation to a degree that is intolerable. A dose of 2.5–5 mg sc (1–2 mg iv) stat, with morphine 5–10 mg sc (2–10 mg iv) should be given, or more if the patient is already receiving regular sedation or opioids. This should be supplemented by an anticholinergic agent if there have been difficulties with retention of secretions. A continuous infusion of about 50 per cent of the bolus doses per hour should be set up and adjusted to achieve the required degree of comfort and sedation. The use of these drugs is also indicated if the patient appears comatose in order to guard against the onset of distress once ventilator settings are changed. Further bolus doses should be available throughout the procedure in case any distress occurs. This is not the place to discuss in detail the technique of ventilator withdrawal, but a process of weaning over 30 to 60 minutes allows prompt control of any distress that might appear after each adjustment of the ventilator without being unduly prolonged.[23]

Antisecretory drugs

Owing to bulbar weakness, retention of secretions in the upper airways is a frequent problem in ALS long before the terminal phase. However, any severely ill patient with reduced ability to cough can accumulate secretions in the upper airways, resulting in noisy breathing which if not always a distress to the patient may well be to attending relatives. At the end of life this problem is one that is best anticipated, as it is not easy to get rid of secretions which have already gathered. If respiratory failure is following on from unsuccessful treatment of a chest infection there are likely also to be purulent exudates present which cannot be prevented, so that it is not possible to stop rattly breathing altogether. Hence the first step in management is to explain to the patient's family the mechanism of the noisy breathing, what is being done and what its limitations are, and reassure them that by this stage of their illness the dying person is unlikely to be nearly as aware of the sounds as they are themselves.

If an anticholinergic agent is already being given by gastrostomy it can be continued and the dose increased if secretion retention is worsening. Atropine tends to be arousing, though, and should dose titration be required it would at this stage be more appropriate to change to a more neutral drug, such as hyoscine butyl bromide or glycopyrronium bromide, or hysocine hydrobromide which is usually sedating. Any of these can be given subcutaneously by syringe driver in combination with morphine and midazolam or levomepromazine.[20] In Britain, the first two are significantly cheaper than the third.

Dose ranges are:

- hyoscine butylbromide: 20 mg stat s.c.; 60–240 mg/24 hours by s.c. infusion.
- glycopyrronium bromide: 0.2–0.4 mg stat s.c.; 0.6–1.2 mg/24 hours by s.c. infusion.
- hysocine hydrobromide: 0.4–0.8 mg stat s.c.; 1.2–2.4 mg/24 hours by s.c. infusion.

Hyoscine butylbromide is very poorly absorbed enterally; the other drugs can be given in their injectable form via a gastrostomy. Neither has a licence for this pattern of use nor, in common with most drugs used in palliative care, for use in a syringe driver.

Conclusion

Care at the end of life is a crucial part of palliative care because it provides some of the most powerful memories for those who are left behind. The future attitudes of the patient's family and friends towards severe illness in themselves or others, and towards death itself, will be moulded by this experience, which in the first world today is rare for anyone below advanced middle age. Good symptom control and good communication with the patient as long as this is possible, and with the family, are crucial not only for their direct benefit to the person with ALS who is dying but also as a public health measure for all those left behind who have been close to him.

References

1. Leigh P. N., Ray-Chaudhuri K. (1994) Motor neuron disease. *Journal of Neurology, Neurosurgery and Psychiatry* 57: 886–96.
2. O'Brien T, Kelly M, Saunders C. (1992) Motor neurone disease: a hospice perspective. *British Medical Journal*, 304: 471–473.
3. Aboussouan L. S., Khan S. U., Meeker D. P., Stehnach K., Mitsumoto H. (1997) Effect of non-invasive positive pressure ventilation on survival in ALS. *Annals of Internal Medicine* 127: 450–3.

4. Calman K. C. (1984) Quality of life in cancer patients – an hypothesis. *Journal of Medical Ethics* 10: 124–7.

5. Hinton J. (1963) The physical and mental distress of the dying. *Quarterly Journal of Medicine* 32: 1–21.

6. Bromberg M. N., Liow M., Forshew D. A., Swenson M. (1998) A time line for predicting durable medical equipment needs for ALS/MND patients. *Proceedings of the 9th International Symposium on ALS/MND*. Munich: International Alliance of ALS/MND Associations.

7. Herth K. (1990) Fostering hope in terminally ill people. *Journal of Advanced Nursing* 15: 1250–9.

8. Neudert C., Oliver D., Wasner M., Borasio G. D. (2001) The course of the terminal phase in patients with amyotrophic lateral sclerosis. *Journal of Neurology* 248: 612–16.

9. McGoldrick M., Gerson R. (1985) *Genograms in Family Assessment.* New York: Norton.

10. Kaub-Wittemer D., von Steinbuchel N., Wasner M., Laier-Groeneveld G., Borasio G. D. (2003) Quality of life and psychosocial issues in ventilated patients with amyotrophic lateral sclerosis and their caregivers. *Journal of Pain and Symptom Management* 26: 890–6.

11. Oppenheimer E. A. (1993) Decision-making in the respiratory care of amyotrophic lateral sclerosis: should home mechanical ventilation be used? *Palliative Medicine* 7: 49–64.

12. National Institute for Clinical Excellence (2004) *Improving Supportive and Palliative Care for Adults with Cancer*. London: NICE.

13. Department of Health (2005) Quality requirement 9: palliative care. In *Department of Health. National Service Framework for Long-term Conditions*, pp. 51–4. London: Department of Health.

14. Dunlop R. J., Hockley J. M., Davies R. J. (1989) Preferred versus actual place of death – a Hospital Terminal Care Support Team experience. *Palliative Medicine* 3: 197–201.

15. Hinton J. (1994) Which patients with terminal cancer are admitted from home care? *Palliative Medicine* 8: 197–210.

16. Pemberton C., Storey L., Howard A. (2003) The preferred place of care document: an opportunity for communication. *International Journal of Palliative Nursing* 9: 439–41.

17. Oliver D (2002) Palliative care for motor neurone disease. *Practical Neurology* 2, 68–79.

18. Ellershaw J., Ward C. (2003) *Care of the Dying: A Pathway to Excellence*. Oxford: Oxford University Press.

19. Oliver D. (1998) Opioid medication in the palliative care of motor neurone disease. *Palliative Medicine* 12: 113–15.

20. Dickman A., Schneider J., Varga J. (2005) *The Syringe Driver: Continuous Subcutaneous Infusions in Palliative Care*. Oxford: Oxford University Press.

21. Portenoy R. K., Southam M. A., Gupta S. K. *et al.* (1993) Transdermal fentanyl for cancer pain. *Anesthesiology* 78: 36–43.

22. Ventafridda V., Spoldi E., De Conno F. (1990) Control of dyspnoea in advanced cancer patients. *Chest* 6: 1544–5.

23. Von Gunten C., Weissman D. E. (2003) Ventilator withdrawal protocol (Part 1). *Journal of Palliative Medicine* 6: 773–6.

Chapter 10

Bereavement

Ann McMurray and Amanda Harris

Summary

For each person the bereavement experience is personal and unique. Contemporary bereavement models may offer a framework to understand the common characteristics of the bereaved person's experience. In ALS, there may be a lengthy period of anticipation of the death that may affect the process and outcome of the bereavement. A range of support should be offered according to the individual needs of the bereaved. Adults and children may be encouraged to retain positive links and memories with the deceased. There is a need for further research to determine whether there are significant differences in responses for people affected by ALS related bereavement.

Introduction

Our sweetest songs are those that tell of saddest thought.
Percy Bysshe Shelley, *To a Skylark*

Bereavement has been defined as the loss of a close relationship by death, a tragedy unequalled by any other for most individuals.[1] ALS-related bereavement begins with the diagnosis, is progressive until the end of life and continues into the post-death period. The bereaved person, who has cared for someone with ALS, will have faced a succession of major losses. This disease presents physical, social, spiritual, emotional and psychological challenges, which may deplete the carer's personal resources. Carers may witness a lingering, prolonged period of dying in the knowledge that there is no cure for this disease.[2]

A network of family and friends, who are individually and collectively affected by the loss and consequently will have a unique experience of bereavement, survives each bereaved person. The various models of grief will be explored below, making connections with the ALS carer's experience of loss. The human response will be considered and interventions suggested that might be effective and supportive for adults and children.

Anticipatory grief

There are no substantive studies concerning the impact of anticipatory grief and bereavement specifically for patients with ALS and their families. Consequently, most evidence is anecdotal or extrapolated from other sources, such as studies relating to people facing death through other illnesses, for example, cancer or multiple sclerosis. Whilst acknowledging this deficit in comparative studies, the following section attempts to examine some of the potential issues for ALS patients and their families in the hope that it may prompt future research.

> Some days I think about the future and want to curl up in a ball and give up because of all that I have already lost. On better days I can get up and go out forcing a smile hoping today *will* be better than I feel.
>
> Lorna, aged 43, caring for her husband who has ALS

Anticipatory grief or preparing for a future loss can be a demanding and exhausting process. However, some sources have even criticized its value as a clinical notion or its presumed positive adaptive value.[3] Others document cases where the family is not able or willing to anticipate a loss until the actual event occurs.[4] However, it has importance for an individual facing the impending loss of a person to whom they have become attached. Alongside the physical responses engendered by ALS are the emotional, psychological and spiritual adjustments necessary to deal with the evolving roles and relationships within the immediate and extended family.

Theoretically, a period of anticipatory grief should enable a patient, their family and extended network to adjust to the reality of the patient's impending death and subsequent loss of a meaningful relationship. This preparatory work may reduce the intensity and duration of the grief experience once the death has occurred. Additionally, a period of anticipating loss may contribute towards a reduction in feelings of guilt, regret and self-reproach following the death and thereby be a positive influence on the bereavement outcome. The experience of grief at the death may be less intense than expected and the period of acute grief more truncated than for survivors of a sudden death. One daughter of an ALS patient summed it up this way:

> We'd done all our crying long before Dad died. I'd already said goodbye to him a long time ago in my mind's eye. He was a shell of the man I remember when I was growing up. I'd lost him even before he finally went.
>
> Janet, aged 27

Adaptation to subsidiary losses along the way, such as loss of employment, may also help the process as adjustments are made incrementally to the family lifestyle. Concurrently, psychological adjustments may be made, feelings expressed and new strengths discovered in the individual or family system. Critically, a quick succession of losses for some families leaves little or no time for readjustment before they are facing an additional change.[5]

As one carer comments:

> We've got the lift installed but now she can't get into the bathroom with her wheelchair. It seems each day brings something new and you have to think ahead to be ready for whatever next.
>
> Fred, husband and carer, aged 44

For some families facing an ALS diagnosis late in the process of the disease means they have only a short period to adjust to the idea of the potential loss of a loved one and may struggle with disbelief and shock until the actual death. For others, the family may live with the underlying anxiety of the impending loss of a relationship for a much longer time. Palliative care studies provide some evidence that suggests there may be negative effects both emotionally and physically on the bereavement of survivors where the anticipation of the death exceeds six months.[6,7] The caregiver may withdraw emotionally from the dying person, causing an imbalance in their relationship that is unfamiliar and uncomfortable. It is not uncommon for caregivers to experience a sense of wishing the ill relative dead if the burden of continual care is too exhausting.[8]

Patients may suffer from increasing anxiety or depression as their illness progresses[9] and mothers in particular may feel isolated and depressed as they lose their physical roles, some as caregivers to children. As Katy comments in Michele Angelo Petrone's[10] collection of pictures and words by people affected by cancer:

> Life is full of challenges: Motor Neurone Disease (ALS) has been my hardest. I hate what it's done to my body, taken my '*doing*' roles, changed my life, forcing me to be dependant when I was so competent; but I still give of myself.

Sensitive social support may be offered to effectively reduce distress[11] whilst acknowledging that patients and caregivers have different and varying responses to their diagnosis of ALS and subsequent coping styles.[12] Bereavement outcomes should prove more positive if such support is offered prior to death of the patient.

Family theorists have emphasized the effects of stress in one part of the family system on others in the same system, some studies going so far as to class carers as 'second-order patients'.[13] Care should be taken not to treat relatives and carers 'merely as an appendage'[14] but as individuals with their own needs. As Tony Smith, a carer for his wife Jean commented at a MND Association seminar in 1990:[15]

I got so depressed that when I went out to play bowls I didn't want to go home, and when I went to bed at night didn't know how I was going to face another day, and wished time after time that I would not wake up again....

A carer's needs should be individually assessed and met both before and after the death of the patient. In some circumstances, a caregiver overloaded with responsibility for the patient may delegate care for younger children to their older siblings then feel guilty about burdening the children. Anxiety may be passed around in a similar way.[16]

Emotional lability, with uncontrollable laughter or crying, is a significant problem for many ALS patients. Communication difficulties may become exacerbated[17] with patients and family withdrawing from local socially supportive situations:

'We only visit gardens and such like away from our home area. Isabel is too embarrassed by her crying and being seen in a wheelchair.'

Ray, husband and carer, aged 51, at a clinic.

This may increase the carer's and family isolation following the death of the patient. For some families, ALS support groups may mitigate some of the effects of isolation before death and during bereavement. The MND Association UK issues a magazine called *Thumb Print*[18] that provides contact for patients and their carers. Additionally, *Build-uk*[19] offers a computer Internet service for ALS patients and carers to help alleviate the difficulties of communication and social isolation.

One study, of children with parents facing death through cancer, showed that they were at heightened risk of psychological vulnerability at the terminal phase of the illness.[20] They hypothesized that depression and anxiety would increase and remain elevated if the terminal phase was extended through many months, affecting both relationships with peers and academic performance. This may be the case for ALS patients and their immediate families. Open communication and a range of support services tailored to individual needs may alleviate some of the stress.

Essentially, it is important to assess the child's perception of the situation and the subjective meaning they apply to any event including facing death. In contemporary theory this is increasingly acknowledged as a factor in successful emotional adjustment to stress.[21,22] As Alexander, aged eight, facing his father's death from ALS, comments:

'I know Daddy won't always be here. That makes me sad ... but he'll always be here *(touches his chest)*. That makes me feel warm inside and sort of sad too.'

Other evidence suggests that the age and gender of the child are important factors to be considered when children are facing stressful life events. Older children may consider their stress levels lower than a younger child who finds it harder to distinguish between events they have control over and those they do not.[23] Where differences are reported, female children report greater negative affect in the face of stressful and fearful situations than their male counterparts.[24] As Amy, aged 15 years remarks:

'It's not just me I worry about, it's mum and the little ones ... they don't seem to know what's happening, not properly I mean. I'm scared about Dad dying and if we will have enough money to live on.'

One study of adolescents facing death of a parent through cancer concluded that this age group's cognitive and empathetic capacities allowed them to be more aware of losses and of their parents' physical and emotional pain. However, their capacities to use intellectual defences, to search for meaning, to develop understanding and seek help were important coping abilities. This meant that most adolescents in their study coped with stress without severe acting-out behaviours.[25] This may have consequences for emotional health and family relationships after the patient has died.

Predictability and controllability over negative events have been demonstrated as helpful factors in reducing perceived stress.[26] However, a child facing the impending death of a parent has little control over this or its effect upon themselves. Active, parent-instigated sharing of age-appropriate information concerning the progression of an illness is vital in reducing stress and confusion for a child.[27] Booklets prepared by the MND Association can be helpful with this to address bereavement issues in preparation for the loss of a parent.[28]

Individual and family adjustment to the stress of the impending loss in ALS may vary according to family social patterns and community support such as cultural or religious groups.[29] It is also recognized that socially disadvantaged groups may suffer more stress from traumatic life events than others.[30] Family systems have implicit and explicit rules to deal with emotional expression.[31] Some decide to invest time and resources in one area of grief at the expense of another. Individual family members do not grieve simultaneously. The rules that govern how a family member deals with loss may be successful for some and costly for others.[32] A thorough ongoing assessment of family member's individual needs is essential if they are to be assisted up until and through bereavement.

Models of grief

Theoretical models that help to explain the process of grief will now be explored. The various models offer a way of understanding the uniqueness of the human response to loss.[33] They also contribute to the development of models of assessment and intervention that assist the practitioner in supporting the bereaved. However, the complexity of the loss experience cannot adequately be explained by one model.

Grief models will continue to evolve, balancing the complex interrelationships between social and economic factors, personality and coping. The models can generally be grouped into the traditional 'grief work' models and the more contemporary models that describe grief as a dynamic ongoing process.

Traditional models

These models evolved as a consequence of the work undertaken by Freud[34] and the development of attachment theory as proposed by Bowlby and others.[35–38] They suggest that the psychological grief work task is to resolve the break in attachment to the deceased person. These theorists have provided a body of work concerning attachment theory that helpfully explains the process individuals must undertake to cope with loss and separation. It is suggested that individuals grieve because they have lost someone with whom they have shared a relationship of attachment. Separation produces a variety of behaviours which signal that the attachment has been broken and this in turn provokes a deep level of distress.

These traditional theories have come to be known as the 'phase/stage' models, with the bereaved moving through phases or stages in the process of their grief. First, they advocate that the bereaved person experiences *numbness*, a stage where shock is the overwhelming response and the bereaved person may feel disconnected from the experience. Parkes[39] describes the shock being replaced by intense feelings of *pining* for the person who has died, often accompanied by feelings of anger, guilt and self-reproach. There may follow a period of *despair or disorganization*, with related depression that can lead to a situation where the bereaved person withdraws socially and becomes very isolated. Finally, it is suggested that over time, bereaved people move towards an *adjustment to these responses*, developing new skills and move on with life.

The qualitative research of Kubler-Ross[40] contributed to the development of a five-stage model for understanding pre death loss and bereavement. This model implied that grief had a course, which was largely predictable. Stages described were: denial, anger, depression, bargaining and gradually moving towards an acceptance of the loss.

Worden[41] promoted grief as a normal process and introduced the idea of grief resolution through the tasks of mourning. The tasks were described as follows:

- *Task 1 – to accept the reality of the loss.* This task involves a deep acceptance of the loss at an intellectual and emotional level.

- *Task 2 – to work through the pain of the grief.* During this task the bereaved person is confronted by the trauma of the grief. The rituals of mourning are helpful in this task as they support and facilitate the expression of emotional pain and distress. There may be attempts to avoid the pain by idealizing the dead person or using denial to cut off or minimize painful feelings.

- *Task 3 – to adjust to an environment in which the deceased is missing.* The bereaved person is adjusting to the new roles and challenges that will involve adopting new skills and ways of understanding their environment. Increasing helplessness and social withdrawal usually indicates avoidance of this task.

- *Task 4 – to emotionally relocate the deceased and move on with life.* The bereaved person needs to find an emotional place for the deceased where they can continue to remember them at times of special meaning. The grief no longer interferes with the bereaved person's ability to live their lives, meeting new challenges and making new relationships. Some people avoid this task by maintaining a close unchanged attachment with the deceased.

Whilst the 'phase/stage' models have been particularly influential in providing an understanding of this aspect of human experience, a number of limitations have been identified.[42] Within this model, bereavement responses were considered to be rigid, implying that the bereaved move systematically from one grief stage to the next. They did not allow for the difference and unique character of bereavement related to long-term debilitating illnesses such as ALS to be recognized as distinct from other illness related death such as Alzheimer's disease or sudden unexpected death.

Contemporary models

Dual process model

The dual process model of coping with loss offers a multidimensional frame-work for understanding grief. Stroebe and Schut[43] argue that there are two preferred coping styles involved in adaptation to bereavement: loss orientation and restoration orientation. The bereaved person who is loss orientated will be focused on the loss, feeling intense emotional pain and may be preoccupied with thoughts about the deceased person. If the focus is on restoration, the bereaved person may be engaged with activities that seek to avoid memories that remind them of the loss or any action or thought that seeks to draw them closer into the bereavement experience. Optimally, the bereaved person needs to oscillate between loss and restoration-focused coping, allowing time for both the expression of feelings and distraction from the grief. This model considers the influence of factors, such as, circumstances of the death, gender, personality, individual and family culture as important to the outcome of the bereavement.

Continuing bonds

This model acknowledges that although the death is permanent, the process of adjustment is an ongoing one. It offers hope for continuity of the relationship beyond the grave. Death is not regarded as the end but an invitation to a new relationship. The bereaved person continues to develop and renegotiate their relationship with the dead person over time. Comfort is sought from memories and the bereaved person gradually develops a sense of meaning in the new relationship. The bereavement process involves taking from the relationship what was important and using this through a process of reconstruction to develop a deep meaning in the relationship. It is reassuring for the bereaved person to know that they do not need to give up the dead but may retain their continuing presence as an important and vital relationship that will endure over time.[44]

Narrative models

The continuation of the relationship with the deceased person is the central theme in models that focus on biography and narrative.

Walter[45] suggests that the bereaved should be reassured that they might retain the deceased. He proposes, that in postmodern culture, individualization and rejection of grand theory are central issues to be considered when developing a new model of grief. This model promotes the idea of talking to others who knew the deceased person and through that process a living and enduring biography is created. The bereaved person is then able to integrate the dead person into their ongoing lives. This model places grief within the social context by suggesting that close interpersonal relationships with others who knew the dead person will support the bereaved.

Grief responses

Bereavement and loss are recognized as major sources of stress for individuals and families. The responses to grief will be explored in relation to physiological, psychological, emotional, cognitive and behavioural responses. This approach to understanding the impact of bereavement on individuals is largely derived from the theoretical models of stress and coping.

Physical responses

Bereaved people may experience a wide range of physical responses following the death. Typical responses may include difficulty in going to sleep or waking up during the night, weight loss or gain, low energy, headaches, chest pain and digestive problems. Connections have been made between the range of stresses related to bereavement and responses in the neuroendocrine system.[46] Brown and Harris[47] established a link between bereavement and the development of physical and mental illness through its impact on the body's immune system. Pre-existing conditions may be worsened as the body's immune defences are lowered. Irwin et al. [48] made a connection between suppression of the immune system and disrupted sleep in the bereaved person. Taking care of oneself may be difficult following a loss and the individual may not be able to cope on a practical level without support. In ALS-related bereavement, carers may have neglected their own physical needs whilst focusing on care giving. This may result in exacerbation of pre-existing health problems following the death.

Emotional and psychological responses

The bereaved may experience a range of psychological responses as a reaction to loss. Represented among these responses are sadness, anger, guilt, self-reproach, anxiety, tiredness, helplessness, hopelessness, shock, numbness and loneliness. Memories may be particularly vivid and frighteningly detailed. Payne et al.[49] suggest that these responses can be categorized into three groups: emotional, cognitive and behavioural. Bereaved people describe emotions such as shock where the person feels disconnected from the loss experience. Some people report feeling emotionally frozen in time. There may be a sense of being overwhelmed by sadness and despair. Anger is often expressed and may be directed towards the disease process or professionals involved in the care or the person who has died. This is a time when bereaved people will review the telling of the diagnosis and the management of the illness, especially if they perceive it to be problematic, as part of the process of making sense of the loss.

There may be feelings of helplessness and disempowerment accompanied by hopelessness about the future and loss of direction in life. Anticipating change and assuming new roles often increase anxiety, for example, managing the childcare and finances alone. The bereaved person may have a sense that life is unmanageable. Depression is common and the signs of clinical depression need to be distinguished from the normal and appropriate feelings of sadness experienced by most people who are bereaved.

In situations of chronic or traumatic grief there may be increased risk of developing major depression or anxiety states.[50,51] Clinical depression may be present when there is continued low mood, extreme anguish and despair. The bereaved person is unable to function normally and the grief interferes with their ability to carry out activities of daily living, e.g. caring for self or other dependent children. Depression in bereavement may ebb and flow in intensity depending on the person's exposure to memories. The loneliness and isolation may be particularly acute in ALS-related loss, where much time has been spent providing care for the person who has died. The loss of the professional network may add to the sense of abandonment.

Bereaved people may experience cognitive changes. Some people find it hard to concentrate, are restless and may experience difficulty in making decisions. These changes in thought patterns can fluctuate in strength and prevalence. Confusion and disorientation are common. This can be very disturbing for the bereaved person and increase their anxiety, as the feelings associated with the thought processes are very unfamiliar. People may have a sense that they are unconnected to their current environment. Even family and friends may feel remote. They may not be able to process information as before and this can be worrying for the individual and family members. Bereaved people sometimes report experiencing 'hallucinations'. Vivid memories may be evoked and the bereaved person may see the deceased person as alive and with them.[52,53] These are common experiences and may be comforting or distressing. With ALS-related bereavement, these thoughts may focus on difficult time periods during the illness journey or the events leading up to the death or even the death itself.

Behavioural responses

Common behaviours associated with acute grief are, sleep disturbance, forgetfulness, angry outbursts and social withdrawal.

Crying is by far the most common behaviour and represents the painful emotional expression of loss and separation. Acute mourning may last several months. Bronstein et al.[54] found evidence that 17 per cent of all widows in the study were experiencing acute grief 13 months after the death, including crying episodes and weight loss. Anger at the unfairness of the loss or apportioning blame for the illness may present itself as verbal or physical hostility. Interruption to the normal sleep pattern may occur as the bereaved person may continue in the pre-death pattern of night-time caring. Loss of role, purpose and social withdrawal may be in evidence as the bereaved person struggles with the permanency of the loss. Food avoidance may occur as the bereaved person adjusts to the loss and attempts to move away from the pattern of food preparation they were accustomed to prior to the death. In ALS bereavement, normal focus on daily tasks may be difficult as the survivor surrenders the caring role and searches for a reunion with the person who has died. If swallowing was a problem during the illness, the bereaved person may experience difficulty with appetite or accepting food. The loss of role and subsequent feelings of low self-esteem may make it difficult for the individual to function in terms of decision-making and performing the normal roles of everyday life.

The interplay of the psychological, emotional, physical and behavioural manifestations of grief consumes much energy but gradually the intensity diminishes and gives way to reorganization and reintegration. It is a hallmark of recovery from bereavement when the individual is able to function well enough to meet social expectations and hold on to emotionally significant relationships.[55]

Bereavement interventions

The literature relating to resilience indicates that a large proportion of people recover from short-lived trauma and adversity with little detectable impact or need for intervention. People will experience loss as they progress through the life cycle, with only some experiencing acute distress. Numerous people endure the upheaval of the loss with no evident disruption to their ability to function at work or in relationships, and appear able to move on to new challenges with ease. Bonanno and colleagues[56,57] suggest that resilience, the ability to maintain a stable balance in the face of adverse events, is common following a loss. However, others suggest that chronic and transitional events can be more damaging than acute losses.[58]

Following the death of a person with ALS, it is helpful for professionals to be aware of a range of interventions available to assist the individual, family and social network to grieve the loss of their loved one.[59] The focus should be on facilitating open communication of feelings about the impact of the loss on individual members and an acceptance that individuals grieve and adjust to loss at different rates. This encourages family members to understand the specific needs of others, recognizing that certain members may be at risk of becoming isolated or depressed.[60] Professional intervention should allow for a review of the loss in a safe environment.

Bereavement support

Individual counselling with a bereavement counsellor or trained listener may be helpful for a person bereaved through ALS. Some people may prefer a therapeutic or social group setting. Others may choose a family, faith or community group that is significant for them. Numerous studies have shown the significance of religious or spiritual beliefs and experiences at the time of bereavement and in adapting to loss.[61–63]

ALS may predispose a person to a more difficult experience of bereavement, particularly if protective factors are absent. For someone bereaved by ALS it may be difficult to accept that the illness journey has ended. The following strategies will assist in making real the loss.

Providing an opportunity to view the body

This can be a helpful strategy in promoting a psychological acceptance of the reality of the death. As one relative said:

'It wasn't until I saw Jim and he felt so cold to touch that I truly realized that he was finally dead.'

Jean, bereaved wife

The bereaved person may be fearful of viewing or have never experienced seeing a dead person before. It is important to talk through fears and expectations that may be related to past traumatic events. In this way, the individual may be empowered to make a formal choice about whether or not viewing would be helpful. If there are specific cultural practises or religious differences they should be facilitated.[64,65]

Allowing for the expression of feelings

It is crucial for the bereaved person to be able to identify and express what they feel about the loss.[66] Being able to do so from soon after the death will help the grieving process and minimize distress or complications at a later stage.

As a carer comments:

I felt lost for words. Tears would stream down my face but I had no words to describe the pain and hurt I felt. Talking one-to-one helped me find new words to say how I was feeling. The best thing was I could tell other people too.

Sally, bereaved daughter

As the bereavement process is unique to each individual, so too is the expression of distress. It may or may not be possible for some individuals to actively verbalize their feelings of intense sadness. Verbal skills may be limited or language may not be sufficiently developed to describe any emotions. Feelings, particularly ambivalent ones, may have been suppressed whilst caring for the ALS patient over many months or years. The bereaved may need help to name and understand feelings that are not easily recognizable or uncomfortable to express openly. There may also be a fear of losing control when feelings such as sadness or anger are openly expressed. It is helpful to provide reassurance and a sense of containment during this period of open expression.

For some individuals, visual representations of feelings, such as paintings or pictures, may better facilitate their expression of emotions.[67] For others, written or spoken words such as a feelings diary or poetry are more helpful. Some bereaved people may find physical activity such as gardening, pottery, dancing, singing or shouting relieves tension and enables expression of feeling. Above all, the loss and depth of emotional distress must be acknowledged and reassurance provided that the support will be consistent and appropriate to the bereaved persons needs.

Acknowledging the normality of grief

In the face of overwhelming emotions, the role of the helper must be to communicate to the bereaved person that it is healthy, normal and permissible to grieve. In some communities, pain and distress may be tolerated only for short periods. It may be the view of friends or family members that enough emotional energy has been spent on the grief and that it is time to move on. Talking about the illness, death and memories may cause discomfort in others but failure to do so can result in the expression of grief being prolonged or blocked. The bereaved person may feel inhibited about expressing pain and worried about causing further distress in others. The supporter will be required to enable the bereaved person to create a space for continued grieving.

As a wife remarks:

> Other people seem to have moved on but I'm still stuck here day by day without George. They seem to think that I should be over it by now. But how can you get over 30 years of being man and wife in a few months.
>
> Janet

Review the loss experience

The bereaved person must be allowed to tell their story as they wish. Discussing life before and during the illness and the associated responses can be helpful. The supporter needs to listen attentively to the history and events of the illness and the worries and fears about the future. It is vital to communicate genuineness and empathy when responding to the bereaved person's story.[68]

Provide information and support about the grief process

It is not uncommon for bereaved people to be confused and overwhelmed by the vast range of physical, psychological, emotional and behavioural responses, many of which will be unfamiliar. Providing information about the process of grieving can be therapeutic and reduce anxiety. Such information should be given in a sensitive way appropriate to the needs and stage of grieving. It should include information about the process and intensity of grief, identify common reactions to loss and provide a list of bereavement resources and organizations, for example, Cruse Bereavement Care[69] or local hospice bereavement services.[70] It may not be possible to predict how long the period of adjustment will take, but it is important to inform people that if the illness and death has been complicated, the bereavement experience may be prolonged.

Bereaved people have many practical needs following the death and during the early weeks of the bereavement, such as organizing bereavement benefits or dealing with the estate of the deceased person. It can be helpful to offer support with these tasks to reduce the likelihood of the person feeling overwhelmed.

Anniversaries and memories

In the first year following death, there are many difficult times to be reviewed and remembered. The anniversaries of the date of diagnosis and hospital admissions may bring back painful memories. Other significant events such as birthdays, the first holiday alone and visiting places of particular significance may prove distressing. The bereaved often worry in advance about the anniversary of the death and the funeral. A young person put it this way:

> I was glad that I had thought about what we were going to do. Going to Margate and eating fish and chips like we used to do when Dad was here was great. We smiled, ate chips and cried a bit too. It was okay.
>
> Jessica, aged 13

Each occasion is special to the individual and they need to be able to remember in a way that fits with the family culture of mourning.

Scrutton[60] suggests that these confrontations with the loss may generate feelings of loneliness, which can lead to intense anxiety, distress and other physical symptoms. It can be helpful to be aware of and anticipate significant times for the bereaved person, acknowledge the importance of the event and provide appropriate support.

Secondary losses

To reduce the impact of any additional losses following the death of the person with ALS, sensitivity and care should be exercised when equipment needs to be removed from the home. For example, a Lightwriter that has been the voice of the deceased may be extremely hard to relinquish. One partner comments:

> I was okay until they took it (the Lightwriter) and I realized it had so many memories attached to it. Kevin hated it and its stupid American voice. . . . but then we used to laugh. I know it wasn't Kevin's real voice but it was a big part of him in the end and I miss it.
>
> Jane

Equally, the withdrawal of involved professionals needs to be paced sympathetically and appropriately to the needs of the individual or they may feel further abandonment or rejection. Other sources of support may be introduced for ongoing contact where necessary.

Within the context of contemporary bereavement models, sharing of thoughts, feelings and practical tasks may be undertaken within a family context rather than through individual counselling or group support.

Bereaved families

> Heirlooms we don't have in our family. But stories we got.
>
> Rose Cherin, author

Kissane and Bloch's[71] Australian study of Family Focused Grief Therapy (FFGT) outlines family therapy as a method of support and intervention with family groups who are facing the death of a member. The family is viewed as the central unit of care for the patient and it is suggested that the intervention seeks to support the unit. The family is seen together, issues and feelings are expressed in the group, and the family reflects on its own narrative of events. Through FFGT, the aim is that intervention will 'enhance cohesiveness, communication and conflict resolution' and 'promote the expression of grief'. Families are usually seen for a series of six sessions prior to and after the bereavement.

Kissane and Bloch helpfully outline major themes that develop (Table 4.1, p. 76) and are common to each grieving family, for example, care provision and sharing of responsibility. Emotional distress may be reduced through joint reflection and 'making sense' of suffering through a family's own reflective framework. Cultural and spiritual diversity may be accommodated and validated.[72] Additionally, important issues such as discussing death and saying goodbye can be addressed while there is time to reflect upon the task; reviewing quality of relationships, completing unfinished business and expressing gratitude for the good times shared.[73]

Bereaved children

Parents often have the greatest influence on a child's adjustment to grief[74] and should be included in any plans to support a child. However, if their own grief journey is particularly traumatic, parents may find it hard to connect emotionally with a child.[75] This may be the case for ALS-related bereavement. It is important to engage a parent or caregiver fully in the process of assessment and supporting a bereaved child in order that they do not feel their role has been 'taken over' by professionals.[76]

Worden[77] suggests that interventions with bereaved children and young people may be offered at three different levels: first, to intervene *only* where children display observable levels of emotional and behavioural problems or psychological distress; second, to offer intervention where a child is identified as being *at risk* of a difficult or traumatic bereavement; third, to offer intervention routinely *to all* bereaved children and their families. Sources of support for ALS-bereaved children may vary across each local community depending which model has been chosen. A practitioner working with children will need to assess the particular services needed for each child. It will also be helpful to enlist the support of the child's school with their parent's permission.[78]

Helping with traumatic memories

If an experience of a parent's death is particularly traumatic for a child, it is essential that the intervention carefully balances debriefing for any post-traumatic stress disorder together with creating remembrance of non-traumatic memories.[79]

A range of different interventions may be offered to assist with trauma, such as helping parents and children understand and control traumatic flashbacks, nightmares and persistent negative thoughts. As one child's experiences illustrates:

> 'I have to have the radio on at night-times as all I can hear in my head is Daddy's breathing machine.'
>
> Jasmine, aged 9

Some children will value individual sessions with a play therapist, social worker or bereavement counsellor. Here, a variety of techniques may be used with children to help with their bereavement including visualization, cognitive restructuring, role play, telling their story, music, creative writing, poetry, or completing activity books like *Muddles, Puddles and Sunshine*[80] or *When someone very special dies.*[81]

Nurturing positive memories

A Harvard study concluded that children who maintain good links with the deceased parent seemed better able to express their emotional pain, to talk with others about the death and accept support from family and friends.[77] Therefore, it is desirable to complete practical work with children to support their continuing bond to the deceased. As practitioners, it is also essential to ensure that this is not a way of denying the death of a parent but promoting a proactive bond that continues into the future life of the bereaved child.[82]

In the anticipatory grief phase, it may have been possible for the family to create a memory box for each child. As well as containing biographical details concerning the child's relationship with the ill parent, such as a family tree and history, they might contain photographs, videos, DVDs or letters from the ill parent, all evocative of past memories shared together. Other items to support memories may also be included, such as shells from a beach trip, perfume or aftershave that the parent wore, scarves, cinema tickets, cufflinks, birthday cards and music. In fact, any relevant object that helps the child to tell a good story and evoke a positive memory about their relationship with their parent may be included. For example, one child said:

'When I feel sad and I am frightened that I will forget Mum, I take out my box and smell the perfume she used to wear.'

Jennifer, aged 11

It is important that the container be individualized for each child, reflecting their personality and connection with the dying person. Winston's Wish[83] makes ready prepared boxes but a child and parent may choose to make their own special container together. This organization also provides a series of recommended worksheets with suggested activities for bereaved children to encourage memories of the deceased. If it has not been possible to create a memory box before the death of the parent, one should be started as soon as possible following the death, especially in the case of younger children who will need additional help to maintain their memories of the deceased. Younger children tend to retain more memories of physical attributes whereas older children may recall more subtle personality traits.[76] The boxes' contents may be used to promote true 'storytelling' about the deceased with another child or adult. Alternatively, they may be looked at independently when the child or young person wishes to think about or remember the deceased.

Children and adolescents may find it helpful to read fictional or true stories about other bereaved children or situations. Internet web sites (such as www.rip-rap.org.uk for young people's discussion of issues related to cancer) also provide the possibility for adolescents to share grief stories. Early adolescents may have periods of strong grief reactions then carry on as if nothing has changed.[84] Way and Bremner[85] found that exploration of the dual process model discussed earlier in the chapter particularly helped one young person make sense of her own bereavement journey.

Group work with bereaved children offers a different opportunity to share a child's story of their loss and can reduce the loneliness and isolation that a child or young person may feel.[86] Young Carers' groups may offer support, enhance self-esteem, and help to develop problem-solving skills and foster resilience before and after the death of a parent. Therapeutic groups offer a range of choices to children and their families. In the writer's experience of a local group work programme for bereaved children, it is extremely beneficial to provide a safe space for children to express their feelings and share experiences with other young people who are similarly affected by loss. Furthermore, evaluation by children and carers found that the experience enabled them to talk more freely with their carer about the loss and facilitated more open communication within the family.

Developing resilience in children and young people

Factors that support and foster resilience in children and young people are: strong social support networks, the presence of at least one loving relationship, having a mentor outside the immediate family with whom the child can have a relationship of trust, having a sense of belief and value that actions will make a difference and a positive school experience. Bereaved children and young people may benefit from opportunities that allow them to develop problem-solving skills and a range of emotional coping strategies.

Conclusion

The impact of loss on the families and caregivers of people with ALS has not been substantially or adequately researched. This needs to be addressed to directly explore the experience of ALS-bereaved people and the best possible practice outcomes. Contemporary bereavement models, particularly the dual process model and narrative therapy offer a helpful way of understanding the bereaved person's experience. The bereaved adult or child may be encouraged to retain positive connections and memories of the deceased. Practitioners may support the bereaved in a variety of ways depending on the individual needs of the person, including anticipatory grief work, family therapy, individual counselling or group work.

References

1. **Stroebe M. S., Stroebe W., Hansson R. O.** (1993) *Handbook of Bereavement. Theory, Research and Intervention.* Cambridge: Cambridge University Press.

2. **Leach C. F., Delfiner J. S.** (1989) Approaches to loss and bereavement in amyotrophic lateral sclerosis. In Klagsbrun S. C. (ed.) *Preventive Psychiatry: Early Intervention and Situational Crisis Management,* pp. 201–11. Philadelphia, PA: Charles Press.

3. **Siegel K., Weinstein L.** (1983) Anticipatory grief reconsidered. *Journal of Psychosocial Oncology* 1: 61–71.

4. **Ledbetter-Stone M.** (1999) Family intervention strategies when dealing with futility of treatment issues: a case study. *Critical Care Nursing Quarterly.* 22 (3): 45–50.

5. **Demmer C.** (2001) Dealing with AIDS-related loss and grief in a time of treatment advances. *Am J Hosp Pall Care* 18 (1): 35–41.

6. **Schwab J., Chalmers J., Conroy S., Farris P., Markash R.** (1975) Studies in grief: a preliminary report. In Schoenber B., Gerber I., Wiener A., Kitscher A., Peretz D., Carr A. (eds) *Bereavement; Its Psychosocial Aspects.* pp. 78–87. New York: Columbia University Press.

7. **Higginson I., Wade A., McCarthy M.** (1990) Palliative care: views of patients and their families. *BMJ* 1: 277–81.

8. **Middleton W., Raphael B., Martinek N., Misso V.** (1993) Pathological grief reactions. In Stroebe M., Stroebe W., Hansson R. O. (eds) *Handbook of Bereavement. Theory Research and Intervention.* pp. 44–61. Cambridge: Cambridge University Press.

9. **Vachon M. L. S., Kristjanson L., Higginson I.** (1995) Psychosocial issues in palliative care: the patient, the family and the process and outcome of care. *Journal of Pain and Symptom Management* 10 (2): 142–50.

10. **Petrone M. A.** (1999) *Touching the Rainbow – Pictures and Words by People Affected by Cancer.* East Sussex/Brighton and Hove Health Authority: NHS Health Promotion Department.

11. **Harrison T., Stuifbergen A.** (2002) Disability, social support and concern for children: depression in mothers with multiple sclerosis. *Journal of Obstetric, Gynecologic and Neonatal Nursing* 31: 444–53.

12. **Bolmsjo I., Hermeren G.** (2001) Interviews with patients, family and caregivers in amyotrophic lateral sclerosis: comparing needs. *Journal of Palliative Care* 17 (4): 236–40.

13. **Rait D., Lederberg M. S.** (1989) The family of the cancer patient. In Holland J. C., Rowland J. (eds) *Handbook of Psycho Oncology, Psychological Care of the Patient with Cancer,* pp. 585–97. New York: Oxford University Press.

14. **Spackman A.** (1991) *The Health of Informal Carers.* Southampton: Institute of Health Policy Studies, University of Southampton.

15. Smith T. (1990) *Coping with MND in the home* 'Carer's Perspective' talk given by Tony Smith at the one day seminar 1 May 1990, Motor Neurone Disease Association, Northampton.

16. Heiney S. P., Bryant L. H., Walker S., Parrish R. S., Provenzano J., Kelly K. E. (1997) *Oncology Nursing Forum* 24 (4): 655–61.

17. Murphy J. (2004) Communication strategies of people with ALS and their partners. *ALS and Other Motor Neurone Disorders* 5: 121–6.

18. *Thumb Print*, the quarterly magazine of the Motor Neurone Disease Association UK, PO Box 246, Northampton, NN1 2PR.

19. www.build-uk.net – building a motor neurone disease network for the UK. This web site forum can be used to contact others with a similar interest in MND – to decide what information and services should be provided, to tell others what people would like and to share information. There are voting pages and a chat room.

20. Siegel K., Karus D., Raveis V. H. (1996) Adjustment of children facing the death of a parent due to cancer. *J Am Acad Child Adolesc Psychiatry* 35 (4): 442–50.

21. Goodyer I. (1990) *Life Experiences, Development and Childhood Psychopathology.* Chichester: Wiley.

22. Sandberg S., Rutter M., Giles S., Owen A., Champion L., Nicholls J., Prior V., McGuinness D., Drinnan D. (1993) Assessment of psychological issues in childhood; methodological issues and some substantive findings. *Journal of Child Psychology and Psychiatry* 34: 879–97.

23. McWhirter L. (1984) Is getting caught in a riot more stressful for children than seeing a scary film or moving to a new school? Paper presented to the Annual Conference of the Northern Ireland Branch of the B. P. S. Port Ballintrae, May 1984.

24. Brody L. R., Lovas G. S., Hay D. H. (1995) Gender differences in anger and fear as a function of situational context. *Sex Roles* 32: 47–78.

25. Christ G. H., Siegel K., Sperker D. (1994) Impact of parental terminal cancer on adolescents in *Am J Orthopsychiatry* 64: 604–13.

26. Lazarus R. S., Folkman S. (1984) *Stress Appraisal and Coping.* New York: Springer.

27. Hooper Zahlis E. (2001) The child's worries about the mother's breast cancer: sources of distress in school-age children. *Oncology Nursing Forum* 28 (6): 1019–25.

28. MND Association (UK) (1995) *When Your Parent has Motor Neurone Disease.* Booklet, obtainable from MND Association (UK) PO Box 246, Northampton NN1 2PR, UK.

29. Muldoon O. T. (2003) Perceptions of stressful life events in Northern Irish school children: a longitudinal study. *Journal of Child Psychology and Psychiatry* 44 (2): 193–201.

30. Silverman W. K., La Greca A. M., Wasserstein S. (1995) What do children worry about; Worries and relation to anxiety. *Child Development* 66: 672–86.

31. Ford F. (1983) Rules: the invisible family. *Family Process* 22: 135–45.

32. Rosenblatt P. C., Wright S. E. (1984) Shadow realities in close relationships. *American Journal of Family Therapy* 12 (2): 45–54.

33. Stroebe M. S., Schut H. (2001) Models of coping with bereavement: a review. In Stroebe M. S., Hansson R. O., Stroebe W., Schut H. (eds) *Handbook of Bereavement Research. Consequences, Coping and Care.* Washington, DC: American Psychological Association.

34. Freud S. (1957) *Mourning and Melancholia* (1917), Standard Edition, vol XIV. London: Hogarth.

35. Bowlby J. (1969) *Attachment and Loss: Attachment*, vol 1. New York: Basic Books.

36. Bowlby J. (1973) *Attachment and Loss: Separation, Anxiety and Anger*, vol II. New York: Basic Books.

37. Bowlby J. (1980) *Attchment and Loss: Loss, Sadness and Depression*, vol III. New York: Basic Books.

38. Ainsworth M. D., Eichberg C. (1991) Effects on infant-mother attachments of mother's unresolved loss of an attachment figure or other traumatic experience. In Parkes C. M., Stevenson-Hinde J., Morris P. (eds) *Attachment Across the Life Cycle*, pp. 160–183. London: Tavistock.

39. Parkes C. M. (1996) *Bereavement: Studies of Grief in Adult Life*, 3rd edn. London: Routledge.

40. Kubler-Ross, E. (1969) *On Death and Dying*. London: Tavistock.

41. Worden J. W. (1983/1991) *Grief Counselling and Grief Therapy. A Handbook for the Mental Health Practitioner*, 2nd edn. London: Tavistock/Routledge.

42. Bugen L. (1979) *Death and Dying: Theory, Research, Practice*. Dubuque, IA: W. C Brown, Co.

43. Stroebe M. S., Schut H. (1999) The dual process model of coping with bereavement: rationale and description. *Death Studies* 23: 197–224.

44. Klass D., Silverman P. R., Nickman S. L. (1996) *Continuing Bonds: New Understandings of Grief.* Washington, DC: Taylor & Francis.

45. Walter T. (1996) Bereavement models. In *Progress in Palliative Care*, 4: 179–200.

46. Kim K., Jacobs S. (1993) Neuroendocrine changes following bereavement. In Stroebe M. S., Stroebe W., Hansson R. O. (eds) *Handbook of Bereavement. Theory, Research and Intervention*, pp. 143–158 Cambridge: Cambridge University Press.

47. Brown G. W., Harris T. O. (1989) *Life Events and Illness*. London: Guilford.

48. Irwin M., McClintick J., Costlow C., Fortner M., White J., Gillin J. C. (1996) Partial night sleep deprivation reduces killer cell activity during bereavement. *Biological Psychiatry* 24: 173–8.

49. Payne S., Horn S., Relf M. (1999) *Loss and Bereavement*. Buckingham, UK, Open University Press.

50. Horowitz M. J., Siegal B., Holen A., Bonanno G., Milbrath C., Stinson C. H. (1997) Diagnostic criteria for complicated grief disorder. *American Journal of Psychiatry* 154: 904–10.

51. Prigerson H. G., Shear M. K., Newsom J. T., Frank E., Reynolds C. F., Macijewski P. K., Houch P. R., Bierhals A. J., Kupfer D. J. (1996) Anxiety among widowed elders: is it distinct from depression and grief? *Anxiety* 2: 1–12.

52. Conant R. D. (1996) Memories of the death and life of a spouse: the role of images and sense of presence in grief. In Klass D., Silverman P., Nickman S. L. (eds) *Continuing Bonds*. Philadelphia, PA: Taylor and Francis.

53. Young M., Cullen L. (1996) *A Good Death*. London: Routledge.

54. Bronstein P. E., Clayton P. J., Halikas J. A., Maurice W. L., Robins E. (1973) The depression of widowhood after thirteen months. *British Journal Psychiatry* 122: 561–6.

55. Weiss R. S. (1993) Loss and recovery. In Stroebe M. S., Stroebe W., Hansson R. O. (eds) *Handbook of Bereavement. Theory, Research and Intervention*, pp. 271–84. Cambridge: Cambridge University Press.

56. Bonanno G. A., Wortman C. B., Lehman D. R., Tweed R. G., Haring M., Sonnega J. (2002) Resilience to loss and chronic grief: a prospective study from pre-loss to 18 months post-loss. *Journal of Personality and Social Psychology* **83**: 1150–64.

57. Bonanno G. A. (2004) Loss, trauma and human resilience. *American Psychologist* **59**: 20–8.

58. Ribbens McCarthy J. (2005) *Young People, Bereavement and Loss. Disruptive Transitions?* London: Joseph Rowntree Foundation/NCH.

59. Bloch S. (1991) *Research Studies into Family Grief.* Melbourne: University of Melbourne.

60. Scrutton S. (1995) *Bereavement and Grief: Supporting Older People Through Loss.* London: Age Concern.

61. Parkes C. M., Weiss R. S. (1983) *Recovery from Bereavement.* New York: Basic Books.

62. Richards A., Folkman S. (1997) Spiritual aspects of bereavement among partners of men who died from AIDS. *Death Studies* **21**: 527–52.

63. Zur J. N. (1998) *Violent Memories: Mayan War Widows in Guatemala.* Boulder, CO: Westview.

64. Firth S. (2004) Minority ethnic communities and religious groups. In Oliviere D., Monroe B. (eds) *Death, Dying and Social Differences*, pp. 25–41. Oxford: Oxford University Press.

65. Neuberger J. (2004) *Caring for Dying People of Different Faiths*, 3rd edn. Oxon: Radcliffe Medical Press Ltd.

66. Cook A. S., Oltjenbruns K. A. (1998) *Dying and Grieving: Lifespan and Family Perspectives*, 2nd edn. Fort Worth, TX: Harcourt Brace.

67. Connell C. (1998) *Something Understood – Art Therapy in Cancer Care.* Wrexham: Wrexham Publications.

68. Rogers C. R. (1967) *On Becoming a Person.* London: Constable.

69. Cruse Bereavement Care – www.crusebereavementcare.org.uk. A web site for details of local UK service provision.

70. Hospice Bereavement Services – www.hospiceinformation.info/. A web site on which to find local services.

71. Kissane D. W., Bloch S. (2002) Facing Death Series. Family-focused grief therapy: a model of family-centred care during palliative care and bereavement. Buckingham, UK, Open University Press.

72. Schofield H., Bloch S., Herman H., Murphy B., Nankervis J., Singh B. (1998) *Family Caregivers. Disability, Illness and Ageing.* St Leonards: Allen & Unwin.

73. Meares R. (1981) *On saying goodbye before death. Journal of the American Medical Association* **246**: 1227–9.

74. Silverman P. R. (2000) *Never too Young to Know: Death in Children's Lives.* New York: Oxford University Press.

75. Dyregrov A. (1991) *Grief in Children: A Handbook for Adults.* London: Jessica Kingsley Publishers.

76. Stokes J. A. (2004) *Then, now and always – supporting children as they journey through grief: a guide for practitioners.* Cheltenham, UK, Winston's Wish Publishers.

77. Worden J. W. (1996) *Children and Grief – When a Parent Dies.* New York: The Guilford Press.

78. Rowling L. (2003) *Grief in School Communities. Effective Support Strategies.* Buckinghamshire: Open University Press.

79. Yule W. (2005) Working with traumatically bereaved children. In Monroe B., Kraus F. (eds) *Brief Interventions with Bereaved Children.* Oxford: Oxford University Press.

80. Crossley D. (2000) *Muddles Puddles and Sunshine.* Gloucestershire: Hawthorn Press/Winston's Wish.

81. Heegaard M. (1991) *When Someone Very Special Dies – Children Can Learn to Cope With Grief,* p. 424, Minneapolis MNSS Fairview Press.

82. Gal-Oz E., Field N. (2002). Do continuing bonds always help with adjustments to loss? *Bereavement Care* 21 (3): 42–3.

83. Winston's Wish – www.winstonswish.org.uk. A web site for children, families and professionals concerning childhood bereavement.

84. Christ G. H. (2000) *Healing Children's Grief: Surviving a Parent's Death from Cancer.* Oxford: Oxford University Press.

85. Way P., Bremner I. (2005) Therapeutic interventions. In Monroe B., Kraus F. (eds) *Brief Interventions with Bereaved Children.* Oxford: Oxford University Press.

86. Haasl B., Marnocha J. (2000) *Bereavement Support Group Program for Children,* 2nd edn. Philadelphia, PA, USA: Taylor and Francis.

Chapter 11a

Personal experiences

One day at a time: the experience of an ALS caregiver

Linda Centers

I will never forget the day I learned of the existence of ALS. I was an occupational therapy student and had just heard an absurdly short – possibly only ten minute – lecture on the disease. I sat, very disturbed by the symptoms and prognosis, wondering why we were given no information about treatments or interventions. I remember becoming tearful in class. It is interesting that my reaction was so powerful. I had never been so shocked and moved by a diagnosis. I thought, 'Thank God this is such a rare disease. If anyone I loved ever got it, I couldn't take it.'

Years later, I did 'take it'. My mother, Elaine, who was truly my best friend and closest confidant, was diagnosed with ALS in the spring of 1996. She died in the summer of 1998, at the age of 61. With a sense of grief but also pride, I refer to myself as an 'ALS survivor' and consider myself a diplomatic messenger of sorts, sharing with professionals my personal experiences of ALS and sharing with ALS patients and caregivers both my professional and personal experiences.

Mother Teresa said, 'I know God won't give me anything I can't handle. I just wish He didn't trust me so much.' This quote hung on my refrigerator throughout most of my mother's illness. I have left it there, sort of as a reminder of my mother. There are many seemingly trivial reminders of my mother around my house that I have been unable to discard – little scraps of paper with her handwritten notes and lists, unused bags and syringes for tube feedings, the hook that I hung her feeding bag from, an answering machine recording made when she could still speak, the last book she read, a 'tic-tac-toe' game she had played with my son.

I am only one of countless ALS caregivers, and can only speak as candidly as possible about my own experiences. I believe our experience of ALS was both easier and more difficult than 'typical'. My mother was cared for by a physician who is not only an ALS expert, but also one of the most approachable, available, and positive people I have known. On the down side, my mother had a rather rapid, quite bulbar course of ALS (but was also quadriplegic for the last several months of her life). She also had a daughter who worked in healthcare and who knew just enough to be completely overwhelmed and engulfed by the gravity of the situation. Not to mention this daughter's tendency to feel responsible for everything and everyone and responsible for making everything 'all right'. Not an easy task in ALS, to be sure.

I hope to provide a view that is both intimate and pragmatic. I would like to share with you my experiences and suggestions related to such issues as profound loss and the experiences of abandonment. Non-abandonment is frequently mentioned as a virtue in ALS literature, but the many facets of this construct, which comes to have many meanings to the patient and family, have not been appropriately explored or illuminated.

In attempting to recall my ALS experiences, I am reminded of several things. Of the true horror and panic followed by numbness and disbelief on receiving the diagnosis. Of telling my father and brother of the diagnosis (and seeing my father cry, something I had never witnessed). Wondering, 'Will this be our last Christmas, our last Mother's Day, our last smile of unspoken understanding, our last day?' Feelings of fear, isolation, anger – yet knowing my only choice was to go forward, as courageously and lovingly as possible.

Feelings of guilt – about not doing enough, about enjoying my life as she lay in bed, about sometimes hoping death would come quickly, for reasons of finance or limits of human physical and emotional endurance. Lying awake and hearing her strange vocalizations at night. 'Does she need me? Has she lost her call button? Maybe she is cold and cannot cover herself. Maybe her head is out of position and she cannot get a good airway. Maybe she is just making noises in her sleep. She always does that. But maybe I should check.' And then, if the sounds stopped, 'Is she dead?' These were the conversations that took place in my head several times nightly.

Seeing looks of true terror in the eyes of a very courageous woman. It is very unnerving to see a look of longing, fear, or pain in the eyes of a loved one and to have absolutely no idea what is wrong – much less what to do. Augmentative communication is all very well, but is not so effective during the times of intense emotions of fear, panic, or rage.

In trying to provide a description of the experience of caregiving, I am reminded in some ways of caring for my infant children. There is the time spent planning for, packing, and hauling equipment for even short outings, the scheduled feedings, the breathless listening for sounds in the night, the provision of toilet and hygiene, the around-the-clock care during the terminal stages. With an infant, however, there is a sense of joy and anticipation, and the energy that is born of the belief that things will eventually get easier. There is the joy of watching a unique person come into flower. With ALS, there is a sense of sorrow, loss, apprehension, and the knowledge that things can be expected to get worse. Not to mention the pain of seeing your loved one, with whom so many life memories are built, waste away while in complete lucidity. As one of my mother's friends once cried, 'This is like watching an ice cube melt!'

ALS represents not only loss of your loved one, but also a loss of the future and a rather painful shattering of illusions. I thought I would have my mother's love and wise guidance as I raised my children into adulthood. I was wrong. I thought my extended family was very stable, close-knit, and capable of setting aside any petty differences in order to love and nurture my mother in her last days. I was wrong again. Over a year after her death, I am still somewhat shocked by the diagnosis. I still miss her terribly. I still have dreams about her. I still find my emotions to be irrational and out of control at times. I especially notice – [Page No. 184] to my loved ones' great discomfort – a sort of free-floating anger that all too easily find an unsuspecting target.

I have heard other ALS caregivers discuss these feelings. I believe many of these feelings are based on fear and on a feeling of abandonment. It is not so irrational to abandoned in this situation. ALS patients and family members are often abandoned by an one and everyone who is unable to face death – which can be everyone at times. They abandoned by false friends, who are more numerous than one might imagine. They abandoned by family. They are often abandoned by several professionals before finding one who is willing to have a relationship with them.

Much ALS literature mentions the virtues of non-abandonment and the need to assure the patient that he or she will not be abandoned. But I have yet to read a discussion on what exactly this means. I don't believe it is simply physical non-abandonment that is being referred to. No, it is actually a *spiritual and emotional non-abandonment* that the ALS patient and caregiver need. Non-abandonment in this sense comes to mean many things. It means fidelity, trust, honesty, reliability, genuineness, beneficence, availability, and love – among others. Non-abandonment beings at the time of diagnosis, and can be sensed by the patient and family in the way the diagnosis is disclosed.

Anyone who works with ALS has heard horror stories of patients receiving the diagnosis in a callous manner. My mother was out of town, all alone, when she received her diagnosis. She had been told she was simply going for tests and that her general neurologist would review the results with her. On the day of testing, a neurologist she had never seen before, and did not see again, walked in and said, 'I'm sorry. You have ALS. Do you have any questions?' She was then released to drive herself home.

I do not understand why these things happen. It seems that certain considerations should be common sense when disclosing such a diagnosis. The patient should be warned and prepared ahead of time for the diagnosis, having loved ones close by if the patient so desires. He or she should be scheduled for follow-up with a professional within a few days of receiving the diagnosis. Nobody can think of intelligent questions after having received such news. That is the benefit of having well-selected literature and resources for the patient, not just at diagnosis but throughout the illness. This literature should not be overwhelming, but rather take a hopeful approach, covering the basics of ALS as well as what can be done and what resources and support are available. Of particular importance is sensitive literature on the mode of death. Although it may not be appropriate to provide such information at the time of diagnosis, most patients and caregivers have terrifying misinformation on the death process, and they receive this misinformation rather quickly.

Recognize that acceptance of the diagnosis, or of any loss, cannot happen overnight. Nobody can quickly believe he (or his loved one) is dying of a completely incurable disease. I found that I had to fully understand and believe in the diagnostic process, including which diseases had been ruled out, before having any confidence in even saying 'ALS'. This was not necessarily pleasant for my mother's neurologist. For me, accepting the diagnosis meant accepting her death, and the loss of one of the greatest loves of my life. I could not just blindly accept that information on the authority of anyone – no matter what their title, status, or expertise. Do not be offended if patients and family will not accept the news, or cannot hear all you are saying. One way to show your commitment is to be willing to clarify and explain, over and over again if necessary, not only the diagnosis but any other information. Try not to take it personally.

I think it is most helpful for the ALS professional to consider him or herself more of a consultant, teacher, collaborator, and friend than an omniscient healer. It is very important to provide a calm, compassionate, and reliable presence. I believe this is more important than any of your particular treatments, more important than any of your words. There are several ways to convey your intention not to abandon. Return phone calls quickly, if possible. Provide frequent clinic visits. Give of your time. Slow down and spend time listening, without rushing in with advice and solutions (a difficult task for many physicians, I have observed!). Be available for more than simply meeting medical needs. Show your willingness to listen to expression of feelings, *especially unpleasant ones.* Just listen. Sometimes all the caregiver needs is just a very simple acknowledgment that the job is difficult and painful. Don't give canned advice. Be present. Be human. If you are not comfortable listening to the expression of painful and intense emotions, you are deficient in an essential component of quality caring for the dying and their loved ones.

It is certainly desirable to be positive, upbeat, and hopeful. But try not to always hide behind this. At times, professionals caring for my mother were *so* positive that I felt I was in some macabre play. 'Doesn't anyone notice how nightmarish this is?' I would sometimes wonder. Avoiding negative topics or minimizing unpleasant feelings is a particular form of emotional abandonment.

One of the most poignant and healing moments for me came near the end of a rather mundane telephone consultation with my mother's neurologist. 'Linda,' he said, 'I am sorry your mother has this crummy disease.' I hung up the phone and cried – tears of relief actually. Yes, there are gifts of ALS, there are real reasons for joy, hope, and gratitude. But to pretend it is easy is an injustice and an insult to those experiencing it. The pain, fear, and struggle of ALS are very real and need to be acknowledged. They do not 'go without saying'.

Another method of conveying non-abandonment is to freely support the patient and caregiver's decisions, *regardless of your personal or professional opinions.* Provide the information, give advice, but then step back. ALS involves many heartbreaking losses. The loss of independence, the loss of the ability to hold your loved ones or to say the words 'I love you', the loss of dreams. You, the professional, can only theorize and speculate as to how you would handle these losses. Try to avoid passing judgement when the patient, after being given the necessary information, refuses a particular 'appropriate' intervention.

For example, choosing a PEG is clearly a wise decision, from a clinical standpoint. Most patients are aware of this. However, going on a PEG represents a most unsettling and unusual emotional defeat. It represents not only disease progression, but also the loss of a skill we have had since birth. It heralds the loss of one of the only reliable and consistent pleasures in life. Also, not everyone with ALS wishes to prolong the inevitable: the desire to succumb quickly to ALS is not so unreasonable.

My last piece of advice is not only for the benefit of the caregiver but concerns how you, the professional, can better take care of yourself. When dealing with issues such as death, it is easy to lose sight of your personal boundaries. An example of this would be giving care-givers your home phone number and taking calls at all hours that could have waited until office hours – or spending hours of your personal time on the telephone. I believe this can be a source of professional burnout and resentment. It also gives the caregiver the wrong perception of the relationship.

It is important to recognize that the caregiver is very vulnerable to you and is probably, feeling frightened and insecure. You represent one of the very few ports in the storm and *much more of a source of hope and comfort than you may even imagine.* When comforting someone in times of great emotional crisis, perhaps in death issues particularly, it is easy to cross the line and to move from empathy and compassion and into something less healthy for everyone involved. Watch for and be aware of transference issues, both in yourself and in the caregiver. Although a caregiver certainly may need a shoulder to cry on, and an empathetic and caring professional – needs for certain levels of assistance and consolation should rightfully come from the caregiver's own support system – not from professional, no matter how well-meaning.

So know where to draw the line, not only for the patient and caregiver's emotional benefit, but for your own. When the patient dies, there is often a sense of loss not only of loved one with ALS, but also a loss of the relationship with the professional and even ALS community. Do not make promises that you cannot or will not keep. The patient will die, the caregiver is left to move on, trying to make sense of it all; trying to figure out what the 'lesson' might be.

I had never before been with a dying person. I wasn't sure what to expect or when, exactly, to expect it. I knew, in spite of her neurologist's more optimistic predictions, that my mother was to die soon. I knew this because her eyes stopped smiling. She stopped laughing. Her only visible emotions were fear, sadness, or defeat. My mother died peacefully, however, with my husband holding her hand. I entered the room minutes later, shocked at how unquestionably dead she appeared. Although she had been in a coma for two days, I was surprised at the dramatic difference between life and death at the defining moment.

I approached her bed. 'Well done, Elaine. You go now,' was all I heard myself say. I felt a sense of loss for myself, but also relief and pride for my mother.

I cried as I helped the hospice nurse wash and dress her body. 'Are you okay?' she asked. 'No,' I said. 'Do you want to leave?' she asked. 'Of course not,' I replied.

We gathered together around her bed – those who were present at the moment of death and those who came by having heard the news. We held hands and prayed. We thanked God for her particular influence in each of our lives. We shared stories of how she had touched us. Perhaps the most difficult part was watching strangers carry my mother's body out of her home. I followed along, much like a frightened child, all the way to the hearse. Trying to will time to slow down. Knowing I would not see my hero in this life again.

Personal experiences

Amyotrophic lateral sclerosis and how it affects my life

Phil Hankins

I have had this disease for two and a half years now and it is slowly progressing downhill, my wife has rheumatoid arthritis with myasthenia gravis in remission for many years. My 18-year-old daughter has just started university. I used to be the main carer but obviously I cannot do that any longer. This disease has turned our family upside down with a bad forecast for my future.

My first inclination that I had a problem was trying to hang the washing out and putting keys in locks, this was some two and a half years ago. My body felt out of sequence somehow and when I fell during a children's playscheme breaking my sunglasses and bruising my shoulder I knew I had a problem. After seeing my family doctor he referred me to a consultant neurologist at the local hospital who mentioned ALS but said only time would confirm this. I saw further specialists at King's College Hospital in London who confirmed I had ALS in February 1998. Up to this point nobody would help me but after this confirmation everybody began working towards helping me.

The Motor Neurone Disease Association would only help when I had been confirmed with ALS but after this they became a brilliant organization for me; I was introduced to the Regional Care Adviser and she gives my family and me loads of help.

It became obvious that I would need a bed, shower and toilet downstairs for the future so we spoke to the local council about a grant and extension; this took 15 months to achieve. It came exactly at the right time for me as toileting was becoming a problem. So thank goodness for the Closmat toilet. We also have a hoist in the ceiling ready for use when I need it.

My daily routine is exactly that: a daily routine. Two carers arrive at 6.45 a.m. to get me out of my downstairs bed, put me on the toilet, dress me and give me my breakfast. By 7.40 I am ready for work, a taxi takes me, in my electric wheelchair, to work for 8.00 where I remain until 4.30 p.m. A carer comes at 12.30 to give me my dinner (sandwiches and yoghurt) and then another carer comes at 5.30 to help with our evening meal. At 6.15 I am showered with two carers and then put in my chair for the evening until 10.00 when two carers come to put me to bed.

I am on a ventilator all night and need turning about 8 times a night by my night time carer. I also have a rest with my ventilator twice a day at work and weekends sometimes sleeping for 45 minutes, sometimes just 10 minutes.

I have lower motor neurone nerve damage so statistically I should survive five years (I have had two and a half years already), I am only mobile with an electric wheelchair, I cannot stand unaided, I cannot eat unaided. Basically I can talk although this is becoming more of a problem with breathing becoming more difficult, it takes a lot of effort to go through the day and some people wonder why I still work! The job I have needs me to be able to talk to people and if I didn't work what would I do? Because when my voice goes I will be unable to do my job.

I have worked at Nene Park Trust for 22 years and I am now the head ranger and my general manager has done his utmost to keep me at work. I am very fortunate that the job I have I can still do. Some people I feel think that because I am still at work I cannot be as ill as I am as all I can do is sit in my wheelchair and talk, although my voice isn't very strong these days.

The Access to Work Act has helped me to remain at work with things like ramps, disabled toilets, widening doorways, an electric wheelchair and voice activated computer. I can still manage to sustain the job that I am employed to do for the present with a lot of help from my colleagues. No matter how much help I get, it is my colleagues that give me the encouragement and assistance to carry on with my work.

Lots of other things happen to you with ALS. You lose confidence because of your reduced body abilities, you get scared of being alone with the mask on, but mostly you become withdrawn into your disease and do not want to get involved with things you loved to do. My family is very important to me but sometimes I am more concerned with my disease than I am with them. This makes me very sad and upset because I've been married 24 years to a lovely lady and we have a lovely daughter. Unless you get close to someone with this disease you cannot understand the pain it brings for me and everybody surrounding me.

I am now on a ventilator at night and sometimes during the day. I sleep mostly down stairs away from my wife who has rheumatoid arthritis so she is unable to help me. I used to be her main carer but obviously I am no longer able to help her. We had a meeting at our house some nine weeks ago and everybody agreed that I should have help at night; it took seven weeks to organize this. My relationship with my wife was becoming very difficult and I was getting towards the end of my tether so it was a great relief when the night care finally arrived.

The main frustration with this disease seems to be that people often react too late to cope with my immediate needs, with this disease you are on a plateau one day but the next day you have fallen over the side. When you have fallen off the plateau it is very important that you have faith in the people around you. The MND Association is very aware of my next in my opinion much more aware than the healthcare professionals. I need help and if someone as a healthcare professional offers to provide help it needs to be done as quickly as to possible. Some people who are not disabled do not always understand the frustrations that disabled people have to put up with.

The help that I get from various sources is awesome – the doctors, the hospitals, the Regional Care Adviser, and all my friends and family. Without their help I don't know if I would still be alive.

Phil Hankins died in his local hospice on 15 January 2000.

Appendix 1

SUPPLIERS OF EQUIPMENT

United Kingdom
Most equipment can be obtained from
distributors in the UK, in particular:

Headmaster Collar
Quest Enabling Designs Ltd
1 Prince Alfred Street
Gosport
Hampshire PO12 1QH
www.qedltd.com

Oxford MND Collar
Salt & Sons Ltd
Saltair House
Lord Street
Heartlands
Birmingham B7 4DS
www.salts.co.uk

**Nottingham Rehab Supplies – can supply
most rehabilitation needs**
Victoria Business Park
Pintail Close
Netherfield
Nottingham
NE4 2PE
www.nrs-uk.co.uk

Neater Eater
Neater Solutions Ltd
13 Spencer Road
Buxton
Derbyshire
SK17 9DX
www.neater.co.uk

USA

With the exception of some of the collars, most equipment
can be obtained in the United States from the following distributors:
Sammons Preston Rolyan
270 Remington Boulevard, Suite C
Bolingbrook
Illinois 60440-3593
USA

630 226 1300
www.sammonspreston.com

North Coast Medical Inc.
18305 Sutter Boulevard
Morgan Hill
California 95037-2845

(800) 235 7054

www.ncmedical.com
www.beabletodo.com

Aspen Collar:
Aspen Medical products
6481 Oak Canyon
Irvine
California 92618–5202

www.aspencollar.com

Other contacts

The ALS/MND Associations will often be able to provide further
information on the local availability of equipment
Helpful websites include:
www.dlf.org.uk
www.ilc.com.au

Appendix 2

List of useful websites for ALS patients

Please note: there are thousands of websites which claim to contain information relevant to ALS patients. However, in many cases the information has not been reviewed for accuracy and may sometimes be misleading or even directly aimed at obtaining financial profit by offering "miracle drugs" or other devices with no proven benefit. Therefore, some degree of caution is advisable when surfing the net for information on ALS.

The following websites all have a very high standard and offer reliable information, addresses and links to other websites of interest. This list, of course, is by no means exhaustive.

www.wfnals.org– the World Federation of Neurology ALS site. An excellent site with regularly updated clinico-scientific news on ALS and a worldwide list of ALS specialists and centres.

www.alsmndalliance.org – the International Alliance of ALS/MND Associations. Includes a directory of ALS societies worldwide.

www.alsa.org – the American ALS Association. This site has a great deal of relevant information.

www.mda.org – the American Muscular Dystrophy Association, which also runs a strong ALS care program.

www.lesturnerals.org – the Les Turner ALS Foundation (Chicago).

www.als.ca – the Canadian ALS Association.

www.mndassociation.org – the UK Motor Neurone Disease Association.

www.scotmnd.org.uk – the Scottish Motor Neurone Disease Association.

www.imnda.ie – the Irish Motor Neurone Disease Association.

www.dgm.org – the German Neuromuscular Disease Association.

www.alslinks.com – an Internet portal for ALS

www.alsnetwork.com – award-winning website dedicated to providing information to ALS patients.

www.focusonals.com – a well-designed website for ALS patients, run by an ALS patient.

www.als-tdf.org – The ALS Therapy Development Foundation

www.dunitz.co.uk – contents and abstracts of each issue of the journal, "ALS and other motor neurone disorders".

www.caregiver.org – the website of the Family Caregiver Alliance

www.partnershipforcaring.org – the website of the Partnership for Caring, for carers

www.ninds.nih.gov – the website of the National Institute of Health Neurologic Institute

Index